Piyush Gupta's
PEDIATRIC
DRUG COMPANION

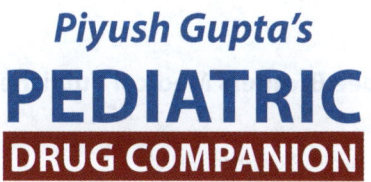

Piyush Gupta's
PEDIATRIC DRUG COMPANION

Nidhi Bedi
MD
Professor
Department of Pediatrics
Faculty of Medicine and Health Sciences
(Formerly SGT Medical College Hospital and Research Institute)
Gurugram, Haryana, India

Piyush Gupta
MD FIAP FNNF FAMS FRCPCH
Professor
Department of Pediatrics
Principal
University College of Medical Sciences
New Delhi, India
President, Indian Academy of Pediatrics (2021)

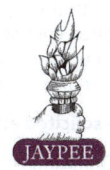

JAYPEE BROTHERS MEDICAL PUBLISHERS
The Health Sciences Publisher
New Delhi | London

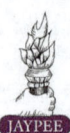 **Jaypee Brothers Medical Publishers (P) Ltd.**

Headquarters
Jaypee Brothers Medical Publishers (P) Ltd
EMCA House, 23/23-B
Ansari Road, Daryaganj
New Delhi 110 002, India
Landline: +91-11-23272143, +91-11-23272703
+91-11-23282021, +91-11-23245672
Email: jaypee@jaypeebrothers.com

Corporate Office
Jaypee Brothers Medical Publishers (P) Ltd
4838/24, Ansari Road, Daryaganj
New Delhi 110 002, India
Phone: +91-11-43574357
Fax: +91-11-43574314
Email: jaypee@jaypeebrothers.com

Overseas Office
JP Medical Ltd.
83, Victoria Street, London
SW1H 0HW (UK)
Phone: +44 20 3170 8910
Fax: +44 (0)20 3008 6180
Email: info@jpmedpub.com

Website: www.jaypeebrothers.com
Website: www.jaypeedigital.com

© 2024, Piyush Gupta

The views and opinions expressed in this book are solely those of the original contributor(s)/author(s) and do not necessarily represent those of editor(s) or publisher of the book.

All rights reserved. No part of this publication may be reproduced, stored or transmitted in any form or by any means, electronic, mechanical, photo copying, recording or otherwise, without the prior permission in writing of the publishers.

All brand names and product names used in this book are trade names, service marks, trademarks or registered trademarks of their respective owners. The publisher is not associated with any product or vendor mentioned in this book.

Medical knowledge and practice change constantly. This book is designed to provide accurate, authoritative information about the subject matter in question. However, readers are advised to check the most current information available on procedures included and check information from the manufacturer of each product to be administered, to verify the recommended dose, formula, method and duration of administration, adverse effects and contra indications. It is the responsibility of the practitioner to take all appropriate safety precautions. Neither the publisher nor the author(s)/editor(s) assume any liability for any injury and/or damage to persons or property arising from or related to use of material in this book.

This book is sold on the understanding that the publisher is not engaged in providing professional medical services. If such advice or services are required, the services of a competent medical professional should be sought.

Every effort has been made where necessary to contact holders of copyright to obtain permission to reproduce copyright material. If any have been inadvertently overlooked, the publisher will be pleased to make the necessary arrangements at the first opportunity.

Inquiries for bulk sales may be solicited at: jaypee@jaypeebrothers.com

Piyush Gupta's Pediatric Drug Companion

First Edition: **2024**

ISBN: 978-93-5696-677-2

Printed at: Samrat Offset Pvt. Ltd.

Dedicated to

Children of India, their parents, and those health personnel who take care of them.

Preface

Someone rightly said, *'A drug is like a holy book. The more you read, the better you treat'*. Drug therapy remains the key element of research in the ongoing era of evidence-based practice. It is essential for every medical personnel to be constantly aware of revised drug updates extending to but not limited to the dose and route of a drug. A good knowledge of the pharmacodynamics and pharmacokinetics of any drug goes a long way in ensuring optimal patient care. We understand that it takes plenty of time, effort, and resources to acquire and assimilate such knowledge and this is where our book can come in handy. This is a complete drug book, covering more than 400 drugs used in pediatric practice, presented alphabetically. The detailed information for each drug has been categorized under individual headings as: Category, Route, Strength, Brands, Mechanism of action, Pharmacokinetics, Indications, Does as per indications, Maximum dosage, Dose adjustments, Adverse effects, Contraindications, and Drug interactions. "One page, one drug" format gives easy access and understanding to readers. The book has been written in simple, clear language for easy understanding and intended for nursing staff, undergraduates, postgraduates, private practitioners, and pharmacists.

All in all, it is a 'must read' complete handbook which can be carried anywhere. We welcome any comments, suggestions and constructive reviews on this project and sincerely hope you enjoy reading (and using) the book, in your day-to-day practice!

Nidhi Bedi
Piyush Gupta

Acknowledgments

We thank our families, children, friends for their support, Dr Pooja Dewan for her guidance and help in composing of the book and Ms Anju Kumari for secretarial assistance. We also thank Shri Jitendar P Vij (Group Chairman), Mr Ankit Vij (Managing Director), Ms Chetna Malhotra (Senior Director—Professional Publishing, Marketing, and Business Development), Ms Pallavi A Mehrotra (Development Editor), and the entire team of M/s Jaypee Brothers Medical Publishers (P) Ltd, New Delhi, India, for their efforts.

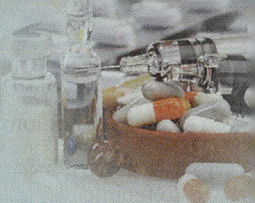

Contents

A

Abacavir 1
Acetazolamide 2
Acetylsalicylic Acid (Aspirin) ... 3
ACTH (Corticotropin) 4
Acyclovir 5
Adefovir Dipivoxil 7
Adenosine 8
Adrenaline (Epinephrine) 9
Albendazole 11
Albumin 13
Alfacalcidol 14
Allopurinol 15
Alprostadil 16
Amantadine 17
Amikacin 18
Aminophylline 19
Amiodarone 20
Amitriptyline 21
Amlodipine 22
Amodiaquine 23
Amoxicillin 24
Amoxicillin-clavulanic Acid .. 25
Amphetamine 26
Amphotericin B 27
Ampicillin 28
Ampicillin with Sulbactam ... 29
Amrinone 30
Anidulafungin 31
Anti-RhD Immunoglobulin ... 32
Antisnake Venom Serum (Polyvalent) 33
Antithymocyte Globulin (Equine) 34
Artemether 35
Artesunate 37
Ascorbic Acid (Vitamin C) 38
Astemizole 39

Atazanavir (ATV) 40
Atenolol 41
Atomoxetine 42
Atorvastatin 43
Atropine Sulfate 44
Azathioprine 45
Azithromycin 46
Aztreonam 47

B

Baclofen 48
Beclomethasone Dipropionate 49
Bedaquiline (BDP) 50
Benzathine Penicillin 51
Benzyl Penicillin 52
Bevacizumab 53
Bisacodyl 54
Bleomycin 55
Budesonide 56
Budesonide with Formoterol 57
Bumetanide 59
Busulfan 60

C

Caffeine Citrate 61
Calcium Carbonate 62
Calcium Gluconate 63
Capreomycin 64
Captopril 65
Carbamazepine 66
Carbenicillin 67
Carbimazole 68
Carnitine 69
Carvedilol 70
Caspofungin Acetate 71
Cefaclor 72
Cefadroxil 73

Cefazolin Sodium 74	Dexamethasone 116
Cefdinir 75	Dextromethorphan 117
Cefepime 76	Diaminodiphenyl Sulfone (DDS) 118
Cefixime 77	Diazepam 119
Cefoperazone-sulbactam 78	Diazoxide 120
Cefotaxime 79	Diclofenac 121
Cefoxitin 80	Dicyclomine 122
Cefpodoxime Proxetil 81	Didanosine 123
Cefprozil 82	Diethylcarbamazine (DEC) 124
Ceftazidime 83	Digoxin 125
Ceftriaxone Sodium 84	Dimenhydrinate 126
Cefuroxime Axetil 85	Dimercaprol 127
Cephalexin 86	Diphenhydramine 128
Cetirizine Dihydrochloride 87	Disopyramide 129
Chloral Hydrate 88	Dobutamine 130
Chloramphenicol 89	Dolutegravir (DTG) 131
Chloroquine Phosphate 90	Domperidone 132
Chlorothiazide 91	Dopamine 133
Chlorpheniramine Maleate ... 92	Doripenem 134
Chlorpromazine 93	Doxapram 135
Cholecalciferol 94	Doxycycline 136
Cholestyramine 95	D-penicillamine 137
Ciprofloxacin 96	Drotaverine 138
Clarithromycin 97	
Clindamycin 98	**E**
Clobazam 99	
Clonazepam 100	Edrophonium 139
Clonidine Hydrochloride 101	Efavirenz (EFV) 140
Cloxacillin 102	Emtricitabine (FTC) 141
Codeine Phosphate 103	Enalapril Maleate 142
Colistimethate Sodium (Colistin) 104	Enoxaparin 143
Cycloserine 105	Ergotamine Tartrate 144
Cyclosporine 106	Erythropoietin c 145
Cyproheptadine Hydrochloride 107	Esmolol Hydrochloride 146
	Etanercept 147
D	Ethambutol 148
	Ethionamide 149
Daptomycin 108	Ethosuximide 150
Darunavir (DRV) 109	
Deferasirox 110	**F**
Deferiprone 111	
Deflazacort 112	Famotidine 151
Desferrioxamine 113	Faropenem 152
Desloratadine 114	Fentanyl 153
Desmopressin 115	Ferrous Sulfate/Fumarate/ Gluconate/Ascorbate 154

Fexofenadine Hydrochloride 155
Fluconazole 156
Flucytosine 157
Fludrocortisone Acetate 158
Flumazenil 159
Flunarizine 160
Fluoxetine 161
Fluticasone Propionate 162
Folic Acid 163
Formoterol Fumarate 164
Foscarnet 165
Fosphenytoin 166
Furosemide 167

G

Gabapentin 168
Ganciclovir 169
Gatifloxacin 170
Gentamicin Sulfate 171
Glucagon Hydrochloride ... 172
Granisetron 173
Granulocyte Colony-Stimulating Factor (G-CSF) 174
Griseofulvin 175

H

Haloperidol 176
Heparin Sodium (Unfractionated) 178
Heparin, Low Molecular Weight (Enoxaparin) 180
Hepatitis B Immunoglobulin (HBIG) 181
Human Milk Fortifier 182
Hydralazine Hydrochloride .. 183
Hydrochlorothiazide 184
Hydrocortisone Sodium Succinate 185
Hydroxyzine Hydrochloride 186
Hyoscine Butylbromide 187

I

Ibuprofen 188
IgM Enriched Immunoglobulin 189
Imipenem-Cilastatin 190
Imipramine Hydrochloride 191
Indinavir 192
Indomethacin 193
Insulin 194
Intravenous Immunoglobulin (IVIG) 195
Ipratropium Bromide 196
Isoniazid 197
Isoprinosine (Inosine Pranobex) 198
Isosorbide Dinitrate 199
Itraconazole 200
Ivermectin 201

K

Kanamycin 202
Ketamine 203
Ketoconazole 204
Ketotifen 205

L

Labetalol 206
Lactulose 207
Lamivudine (3TC) 208
Lamotrigine 209
Lansoprazole Junior 210
Ledipasvir/Sofosbuvir Oral 211
Leuprolide Acetate 212
Levamisole Hydrochloride .. 213
Levetiracetam 214
Levocetirizine 215
Levofloxacin 216
Levosalbutamol 217
Levothyroxine 218
Lignocaine Hydrochloride 219
Lincomycin 220
Linezolid 221
Lisinopril 222
Lithium 223
Lopinavir/Ritonavir (LPV/r) 224
Loratadine 225
Lorazepam 226
Losartan 227

M

Magnesium Sulfate	228
Mannitol	229
Mebendazole	230
Mefenamic Acid	231
Mefloquine Hydrochloride	232
Melatonin	233
Meropenem	234
Metformin	235
Methadone	236
Methimazole	237
Methotrexate	238
Methylcobalamin	239
Methylene Blue	241
Methylphenidate	242
Methylprednisolone	243
Metoclopramide Hydrochloride	244
Metoprolol	245
Metronidazole	246
Mexiletine	247
Micafungin	248
Midazolam	249
Milrinone	250
Miltefosine	251
Minocycline	252
Minoxidil	253
Mometasone	254
Montelukast Sodium	255
Morphine Sulfate	256
Moxifloxacin	258
Mycophenolate Mofetil	259

N

N-acetylcysteine	260
Nalidixic Acid	261
Naloxone Hydrochloride	262
Naproxen	263
Nelfinavir (NFV)	264
Neomycin Sulfate	265
Neostigmine	266
Netilmicin Sulfate	267
Nevirapine (NVP)	268
Niclosamide	269
Nifedipine	270
Nitazoxanide	271
Nitrazepam	272
Nitrofurantoin	273
Nitroprusside	274
Nizatidine	275
Norepinephrine	276
Norfloxacin	277
Nystatin	278

O

Octreotide	279
Ofloxacin	280
Olanzapine	281
Olmesartan	282
Omalizumab	283
Omeprazole	285
Ondansetron Hydrochloride	286
Oral Rehydration Salt (ORS)	287
Ornidazole	288
Oseltamivir	289
Oxcarbazepine	290

P

Palonosetron	291
Pancuronium	292
Pantoprazole	293
Para-amino Salicylic Acid	294
Paracetamol (PCM)	295
Paraldehyde	296
Paromomycin Sulfate	297
Pefloxacin	298
Penicillin G Aqueous	299
Penicillin G Benzathine	300
Penicillin V Potassium (Phenoxymethyl-penicillin)	301
Pentamidine	302
Pentazocine Hydrochloride	303
Permethrin	304
Pethidine Hydrochloride	305
Pheniramine Maleate	306
Phenobarbitone Sodium	307
Phenytoin Sodium	309

Physostigmine 310	Ranitidine 349
Pimozide 311	Rasburicase 350
Piperacillin 312	Remdesivir 351
Piperacillin-tazobactam 313	Respiratory Syncytial Virus (RSV) IG 352
Piperazine 314	Ribavirin 353
Piracetam 315	Riboflavin 354
Piroxicam 316	Rifampicin 355
Polyethylene Glycol (PEG) 317	Ritonavir (RTV) 356
Polymyxin B 318	Rituximab 357
Potassium Chloride 319	Rizatriptan Benzoate 358
Pralidoxime 320	Roxithromycin 359
Praziquantel 321	
Prednisolone 322	**S**
Pregabalin 323	Salbutamol (Albuterol) 360
Primaquine 324	Salmeterol (MDI) 361
Probenecid 325	Saquinavir (SQV) 362
Procainamide Hydrochloride 326	Sevelamer 363
Procaine Penicillin 327	Sildenafil 364
Prochlorperazine 328	Simethicone 365
Promethazine Hydrochloride 329	Sodium Benzoate/ Sodium Phenylacetate 366
Propranolol 330	Sodium Bicarbonate 367
Propylthiouracil 332	Sodium Nitroprusside 368
Protamine 333	Sodium Picosulfate 369
Pseudoephedrine 334	Somatropin 370
Pyrantel Pamoate 335	Spironolactone 371
Pyridostigmine 336	Stavudine (d4T) 372
Pyridoxine 337	Streptomycin 373
Pyrimethamine-Sulfadoxine 338	Sucralfate 374
	Sumatriptan 375
	Surfactant 376
Q	
Quinidine 340	**T**
Quinine Dihydrochloride ...341	Tacrolimus 377
Quinine Sulfate 342	Teicoplanin 378
Quinupristin/Dalfopristin 343	Terbinafine Hydrochloride 379
R	Terbutaline 380
Rabeprazole 344	Tetanus Immunoglobulin (TIG) 381
Rabies Human Monoclonal Antibody 345	Tetracycline Hydrochloride 382
Rabies Immunoglobulin (RIG) 346	Theophylline 383
Racecadotril 347	
Ramipril 348	Thiabendazole 385

Thiamine	386
Thiopental	387
Ticarcillin Disodium/ Clavulanate	388
Tigecycline	389
Tinidazole	390
Tiotropium	391
Tobramycin	392
Tocopherol	393
Tolazoline Hydrochloride	394
Topiramate	395
Tramadol	396
Triamcinolone	397
Triamterene	398
Triclofos Sodium	399
Trifluoperazine Hydrochloride	400
Trimethoprim Sulfamethoxazole	401
Triprolidine Hydrochloride	402
Triptorelin	403

U

Ursodeoxycholic Acid (Ursodiol)	404

V

Valganciclovir	405
Valproate	406
Vancomycin Hydrochloride	407
Varicella-Zoster Immunoglobulin (VZIG)	408
Vasopressin	409
Vecuronium	410
Verapamil	411
Vigabatrin	412
Vincristine Sulfate	413
Vitamin A	414
Vitamin K	415
Voriconazole	416

W

Warfarin	418

Z

Zalcitabine (ddC)	419
Zafirlukast	420
Zanamivir	421
Zidovudine (AZT/ZDV)	422
Zinc Sulfate	423
Index	*425*

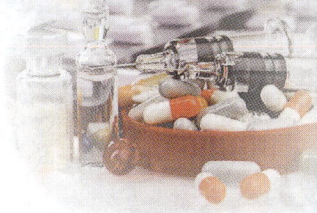

Abacavir

Drug name	Abacavir
Category	Antiretroviral
Route	Oral
Strength	Tab (300 mg)
Brands	Abamune (Tab), Abec (Tab), Virol (Tab)
Mechanism of action	It is a nucleoside analog. Abacavir is converted to carbovir triphosphate (CBV-TP) which inhibits HIV-1 reverse transcriptase
Pharmacokinetics	Rapidly and extensively absorbed, metabolized in liver, excreted primarily in urine. *Half-life:* Around 2 hours
Indications	HIV infection
Dosage as per indications	16 mg/kg/day in 2 divided doses
Maximum dosage	600 mg/day
Dose adjustments	In hepatic derangement
Adverse effects	Malaise, nausea, fatigue, chills, rash, immune reconstitution syndrome, lactic acidosis
Contraindications	Hypersensitivity, children <3 months of age, severe hepatic derangement
Drug interactions	Methadone

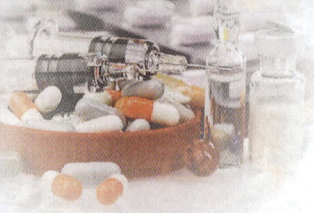

Acetazolamide

Drug name	Acetazolamide
Category	Carbonic anhydrase inhibitor
Route	Oral, Intravenous
Strength	Tab (250 mg); Inj (500 mg powder for sol); Syp (100 mg/100 mL)
Brands	Diamox (Tab), Mazetol (Tab, Syp)
Mechanism of action	Inhibits carbonic anhydrase enzyme
Pharmacokinetics	Rapidly absorbed orally with peak concentration in 2–4 hours; on intravenous administration action starts in 2 minutes and peaks in 15 minutes. Mostly excreted via renal route
Indications	Raised intracranial tension; Seizures; Glaucoma; Altitude sickness
Dosage as per indications	• *For raised intracranial tension:* 5 mg/kg/dose q 8 h • *As diuretic:* 50–70 mg/kg/day q 8 h • *Altitude sickness:* 2.5 mg/kg/dose orally 8–12 hourly
Maximum dosage	1,000 mg/day
Dose adjustments	Dosing interval to be increased to 12 hourly in conditions with creatinine clearance (CrCL) 10–50 mL/min
Adverse effects	Metabolic acidosis, flushing, drowsiness, vertigo, Stevens–Johnson syndrome, hypokalemia, decreased urate excretion
Contraindications	Severe liver/kidney dysfunction, hyperchloremic acidosis
Drug interactions	Diuretics
Remarks	Not to be used intramuscularly

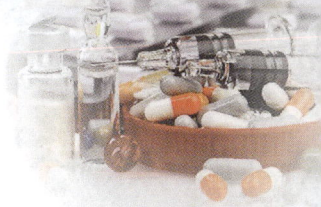

Acetylsalicylic Acid (Aspirin)

Drug name	Acetylsalicylic acid (Aspirin)
Category	Nonsteroidal anti-inflammatory drug (NSAID), antipyretic, antiplatelet agent
Route	Oral
Strength	Tab (75 mg, 100 mg, 325 mg, 650 mg)
Brands	ASA (Tab), Aspirin (Tab), Ecosprin (Tab)
Mechanism of action	Inhibits prostaglandin synthesis by irreversible inactivation of the enzyme cyclooxygenase-1 (COX-1). This inhibits conversion of arachidonic acid to thromboxane A2 (TXA2) leading to irreversible inhibition of platelet aggregation
Pharmacokinetics	Orally absorbed with peak levels obtained in 20–60 minutes, hydrolyzed in plasma, conjugated in liver and metabolites eliminated via urine. *Plasma half-life:* 1–1.5 hours
Indications	As an analgesic/antipyretic; As anti-inflammatory in Kawasaki disease and acute rheumatic fever; As antiplatelet in thrombosis prophylaxis after cardiac surgery
Dosage as per indications	• *Fever:* 10–15 mg/kg/dose 4–6 times/day • *Anti-inflammatory dose:* 80–100 mg/kg/day in 3–4 divided doses • *Kawasaki disease:* 25 mg/kg/dose QID • *Antiplatelet dose:* 3–5 mg/kg/day OD • *Rheumatic fever:* 100 mg/kg/day for 2–3 weeks followed by 60 mg/kg/day for the next 9–12 weeks
Maximum dosage	4 g/24 h
Dose adjustments	In hepatic and renal dysfunction
Adverse effects	Gastrointestinal (GI) disturbance, headache, dizziness. Do not use for treatment of varicella or flu-like symptoms as it may cause Reye syndrome
Contraindications	Hypersensitivity
Drug interactions	Renin angiotensin system (RAS) inhibitors, anticoagulants, NSAIDs

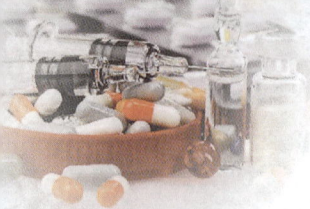

ACTH (Corticotropin)

Drug name	ACTH (Corticotropin)
Category	Hormone
Route	Intramuscular, Subcutaneous
Strength	Inj (25 U/mL, 40 U/mL, 60 U/mL per vial); Gel (40 U/mL, 80 U/mL)
Brands	Acthar (Inj), Acton (Inj), Prolongatum (Inj)
Mechanism of action	Acts like natural ACTH
Pharmacokinetics	Peak levels found in 2–3 hours of administration, levels near normal in 6 hours
Indications	Infantile spasm; West syndrome
Dosage as per indications	20–40 units SC/IM daily for 4 weeks tapered over next 2 weeks
Maximum dosage	Not known
Dose adjustments	Not known
Adverse effects	Hypersensitivity, other side effects like steroids
Contraindications	Congestive heart failure, active severe infections, acute psychosis, peptic ulcer, recent surgery
Drug interactions	Diuretics
Remarks	Protect from light, do not freeze, maintain between 2 and 8°C

Acyclovir

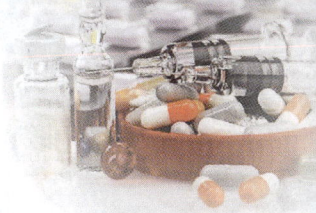

Drug name	Acyclovir
Category	Antiviral
Route	Oral, Intravenous
Strength	Tab (200 mg, 400 mg, 800 mg); Susp (400 mg/5 mL); Inj (250 mg/mL)
Brands	Acivir (Inj, Tab, Syp), Zovirax (Inj, Tab, Syp)
Mechanism of action	Interferes with the viral DNA polymerase and inhibits viral DNA replication
Pharmacokinetics	*Half-life:* 2.5–3 hours, partially absorbed from gut. Mostly eliminated from renal tubular secretion
Indications	HSV infection; Chickenpox (varicella); Varicella zoster infection

Dosage as per indications	• *Neonatal HSV/HSV encephalitis:* Given intravenous for 14–21 days
	  – *Birth to 3 months:*
	    - *<30-week gestation:* 40 mg/kg/day q 8 hourly
	    - *≥30-week gestation:* 60 mg/kg/day q 8 hourly
	  – *3 months to 12 years:* 45–60 mg/kg/day q 8 hourly
	  – *≥12 years:* 30 mg/kg/day q 8 hourly
	• *Mucocutaneous/genital HSV*
	  – *>12 years:*
	    - *Oral:* 1,000–1,200 mg/day in 3–5 divided doses × 7–10 days
	    - *IV:* 5 mg/kg/dose 8 hourly × 5–7 days
	  – *<12 years:* 10–20 mg/kg/dose (max 250 mg/dose) 6 hourly × 5–10 days
	• *Zoster:*
	  – *Oral for children >12 years:* 800 mg 5 times/day × 5–7 days
	  – *IV:* 10 mg/kg/dose 8 hourly for 7–10 days
	• *Varicella:*
	  – *Oral:* >2 years—20 mg/kg/dose (max 800 mg/dose) 6 hourly × 5 days
	  – *IV:* 10 mg/kg/dose 8 hourly (1,500 mg/m^2/24 h) × 7–10 days

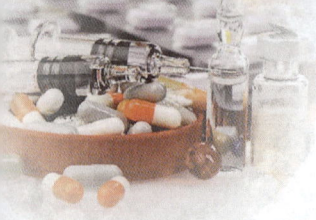

A	Maximum dosage	80 mg/kg/day or 3,200 mg/day
	Dose adjustments	Dose adjustment needed in renal derangement
	Adverse effects	Headache, dizziness, nausea, vomiting, diarrhea, pain abdomen
	Contraindications	Hypersensitivity
	Drug interactions	Probenecid, cimetidine (reduces renal clearance)
	Remarks	Adequate hydration to avoid renal damage

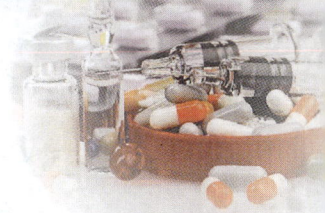

Adefovir Dipivoxil

Drug name	Adefovir dipivoxil
Category	Antiviral
Route	Oral
Strength	Cap/Tab (10 mg)
Brands	Adesera (Cap), Adfovir (Tab), Adheb (Tab)
Mechanism of action	Adefovir is phosphorylated to diphosphate which acts by inhibiting HBV DNA polymerase
Pharmacokinetics	Oral bioavailability around 50–60%. *Half-life:* 8–9 hours, rapidly converted to adefovir which is excreted in urine via glomerular filtration and tubular secretion
Indications	Hepatitis B infection (chronic, lamivudine resistant)
Dosage as per indications	*>12 years of age:* 10 mg/day
Maximum dosage	10 mg/day
Dose adjustments	In renal impairment
Adverse effects	Asthenia, renal injury
Contraindications	Hypersensitivity
Drug interactions	Nephrotoxic drugs

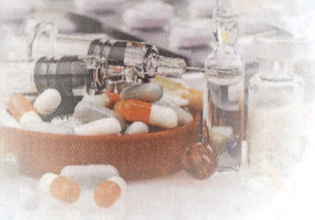

Adenosine

Drug name	Adenosine
Category	Antiarrhythmic
Route	Intravenous
Strength	Inj (3 mg/mL ampoule)
Brands	Adnet (Inj), Adenoject (Inj)
Mechanism of action	Vasodilatory, antiadrenergic, negative chronotropic effects leading to decreased oxygen demand, sinus bradycardia, AV nodal blockade and reduction of accessory pathway
Pharmacokinetics	After IV administration, rapidly cleared from circulation by erythrocyte uptake, further rapidly metabolized. *Half-life:* 10 seconds
Indications	Supraventricular tachycardia
Dosage as per indications	0.1–0.2 mg/kg rapid intravenous push over 1–2 seconds. May increase bolus dose by 0.05 mg/kg every 2 minutes till clinical response or maximum of 12 mg (0.25 mg/kg)
Maximum dosage	• Initial max first dose: 6 mg • Subsequent max dose: 12 mg
Dose adjustments	Not needed in hepatic/renal derangement
Adverse effects	Bronchoconstriction, facial flushing, headache, chest pain, dyspnea
Contraindications	Second/third-degree AV block
Drug interactions	Methylxanthine
Remarks	IV administration should always be followed by rapid saline flush

Adrenaline (Epinephrine)

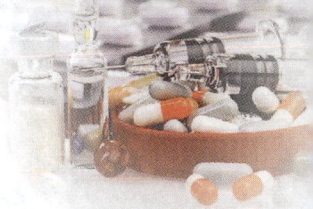

Drug name	Adrenaline (Epinephrine)
Category	Sympathomimetic
Route	Intravenous, Subcutaneous, Endotracheal (ET), Intramuscular
Strength	Inj (1:1,000; 1 mg/mL ampoule)
Brands	Adrena (Inj), Adrenaline Tartrate (Inj), Enatrate (Inj), Vasocon (Inj)
Mechanism of action	Potent stimulant of both alpha and beta adrenergic receptors, leading to vasoconstriction and bronchodilation
Pharmacokinetics	Rapid onset of action, *Half-life:* 2–3 minutes, rapidly inactivated in liver
Indications	Cardiac arrest; Bronchodilation; Shock; Anaphylaxis; For nebulization in croup
Dosage as per indications	• *For cardiac arrest:* 0.1 mL/kg of 1:10,000 diluted intravenous or intratracheal q 3–5 min • *For resuscitation in neonates:* 1:10,000 dilution 0.1–0.3 mL/kg IV q 3–5 min or 0.3–0.5 mL/kg ET • *For CPR in older children:* 0.1 mg/kg IV/ET of 1:1,000 dilution q 3–5 min • *For shock:* 0.05–0.5 µg/kg/min IV infusion • *For bronchodilation:* 1:1000 dilution, 0.01 mg/kg/dose SC, q 15 min × 3–4 doses • *For nebulization:* 0.5 mL/kg of 1:1,000 solution diluted in 3 mL normal saline (max dose in ≤4 years: 2.5 mL/dose and in older children: 5 mL/dose) • *Anaphylaxis:* 0.01 mL/kg 1:1,000 solution SC or IM, max 0.5 mL per dose
Maximum dosage	0.5 mL/dose
Dose adjustments	As per the response
Adverse effects	Tachycardia, hypertension, arrhythmias, headache, nervousness
Contraindications	During labor, with local anesthesia of peripheral structures

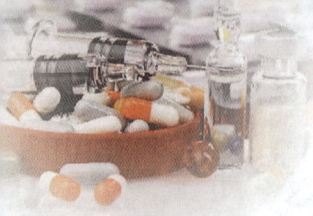

Drug interactions	Inotropes/vasoconstrictors, amitriptyline/beta blocker
Remarks	• Protect from air and light • Can lead to ventricular fibrillation when used along with halothane, sympathomimetic drugs

Adrenaline (Epinephrine)

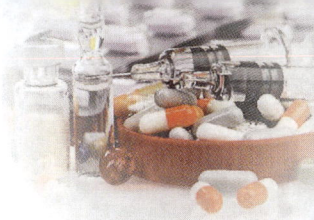

Albendazole

Drug name	Albendazole
Category	Antihelminthic
Route	Oral
Strength	Syp (200 mg/5 mL); Tab (200 mg, 400 mg)
Brands	Bandy (Tab, Syp), Bendex (Tab, Syp), Zentel (Tab, Syp)
Mechanism of action	Inhibits polymerization of tubulin and microtubule, damages cytoplasmic microtubules in the absorptive and intestinal cells of nematodes
Pharmacokinetics	*Half-life:* 8–12 hours, poorly absorbed from gut, >50% plasma protein bound, metabolized, and excreted mainly by hepatobiliary route
Indications	Worm infestation; Taeniasis; Neurocysticercosis; Hydatid cyst
Dosage as per indications	• *For pinworms, roundworms, or hookworms:* Single oral dose of 200 mg in children aged 1–2 years and single oral dose of 400 mg in children >2 years; to be repeated after 2 weeks for roundworm • *Strongyloidiasis and taeniasis:* 400 mg OD for 3 days • *Giardiasis, trichinosis:* 400 mg OD for 5 days • *Neurocysticercosis (NCC):* 15 mg/kg/d for 2–4 weeks with corticosteroids for 5 days to reduce edema. Albendazole is started on day 3 of steroids • *Hydatid cyst:* 400 mg BD for 4 weeks, to be taken with fatty meals. A total of three cycles repeated every 14 days for eradication of hydatid cysts
Maximum dosage	800 mg/day
Dose adjustments	• *Renal:* No adjustments • Hepatic-dose adjustment needed as elimination prolonged in those with altered liver enzymes or with extrahepatic biliary obstruction
Adverse effects	Nausea, vomiting, headache, transaminitis, bone marrow suppression

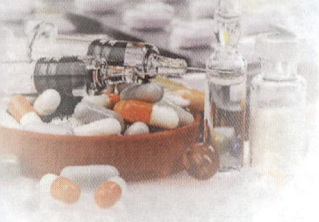

Albendazole

Contraindications	Intraventricular or ocular cysticercosis, cysticercal encephalitis, disseminated NCC, starry sky NCC, biliary obstruction
Drug interactions	Dexamethasone, praziquantel, theophylline, cimetidine
Remarks	It should be preceded with a course of steroids in active NCC to decrease the cytotoxic inflammation expected on albendazole administration

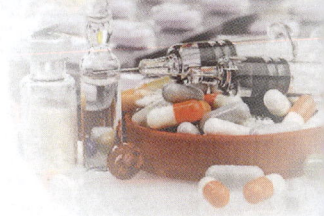

Albumin

Drug name	Albumin
Category	Colloid
Route	Intravenous
Strength	Inj [5% (250 mL, 500 mL), 10%, 20% (50 mL, 100 mL)]
Brands	Albumed (Inj), Albudac (Inj), Volumin (Inj)
Mechanism of action	Main constituent for maintaining of the osmotic pressure of normal plasma thereby regulating the circulating blood volume
Pharmacokinetics	Mainly distributed in extracellular fluid, *Half-life:* Varying between 13 and 19 days
Indications	Hypoproteinemia; Acute hypovolemic shock
Dosage as per indications	*For hypoproteinemia and acute hypovolemic shock:* 0.5–1 g/kg/dose IV over 2–4 h
Maximum dosage	2 g/kg/day or 25 g/day whichever is less
Dose adjustments	• *Liver disease:* Safe • *Kidney disease:* Use with caution
Adverse effects	Fluid overload, hypernatremia, hypersensitivity
Contraindications	Congestive heart failure (CHF), anemia
Drug interactions	Not known
Remarks	• Do not use sterile water as diluent • Fractionated from blood/plasma of donors

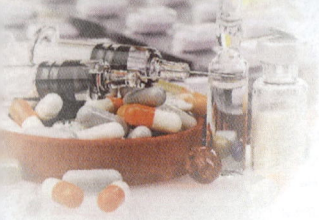

Alfacalcidol

Drug name	Alfacalcidol
Category	Vitamin (1-alpha hydroxycholecalciferol)
Route	Oral
Strength	Cap (0.25 µg)
Brands	Alfacal (Cap), Alfacip (Cap), Alphadol (Cap), One-Alpha (Cap)
Mechanism of action	Increases intestinal calcium absorption, and reabsorption of calcium from bone and kidney
Pharmacokinetics	The drug is absorbed in small intestine, then converted by enzyme 25-hydroxylase in the liver, which is the active form acting on kidneys and bones. *Half-life:* 3–4 hours. Excreted through bile
Indications	Renal osteodystrophy/Chronic renal failure
Dosage as per indications	Hypocalcemia/renal osteodystrophy/secondary hyperparathyroidism in chronic renal failure: 0.04–0.08 µg/kg/day
Maximum dosage	<20 kg: 0.5 µg/day; >20 kg: 1.0 µg/day
Dose adjustments	Not known
Adverse effects	Weakness, headache, fatigue, dry mouth
Contraindications	Hypersensitivity
Drug interactions	Vitamin D supplements, antacids, digoxin, diuretics

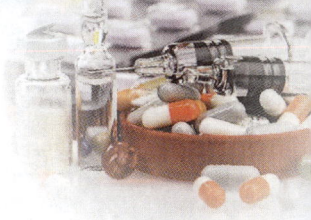

Allopurinol

Drug name	Allopurinol
Category	Antiuric acid (Xanthine oxidase inhibitor)
Route	Oral
Strength	Tab (100 mg)
Brands	Ciploric (Tab), Zyloric (Tab)
Mechanism of action	Both allopurinol and oxipurinol (main metabolite) act by inhibiting xanthine oxidase
Pharmacokinetics	Rapid absorption from gut. Peak levels 1.5 hours after oral administration. *Half-life:* 1–2 hours, 13–30 hours for oxipurinol; thereby providing 24 hours effect
Indications	Tumor lysis syndrome; Hyperuricemia
Dosage as per indications	10 mg/kg/day q 8 h PO
Maximum dosage	800 mg/day
Dose adjustments	Dose adjustment required in renal and hepatic impairment
Adverse effects	Rash, neuritis, hepatotoxic, GI disturbances, bone marrow suppression, Stevens–Johnson syndrome
Contraindications	Hypersensitivity
Drug interactions	6-mercaptopurine (MP), azathioprine, salicylates, coumarin derivatives, diuretics, angiotensin-converting enzyme (ACE) inhibitors, phenytoin
Remarks	Maintain adequate hydration

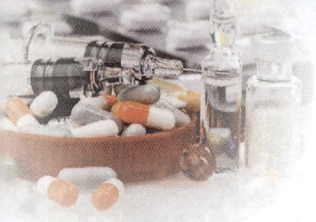

Alprostadil

Drug name	Alprostadil
Category	Prostaglandin E1, vasodilator
Route	Intravenous
Strength	Inj (200 µg/mL, 500 µg/mL, 1,000 µg/mL)
Brands	Alpostin (Inj), Bioglandin (Inj), Prostaver (Inj)
Mechanism of action	Potent vasoactive derivatives of arachidonic acid. Exerts vasomotor, metabolic, and cellular effects on the pulmonary and coronary circulation. The E series of prostaglandins produces vasodilation of the systemic and coronary circulation
Pharmacokinetics	Prostaglandin E1 is rapidly distributed in the body except CNS and very rapidly metabolized. Metabolism and excretion occur mainly in the lung, liver, and kidney
Indications	Ductus-dependent congenital heart disease
Dosage as per indications	*For maintaining patency of ductus arteriosus:* • *Initial dose:* 0.05–0.1 µg/kg/min as continuous IV infusion • *Maintenance dose:* 0.01 µg/kg/min up to 0.4 µg/kg/min
Maximum dosage	Up to 60 µg/24 h have been studied
Dose adjustments	Not studied
Adverse effects	Hypotension, bradycardia, fever, seizures, tissue necrosis and sloughing if extravasated. Weakening of the ductus arteriosus wall and pulmonary artery with prolonged administration
Contraindications	Hypersensitivity
Drug interactions	Not known
Remarks	Titrate dose according to the response. It should be diluted not >20 µg/mL. Prepare fresh solution every 24 hours. It should be put directly into the fluid. Arterial pressure should be monitored. The rate of infusion should be decreased if the pressure falls significantly

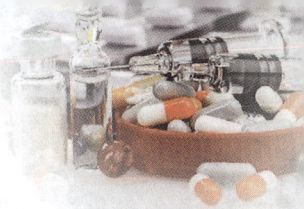

Amantadine

Drug name	Amantadine
Category	Antiviral
Route	Oral
Strength	Cap (100 mg); Syp (50 mg/5 mL)
Brands	Amantrel (Cap), Comantrel (Tab), Parkitidin (Cap)
Mechanism of action	Prevents the release of infectious viral nucleic acid into the host cell by interfering with the function of the transmembrane domain of the viral M2 protein
Pharmacokinetics	Well absorbed orally, primarily excreted unchanged in the urine by glomerular filtration and tubular secretion. Peak levels in 3–4 hours, *Half-life:* 10–25 hours
Indications	Influenza prophylaxis/Treatment
Dosage as per indications	4–8 mg/kg/day in two divided doses for 10 days/24–48 hours off symptoms
Maximum dosage	Maximum dose <10 years: 150 mg/d, >10 years: 200 mg/d
Dose adjustments	Needed in renal and liver derangement
Adverse effects	Dizziness, rash, mental instability, nausea, CHF, edema
Contraindications	Hypersensitivity
Drug interactions	CNS stimulants, anticholinergic drugs, quinidine, quinine
Remarks	For treatment, start as early as possible after onset of symptoms. Neuroleptic malignant syndrome has been reported with abrupt discontinuation or sudden lowering of doses

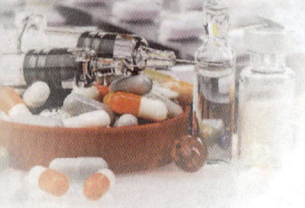

Amikacin

Drug name	Amikacin
Category	Aminoglycoside antibiotic, Bactericidal
Route	Intravenous, Intramuscular
Strength	Inj (50 mg, 100 mg, 250 mg, 500 mg vials)
Brands	Abcin (Inj), Abiox (Inj), Almika (Inj)
Mechanism of action	Binds irreversibly to 30S ribosomal subunit thereby inhibiting protein synthesis
Pharmacokinetics	Rapidly absorbed after intramuscular injection, with a half-life of 2–3 hours. Mostly excreted unchanged within 24 hours
Indications	Gram-negative bacterial infections including UTI
Dosage as per indications	*Neonate:* • *<7 days:* <29 weeks—18 mg/kg 48 hourly; 30–34 weeks—18 mg/kg 36 hourly, >34 weeks—15 mg/kg 24 hourly • *>7 days:* <29 weeks—15 mg/kg 36 hourly till 28 days of life • Others—15 mg/kg 24 hourly *Children:* 15 mg/kg 24 h in 1–2 divided doses
Maximum dosage	1,500 mg/day
Dose adjustments	• *Hepatic:* No adjustment needed • *Renal derangement:* Dose adjustment needed
Adverse effects	Nephrotoxicity, ototoxicity (high frequency deafness), neuromuscular blockade. Risk increases in patients with renal impairment
Contraindications	Drug hypersensitivity
Drug interactions	• Increased risk of ototoxicity and nephrotoxicity with vancomycin, amphotericin, cisplatin, cephalosporin, cyclosporine • Nondepolarizing muscle relaxants increase effects • Neostigmine antagonizes the drug effect
Remarks	Drug to be dissolved in normal saline or 5% dextrose, concentration not >10 mg/mL

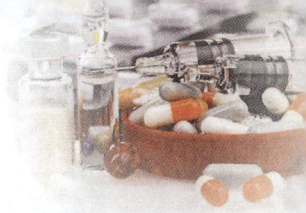

Aminophylline

Drug name	Aminophylline
Category	Bronchodilator
Route	Oral, Intravenous
Strength	Syp (20 mg/5 mL); Inj (250 mg/10 mL)
Brands	Phyllocontin (Tab), Aminophyllim (Inj, Tab)
Mechanism of action	Aminophylline relaxes smooth muscle and relieves bronchial spasm by its theophylline action
Pharmacokinetics	Well absorbed orally, 40–60% bound to plasma. Is metabolized in liver, mainly excreted in urine, *Half-life:* 5–8 hours
Indications	Bronchial asthma; Apnea of prematurity
Dosage as per indications	• *Bronchospasm:* Loading 5 mg/kg IV over 30 minutes followed by maintenance (as per age) – *6 weeks to 6 months:* 0.5 mg/kg/h – *6 months to 1 year:* 0.7 mg/kg/h – *1–9 years:* 1 mg/kg/h – *9–12 years:* 0.9 mg/kg/h • *Apnea of prematurity:* 6 mg/kg IV/PO loading followed by 2 mg/kg/dose q 8–12 h
Maximum dosage	40 mg/kg/d, serum concentrations not to exceed 20 µg/mL
Dose adjustments	Required in renal and hepatic insufficiency
Adverse effects	Tachycardia, restlessness, headache, GI upset, seizures
Contraindications	Hypersensitivity to ethylenediamine, theophylline and caffeine; porphyria
Drug interactions	Beta agonist/antagonist, adenosine, cardiac glycosides, quinolones, allopurinol, macrolides
Remarks	• *Serum therapeutic levels for asthma:* 10–20 mg/L • *For neonatal apnea:* 6–13 mg/L • Monitor serum potassium levels

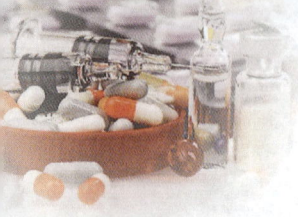

Amiodarone

Drug name	Amiodarone
Category	Antiarrhythmic, Potassium channel blocking agent
Route	Oral, Intravenous
Strength	Tab (100 mg, 200 mg); Inj (150 mg/3 mL)
Brands	Amiodar (Tab), Cordarone (Inj, Tab), Duron (Inj, Tab)
Mechanism of action	It decreases cardiac muscle excitability by reducing action potential and increasing refractory period of cardiac myocytes
Pharmacokinetics	• Pediatric studies not established • In adults, highly protein bound with a half-life of around 50 days. • Mainly metabolized by CYP3A4
Indications	Tachyarrhythmia/Ventricular tachycardia

Dosage as per indications	• *Neonate:*
	  – *IV loading dose:* 5 mg/kg IV infusion over 30–60 minutes
	  – *Maintenance infusion:* Begin with 7 µg/kg/min up to 15 µg/kg/min
	  – *Oral dose:* 5–10 mg/kg/dose q 12 h
	• *Pediatric:*
	  – *IV loading dose:* 5 mg/kg (max dose: 300 mg) over 30 minutes
	  – *Maintenance infusion:* Continuous infusion starting at 5 µg/kg/min up to 15 µg/kg/min
	  – *Oral dose:* 5–7.5 mg/kg/dose q 12 h

Maximum dosage	Loading: 300 mg, infusion: 15 µg/kg/min
Dose adjustments	Dose adjustment in renal impairment
Adverse effects	Bradycardia, rhythm abnormalities, hypotension, thyroid disorders
Contraindications	Sinus bradycardia, sinoatrial heart block, combination of amiodarone with drugs which may induce torsades de pointes, thyroid dysfunction, hypersensitivity, neonate
Drug interactions	Antiarrhythmic drugs
Remarks	For infusions of >1 hour, IV concentrations should not exceed 2 mg/mL unless using a central line. To be diluted in 5% glucose and not normal saline. Use with caution in <3 years old due to severe toxicity and hypersensitivity reactions

Amitriptyline

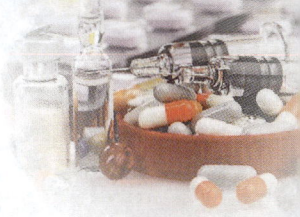

Drug name	Amitriptyline
Category	Antidepressant
Route	Oral
Strength	Tab (10 mg, 25 mg, 50 mg, 75 mg)
Brands	Amiline (Tab), Amitone (Tab), Tryptomer (Tab)
Mechanism of action	Inhibits the membrane pump mechanism responsible for uptake of norepinephrine and serotonin in adrenergic and serotonergic neurons
Pharmacokinetics	Rapidly absorbed, metabolized by P450, excreted in urine
Indications	Depression; Nocturnal enuresis; Migraine prophylaxis

Dosage as per indications	• *Depression:* 1–1.5 mg/kg/day in 2 divided doses, to start from low dose and increase gradually
	• *Nocturnal enuresis:*
	  – *<10 years:* 10–25 mg once at bedtime
	  – *>10 years:* 25–50 mg once at bedtime
	• *For migraine prophylaxis:* Start at 0.25 mg/kg/day and increase gradually every 2–3 weeks to a maximum of 2 mg/kg/day

Maximum dosage	2 mg/kg/day up to 150–200 mg/day
Dose adjustments	In liver derangement
Adverse effects	Cardiovascular (from nonspecific ECG changes to MI), hallucinations, seizures, disorientation, gastritis, nausea, bone marrow suppression, gynecomastia, galactorrhea, testicular swelling
Contraindications	Hypersensitivity, those on MAO inhibitor
Drug interactions	Drugs prolonging QT interval

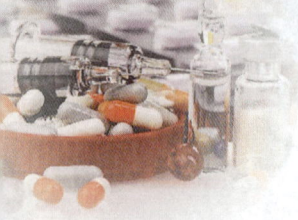

Amlodipine

Drug name	Amlodipine
Category	Calcium channel blocker, Antihypertensive
Route	Oral
Strength	Tab (5 mg)
Brands	Amlong (Tab), Amlopres (Tab), Amlocard (Tab)
Mechanism of action	Amlodipine is a calcium ion influx inhibitor of the dihydropyridine group. It inhibits the transmembrane influx of calcium ions into cardiac and vascular smooth muscle leading to relaxant effect on vascular smooth muscle. Amlodipine dilates peripheral arterioles and coronary vessels
Pharmacokinetics	After oral administration of therapeutic doses, amlodipine is well absorbed with peak blood levels between 6 and 12 hours. Amlodipine is extensively metabolized by the liver. Bioavailability not affected by food
Indications	Hypertension
Dosage as per indications	Starting dose 0.05–0.1 mg/kg/day, may increase to 0.3–0.4 mg/kg/day
Maximum dosage	Starting dose 5 mg/day, can increase up to 0.6 mg/kg/day, max 20 mg/day
Dose adjustments	• No renal adjustment • Start at lowest dose in those with moderate to severe hepatic derangement, titrate gradually
Adverse effects	Palpitations, dizziness, flushing, edema, dizziness
Contraindications	Hypersensitivity to dihydropyridine derivatives, hypotension, shock, obstruction of the outflow tract of the left ventricle
Drug interactions	CYP3A4 inhibitors (protease inhibitors, azole antifungals, macrolides like erythromycin or clarithromycin, verapamil or diltiazem)
Remarks	Titration should be done slowly, at 7–10 days interval

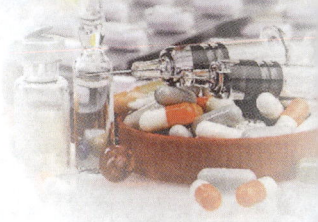

Amodiaquine

Drug name	Amodiaquine
Category	Antimalarial (4-aminoquinolines)
Route	Oral
Strength	Tab (200 mg base); Susp (150 mg base/5 mL)
Brands	Camoquin (Tab), Basoquin (Susp), Amodiaquin (Tab, Susp)
Mechanism of action	Inhibits heme polymerase resulting in free heme accumulation which is toxic to parasites
Pharmacokinetics	After oral administration, amodiaquine hydrochloride is rapidly absorbed. It undergoes rapid and extensive metabolism to desethylamodiaquine which concentrates in red blood cells
Indications	Malaria
Dosage as per indications	10 mg/kg of base stat PO and then 5 mg/kg at 6 hours, 24 hours, 48 hours
Maximum dosage	600 mg/dose
Dose adjustments	In hepatic derangement
Adverse effects	Hepatitis, agranulocytosis, peripheral neuropathy, corneal deposits
Contraindications	Hypersensitivity, severe hepatic derangement
Drug interactions	Efavirenz, nevirapine, zidovudine
Remarks	Used in combination with artesunate

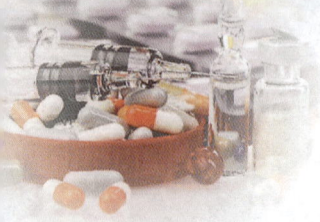

Amoxicillin

Drug name	Amoxicillin
Category	Antibiotic, Penicillin
Route	Oral
Strength	Cap (250 mg, 500 mg); Susp (125 mg/5 mL); Drops (50 mg/mL)
Brands	Mox (Cap, Susp, Drops), Zenmox (Cap, Susp), Novamox (Cap, Susp, Drops)
Mechanism of action	Bactericidal against gram-positive and gram-negative organisms, degraded by β-lactamases. It acts by inhibiting cell wall biosynthesis
Pharmacokinetics	Well absorbed from the gut after oral administration, half-life is around 1 hour. Around 20% bound to plasma protein. Does not penetrate CNS except when inflamed
Indications	Acute respiratory infections; Tonsillitis; Pharyngitis; Otitis media; Lyme disease; Bacterial endocarditis prophylaxis; Urinary tract infection; Enteric fever
Dosage as per indications	• *Acute respiratory infections (ARIs):* 25–50 mg/kg/day q 8 h • *Recurrent otitis media:* 20 mg/kg/dose HS PO • *Tonsillitis/pharyngitis:* 50 mg/kg/day q 8–12 hourly for 10 days • *Bacterial endocarditis prophylaxis:* 50 mg/kg (max 2 g) single dose • *Lyme disease:* 50 mg/kg/day q 8 hourly for 14–21 days
Maximum dosage	ARI: 2–3 g/day, up to 4 g/day have been tried; tonsillitis: 1 g/day, Lyme disease 1.5 g/day
Dose adjustments	Dose adjustment in renal failure
Adverse effects	Diarrhea, vomiting, rash
Contraindications	Hypersensitivity
Drug interactions	Probenecid acid, anticoagulants
Remarks	Administer 1 hour prior to procedure, for endocarditis prophylaxis

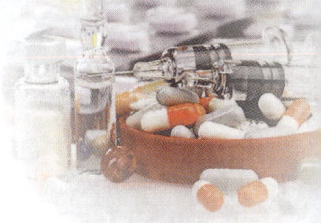

Amoxicillin-clavulanic Acid

Drug name	Amoxicillin-clavulanic acid
Category	Antibiotic, Penicillin
Route	Oral, Intravenous
Strength	Tab (250 mg Amoxicillin with 125 mg Clavulanate, 500 mg Amoxicillin with 125 mg Clavulanate); Syp (200 Amox with 28.5 mg Clavulanate/5 mL, 125 mg Amox with 31.5 mg Clavulanate/5 mL); Inj [150 mg (125 mg Amox), 300 mg (250 mg Amox), 600 mg (500 mg Amox), 1,200 mg (1,000 mg Amox)]
Brands	Advent (Inj, Tab, Syp), Augmentin (Inj, Tab, Syp), Augpen (Inj, Tab, Syp), Clavactum (Inj, Tab, Syp)
Mechanism of action	Amoxicillin component bactericidal against gram-positive and gram-negative organisms. Clavulanic acid is a β-lactam to inactivate β-lactamase enzymes (present in resistant microorganisms)
Pharmacokinetics	Well absorbed from the gut after oral administration, half-life is around 1–1.5 hours for both amoxicillin and clavulanate. Only 20–25% bound to plasma protein. Does not penetrate CNS
Indications	Acute respiratory infections
Dosage as per indications	• *Oral:* 20–40 mg (amox base)/kg/day q 8–12 h • *Intravenous:* 50–100 mg (amox base)/kg/day q 6–8 h
Maximum dosage	*Oral:* 1,000 mg/day amoxicillin, 6.4 mg/kg/day clavulanate
Dose adjustments	Dose adjustment in renal failure. Avoid in hepatic dysfunction
Adverse effects	Diarrhea, rash
Contraindications	Hypersensitivity
Drug interactions	Probenecid acid, anticoagulants, drugs affecting liver enzymes

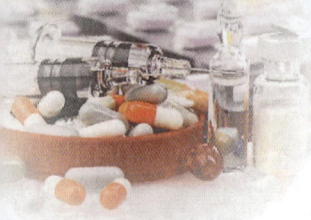

Amphetamine

Drug name	Amphetamine
Category	Stimulant
Route	Oral
Strength	Tab (5 mg, 10 mg, 15 mg, 20 mg, 25 mg, 30 mg)
Brands	Banned in India
Mechanism of action	Blocks the reuptake of norepinephrine and dopamine into the presynaptic neuron and increase the release of these monoamines into the extraneuronal space
Pharmacokinetics	*Half-life:* 10–12 hours, up to 75% excretion via kidneys, rest by hepatic route
Indications	Attention deficit hyperactivity disorder (ADHD)

Dosage as per indications	• *ADHD:* 0.15–0.5 mg/kg/day
	  – *<5 years:* Start at 2.5 mg/day and increase weekly by 2.5 mg/day till response
	  – *>5 years:* Start at 5 mg/day and increase weekly by 5 mg/day

Maximum dosage	40 mg/day
Dose adjustments	In renal and hepatic derangement
Adverse effects	Cardiac sudden events
Contraindications	Hypersensitivity
Drug interactions	Monoamine oxidase (MAO) inhibitors

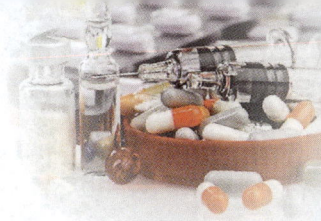

Amphotericin B

Drug name	Amphotericin B
Category	Antifungal
Route	Oral, Intravenous
Strength	Susp (100 mg/mL); Tab (100 mg); Inj (50 mg/vial); Liposomal: (10 mg, 25 mg, 50 mg)
Brands	Ampholip (Inj), Fungisome (Inj), Phosome (Inj)
Mechanism of action	It has fungistatic action. It binds to sterols in the fungal cell membrane causing membrane permeability and leakage of intracellular components. The lipophilic moiety integrates in the lipid bilayer of the liposomes
Pharmacokinetics	*Half-life:* 24 hours, highly bound to plasma proteins, predominantly excreted by the kidneys
Indications	Systemic fungal infection; Kala-azar/Visceral leishmaniasis
Dosage as per indications	Start at 0.25 mg/kg and increase till 1 mg/kg/day OD as infusion in 5% dextrose. • *Liposomal:* 3–5 mg/kg/day OD for *Candida*, *Aspergillus*, and mucormycosis • *Visceral leishmaniasis/kala-azar:* 1 mg/kg every alternate day × 1 month
Maximum dosage	1.5 mg/kg/day
Dose adjustments	Required in renal derangement
Adverse effects	Hypersensitivity, hepatotoxic, renotoxic, neurotoxicity, anemia, agranulocytosis, thrombocytopenia. IV administration may cause chills, fever, vomiting and headache
Contraindications	Hypersensitivity, liposomal not recommended in <1-month-old
Drug interactions	Antineoplastic drugs, digitalis, flucytosine, other nephrotoxic drugs
Remarks	Protect from light, nephrotoxic. Monitor serum potassium levels

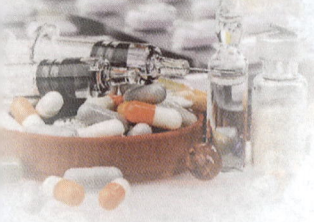

Ampicillin

Drug name	Ampicillin
Category	Antibiotic, Penicillin
Route	Oral, Intravenous
Strength	Cap (250 mg, 500 mg); Syp (125 mg/5 mL); Inj (250 mg, 500 mg)
Brands	Ampicillin (Inj, Cap), Ampipen (Cap, Syp), Biocilin (Inj, Cap/Tab, Syp), Aristocillin (Inj, Cap/Tab, Syp)
Mechanism of action	Inhibits bacterial cell wall synthesis by binding to specific penicillin-binding proteins
Pharmacokinetics	Ampicillin is excreted mainly in the bile and urine with a plasma half-life of 1–2 hours
Indications	Effective against gram-positive and gram-negative bacteria in diseases such as community-acquired pneumonia/Upper respiratory tract infections (URIs); Meningitis; Enteric fever; Subacute bacterial endocarditis (SBE) prophylaxis
Dosage as per indications	• *URI/pneumonia:* 25–50 mg/kg/dose 6 hourly IV; 50–100 mg/kg/day q 6 hourly PO • *Severe infection/meningitis:* 50–100 mg/kg/dose IV 6 hourly • *Enteric fever:* 50 mg/kg/dose q 6 h oral • *SBE prophylaxis:* 50 mg/kg single dose (max 2 g) IV 30 minutes before procedure
Maximum dosage	3 g/dose 6 hourly IV or 1 g/dose 6 hourly oral
Dose adjustments	In the presence of severe renal impairment (creatinine clearance <10 mL/min) a reduction in dose or extension of dose interval should be considered
Adverse effects	Diarrhea, rash, interstitial nephritis, pseudomembranous enterocolitis
Contraindications	Hypersensitivity
Drug interactions	Probenecid acid, allopurinol, oral contraceptives
Remarks	Avoid in patients of infectious mononucleosis/leukemia of lymphoid origin as they tend to develop rash following ampicillin administration

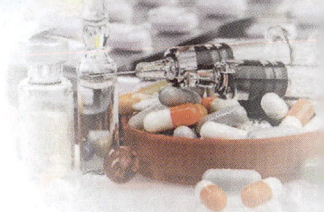

Ampicillin with Sulbactam

Drug name	Ampicillin with sulbactam
Category	Antibiotic
Route	Oral, Intravenous
Strength	Tab (375 mg containing 250 mg Ampicillin); Inj (1 g Ampicillin with 0.5 g Sulbactam vial)
Brands	Ambact (Inj), Ampysul (Inj), Betamp (Inj), Osocillin-S (Inj), Sulbacin (Tab)
Mechanism of action	Inhibits bacterial cell wall synthesis by binding to specific penicillin-binding proteins. Like clavulanic acid, sulbactam inhibits the activity of beta-lactamase
Pharmacokinetics	Both the components are around 30–40% protein bound. Excretion is mainly renal via tubular secretion and glomerular filtration. Elimination half-life is 1 hour
Indications	Severe infections including meningitis. It acts against gram-positive and gram-negative bacteria resistant to ampicillin alone
Dosage as per indications	• *Newborn:* 100 mg/kg/day ampicillin component IV divided every 8 hours in term and 12-hourly in preterm • *Children:* 100–200 mg/kg/day of ampicillin q 6–8 h IV; for meningitis/severe infections: 200–400 mg/kg/day of ampicillin component divided 6 hourly IV
Maximum dosage	2 g/dose ampicillin component
Dose adjustments	Dose adjustment in renal failure and hepatic derangement
Adverse effects	Diarrhea, rash, nausea, tongue discoloration, glossitis, transaminitis, hypersensitivity
Contraindications	Those with jaundice/hepatic dysfunction/hypersensitivity after ampicillin
Drug interactions	Probenecid acid, allopurinol, anticoagulants

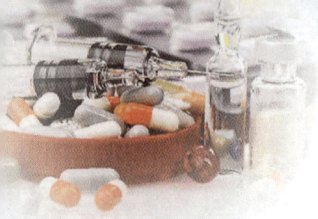

Amrinone

Drug name	Amrinone
Category	Phosphodiesterase inhibitor, Cardiovascular bipyridine, Inotrope, Vasodilator
Route	Intravenous
Strength	Inj (100 mg/20 mL)
Brands	Amicor (Inj), Carditone (Inj)
Mechanism of action	It inhibits c-AMPase thereby increasing cAMP levels and dilates vascular smooth muscles
Pharmacokinetics	Metabolized in liver; 10–20% bound to plasma proteins, primarily excreted in urine, half-life after IV administration: 4–6 hours
Indications	Pulmonary hypertension; Congestive heart failure; Postoperative heart failure
Dosage as per indications	0.75 mg/kg IV bolus over 2–3 minutes followed by 3–5 µg/kg/min in newborns and 5–10 µg/kg/min in children as continuous infusion
Maximum dosage	10 mg/kg cumulative dose
Dose adjustments	Dose adjustments needed in renal and hepatic derangement
Adverse effects	Thrombocytopenia, hypotension, rhythm disturbances, tachycardia
Contraindications	Hypertrophic cardiomyopathy, low platelet counts (<50,000/mL)
Drug interactions	Furosemide should not be injected into intravenous lines carrying amrinone infusions because the drug forms a precipitate when added to amrinone solutions
Remarks	Amrinone is degraded by dextrose and by light. Therefore, amrinone should not be infused in dextrose-containing fluids, and the infusion solution should be protected from light

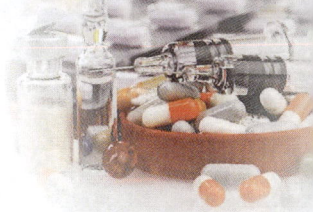

Anidulafungin

Drug name	Anidulafungin
Category	Antifungal, Echinocandins
Route	Intravenous
Strength	Inj (50 mg/vial, 100 mg/vial)
Brands	Eraxis (Inj), Endfung (Inj)
Mechanism of action	*Fungicidal drug:* It inhibits 1,3-β-D glucan synthase, inhibiting formation of 1,3-β-D glucan required for fungal cell wall
Pharmacokinetics	Extensively bound to plasma proteins. *Half-life:* 24 hours
Indications	Systemic candidiasis
Dosage as per indications	*Invasive candidiasis:* • *Neonates:* 3 mg/kg loading dose with 1.5 mg/kg/dose once daily maintenance dose • *Children:* 3 mg/kg loading dose with 1.5 mg/kg/ dose once daily maintenance dose
Maximum dosage	Loading: 200 mg/day; maintenance: 100 mg/day
Dose adjustments	No renal/hepatic adjustments
Adverse effects	Potassium imbalance, thrombocytopenia, increased bilirubin, and liver enzymes
Contraindications	Age <1 month
Drug interactions	Not known
Remarks	The powder is slow to dissolve and may take up to 5 minutes to dissolve. Antifungal therapy should continue for at least 14 days after the last positive culture. Administer at a rate of infusion not >1.1 mg/min

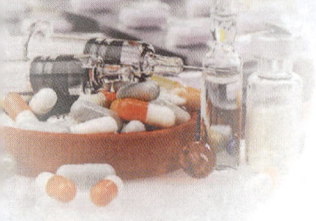

Anti-RhD Immunoglobulin

Drug name	Anti-RhD immunoglobulin
Category	Immunoglobulin
Route	Intramuscular
Strength	Inj (100 µg, 250 µg, 300 µg, 350 µg vials)
Brands	RhoGAM (Inj), Rhoclone (Inj)
Mechanism of action	0.5 mL of packed Rh(D) positive red blood cells (RBCs) or 1 mL of Rh(D) positive blood is neutralized by approximately 10 µg (50 IU) of anti-D immunoglobulin
Pharmacokinetics	High bioavailability. It is slowly absorbed with maximum levels attained in 2–3 days. *Half-life:* 3–4 weeks
Indications	For prophylaxis against Rh isoimmunization in mothers during pregnancy, abortion, amniocentesis; Immune thrombocytopenic purpura
Dosage as per indications	• *For antenatal prophylaxis:* 300 µg single dose IM at 28 weeks and 34 weeks of gestation or within 72 hours of delivery • *For abortion, amniocentesis, version:* 250 µg IM • *For immune thrombocytopenic purpura:* 50–75 µg/kg IV single dose
Maximum dosage	3,000 µg (15,000 IU)/dose
Dose adjustments	Not known
Adverse effects	Fever, RBC breakdown (anemia), pain at injection site, headache. Rarely anaphylaxis
Contraindications	Hypersensitivity
Drug interactions	Live vaccines
Remarks	Live vaccines should be administered at least 3 months after administration of anti-RhD immunoglobulin

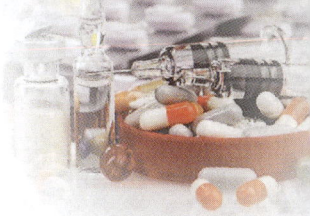

Antisnake Venom Serum (Polyvalent)

Drug name	Antisnake venom serum (Polyvalent)
Category	Immunoglobulin
Route	Intravenous
Strength	Inj (10 mL vial)
Brands	ASVS (Inj)
Mechanism of action	Neutralization of venom is done by neutralization of venom toxin through venom specific F(ab)2 fragments of IgG
Pharmacokinetics	Clear data not available
Indications	Suspected or Xonfirmed venomous snakebite
Dosage as per indications	*Dose of ASV for neuropalytic snakebite:* • ASV 10 vials stat as infusion (diluted in 5–10 mL/kg of normal saline) over 30 minutes followed by 2nd dose of 10 vials after 1 hour, if no improvement within 1st hour *Dose of ASV for vasculotoxic snakebite:* • Low-dose infusion therapy—10 vials for Russell's viper or 6 vials for saw-scaled viper stat as infusion over 30 minutes; followed by 2 vials every 6 hours as infusion in 100 mL of normal saline till clotting time normalizes or for 3 days whichever is earlier • High-dose intermittent bolus therapy—10 vials of polyvalent ASV stat over 30 minutes as infusion, followed by 6 vials 6 hourly as bolus therapy till clotting time normalizes and/or local swelling subsides
Maximum dosage	30 vials
Dose adjustments	Not known
Adverse effects	Dyspnea, hypotension, urticaria, hypersensitivity
Contraindications	No absolute contraindication, should be given with premedication in patients showing hypersensitivity
Drug interactions	Live vaccines
Remarks	Each mL of serum neutralizes standard venom of cobra 0.6 mg, common krait 0.45 mg, Russell's viper 0.6 mg, saw-scaled viper 0.45 mg

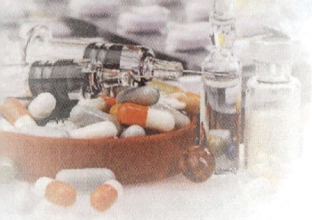

Antithymocyte Globulin (Equine)

Drug name	Antithymocyte globulin (Equine)
Category	Immunosuppressant
Route	Intravenous
Strength	Inj (250 mg/vial)
Brands	Atgam (Inj), Thymogam (Inj)
Mechanism of action	Antibodies which act via selective depletion of T-cells. Antibodies bind to T-cell specific antigens leading to complement-mediated cytotoxicity or apoptosis of T-cells
Pharmacokinetics	T-cell depletion noted within 24 hours. Opsonization mainly in reticuloendothelial system, *Half-life:* 2–3 days
Indications	Renal transplant; Aplastic anemia
Dosage as per indications	• *In renal transplant recipients to prevent rejection and treatment of rejection:* 15 mg/kg IV × 14 days followed by 15 mg/kg IV on alternate days × 14 days (total 21 doses in 28 days) • *Aplastic anemia:* 40 mg/kg IV × 4 days
Maximum dosage	Not known
Dose adjustments	Not known
Adverse effects	Hypersensitivity reaction including fever, and chills and rigors, increased risk of post-transplant lymphoproliferative disorder
Contraindications	Severe hypersensitivity
Drug interactions	Live vaccines
Remarks	Always give a test dose (skin testing with 0.1 mL 1:1,000 dilution given SC) prior to administration. Slow administration over 4 hours recommended

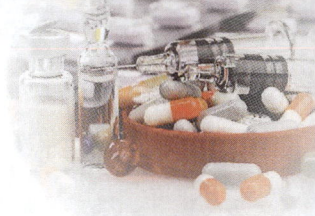

Artemether

Drug name	Artemether
Category	Antimalarial
Route	Oral, Intramuscular
Strength	Tab (20 mg, 40 mg, 80 mg); in combination with Lumefantrine; Syp (20 mg Artemether with 120 mg Lumefantrine per 5 mL); Inj (80 mg/mL, 150 mg/2 mL)
Brands	Larither (Inj, Cap), Lumither (Tab), Lumet (Combination Tab), Combither (Combination Tab)
Mechanism of action	Schizontocidal activity against blood forms of *Plasmodium falciparum* and *P. vivax*. Interferes with the conversion of heme, in the food vacuole of the parasite, to hemozoin which is a malaria pigment. The drug also inhibits nucleic acid and protein synthesis within the malarial parasite
Pharmacokinetics	After intramuscular administration, peak plasma concentrations are achieved in 6 hours. Rapid absorption, with peak plasma levels attained in 2 hours. Rapid clearance with terminal half-life of about 2 hours
Indications	Severe malaria; Uncomplicated falciparum malaria
Dosage as per indications	• *Antimalarial for severe and complicated malaria:* 3.2 mg/kg IM on day 1 followed by 1.6 mg/kg daily for the next 6 days • *For uncomplicated P. falciparum malaria:* The oral dose for fixed dose combination therapy (artemether 20 mg + lumefantrine 120 mg) is as followed: 5–14 kg 1 tablet BD for 3 days; 15–24 kg 2 tablets BD for 3 days; 25–34 kg 3 tablets BD for 3 days; >34 kg 4 tablets BD for 3 days
Maximum dosage	80 mg artemether and 480 mg lumefantrine tablet as per schedule

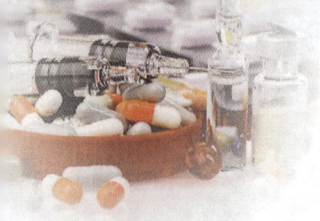

Artemether

Dose adjustments	Caution to be taken in severe hepatic or renal impairment. Close monitoring with ECG and serum potassium should be done
Adverse effects	GI disturbances, agranulocytosis, bradycardia, first degree heart block
Contraindications	Hypersensitivity, drugs causing prolonged QT interval
Drug interactions	Interactions were noted with drugs inhibiting CYP3A4
Remarks	Safety not proven in children weighing <5 kg

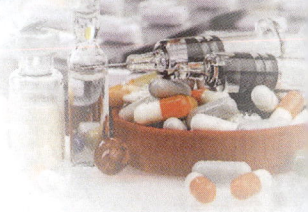

Artesunate

Drug name	Artesunate
Category	Antimalarial
Route	Oral, Intravenous, Intramuscular
Strength	Tab (50 mg, 100 mg, 200 mg); Inj (60 mg, 120 mg vial); also available as part of artesunate combination therapy with mefloquine and sulfadoxine-pyrimethamine
Brands	Falcigo (Inj, Tab), Larinate (Inj, Tab), RTsunate (Inj, Tab)
Mechanism of action	Artesunate and DHA (active metabolite) inhibit protein and nucleic acid synthesis, and interfere with the conversion of heme, in the food vacuole of the parasite, to hemozoin which is a malaria pigment
Pharmacokinetics	Highly protein bound. Half-life: 0.5–1.5 hours. Metabolized to dihydroartemisinin by plasma esterases. Eliminated via urine and feces
Indications	Severe malaria; Uncomplicated falciparum malaria
Dosage as per indications	• *For severe and complicated malaria:* 2.4 mg/kg (3 mg/kg for <20 kg) IV bolus or IM (loading dose) followed by 2.4 mg/kg (3 mg/kg for <20 kg) IV or IM at 12 hours and then OD for 6 days • *For chloroquine resistant uncomplicated falciparum malaria:* Artesunate—4 mg/kg OD × 3 days + sulfadoxine-pyrimethamine (25/1.25 mg/kg) on day 1 OR artesunate—4 mg/kg OD × 3 days + mefloquine 25 mg/kg in two (15 + 10) divided doses on day 2 and day 3 followed by single dose primaquine 0.75 mg/kg
Maximum dosage	Not known
Dose adjustments	None
Adverse effects	Hemolysis, rash, agranulocytosis, first-degree heart block, neurotoxicity, fever
Contraindications	Hypersensitivity
Drug interactions	Drugs which are UDP-glucuronosyltransferase (UGT) inducers or inhibitors
Remarks	The powder for injection should be reconstituted with 5% sodium bicarbonate and diluted in an equal volume of physiological saline or 5% (w/v) glucose

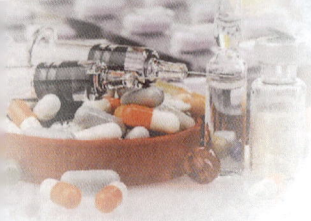

Ascorbic Acid (Vitamin C)

Drug name	Ascorbic acid (Vitamin C)
Category	Vitamin
Route	Oral, Intravenous, Intramuscular
Strength	Inj (500 mg); Tab (100 mg, 500 mg); Drops (100 mg/1 mL; 15 mL, 30 mL)
Brands	Cecon (Drops), Celin (Tab), Malano (Inj)
Mechanism of action	It is required for collagen formation. It also helps in tissue repair by acting as a cofactor. Vitamin C is an important component of oxidation-reduction reactions in body
Pharmacokinetics	Widely distributed, plasma levels nearly same as renal threshold, metabolized to urinary oxalate, when the plasma levels exceed renal threshold, vitamin C is excreted via urine in large amounts, half-life around 15–16 days
Indications	Scurvy
Dosage as per indications	PO/IM/IV • *Child:* 100–300 mg/day once daily or two divided doses • *Adult:* 100–250 mg once daily or two divided doses Give for at least 2 weeks
Maximum dosage	Not known
Dose adjustments	Not known
Adverse effects	Nausea, vomiting, heartburn, flushing, headache, faintness, dizziness, and hyperoxaluria
Contraindications	Hypersensitivity
Drug interactions	Aluminum hydroxide, deferoxamine, amphetamine
Remarks	Use with caution in G6PD patients. Injectable preparation is light sensitive

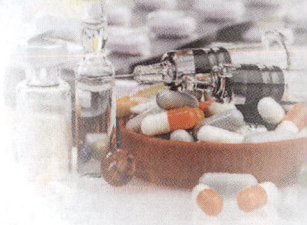

Astemizole

Drug name	Astemizole
Category	Antihistaminic (H1 antagonist)
Route	Oral
Strength	Tab (10 mg); Syp (5 mg/5 mL)
Brands	Stemiz (Tab, Syp), Acemiz (Tab), Histeeze (Tab), Astelong (Tab)
Mechanism of action	It attaches to peripheral (and not central) H1 receptors. Absorption decreases by 60% when taken with meals, rapidly absorbed by GI tract
Pharmacokinetics	Rapidly absorbed from gut, highly protein bound, completely metabolized in liver, excreted in feces, *Half-life:* Around 24 hours
Indications	Allergic rhinitis
Dosage as per indications	<6 years—0.2 mg/kg OD 6–12 years—5 mg OD >12 years—10 mg OD
Maximum dosage	10 mg/day
Dose adjustments	In hepatic derangement
Adverse effects	Can cause drowsiness, low blood pressure, headache, dry mouth, nausea, QT prolongation; and life-threatening arrhythmias, if given with drugs like erythromycin, itraconazole, ketoconazole, cimetidine, ciprofloxacin
Contraindications	Hepatic dysfunction, hypersensitivity
Drug interactions	Drugs affecting liver function, erythromycin, itraconazole, ketoconazole, cimetidine, ciprofloxacin
Remarks	Avoid abrupt discontinuation. *Now banned in India*

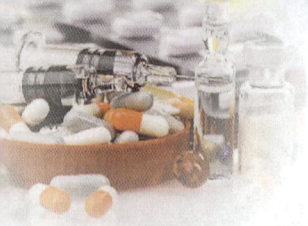

Atazanavir (ATV)

Drug name	Atazanavir (ATV)
Category	Antiretroviral, Protease inhibitor
Route	Oral
Strength	Caps (100 mg, 150 mg, 200 mg, 300 mg)
Brands	Atazor (Cap), Virataz (Cap)
Mechanism of action	Inhibits the virus-specific processing of viral Gag-Pol proteins in HIV-1 infected cells
Pharmacokinetics	Coadministration of atazanavir and ritonavir increases bioavailability of atazanavir. Highly bound to plasma proteins. Metabolized in the liver through CYP3A4
Indications	Acquired immunodeficiency syndrome
Dosage as per indications	• *15–20 kg:* ATV 150 mg + RTV (ritonavir) 100 mg OD with food • *20–39 kg:* ATV 200 mg + RTV 100 mg OD with food • *≥40 kg:* ATV 300 mg + RTV 100 mg OD with food
Maximum dosage	300 mg/day
Dose adjustments	No adjustments in renal derangement, dose adjustment in hepatic derangement
Adverse effects	Jaundice, prolonged PR interval, first-degree symptomatic atrioventricular (AV) block, nephrolithiasis, hyperglycemia, fat maldistribution, rash, raised liver enzymes
Contraindications	Hypersensitivity, liver derangement (moderate to severe), hemodialysis, substrates of CYP3A4
Drug interactions	Simvastatin/lovastatin, rifampicin, sildenafil, drugs affecting CYP3A4
Remarks	Recommended in children >6 years

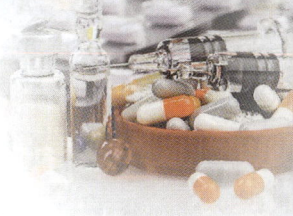

Atenolol

Drug name	Atenolol
Category	Beta blocker
Route	Oral
Strength	Tab (50 mg, 100 mg)
Brands	Acard (Tab), Aten (Tab), Betacard (Tab)
Mechanism of action	Acts on beta-1 adrenergic receptors. Has membrane-stabilizing and negative inotropic effects
Pharmacokinetics	Around 50% absorption on oral administration. Peak plasma concentrations 2–4 hours after oral intake. *Half-life:* 6 hours
Indications	Hypertension
Dosage as per indications	0.8–1.5 mg/kg/day
Maximum dosage	2 mg/kg/day up to 100 mg/day
Dose adjustments	• *Hepatic derangement:* No adjustment • *Renal derangement:* Dose to be decreased
Adverse effects	Hypotension, second- or third-degree block, lethargy, dizziness
Contraindications	Pulmonary edema, cardiogenic shock
Drug interactions	CCBs, digitalis, antiarrhythmic, sympathomimetics, antidiabetics, prostaglandin synthetase inhibiting drugs
Remarks	Should not be stopped suddenly, taper over 2 weeks. It can mask signs of hypoglycemia and thyrotoxicosis

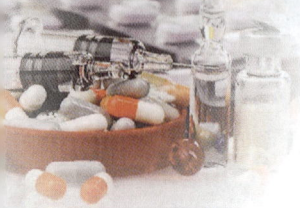

Atomoxetine

Drug name	Atomoxetine
Category	Nonstimulant/Miscellaneous
Route	Oral
Strength	Tab (10 mg, 18 mg, 25 mg, 40 mg, 60 mg)
Brands	Attentrol (Tab), Axepta (Tab), Tomoxetin (Tab)
Mechanism of action	Selective norepinephrine reuptake inhibitor (SNRI)
Pharmacokinetics	Well absorbed orally, *Half-life:* 5 hours, metabolized mainly by CYP2D6 enzymatic pathway, excreted predominantly in urine
Indications	Attention-deficit hyperactivity disorder (ADHD)
Dosage as per indications	0.5 mg/kg/day up to 1.2 mg/kg/day; start and increase gradually
Maximum dosage	1.2 mg/kg/day
Dose adjustments	Renal and hepatic derangement
Adverse effects	Vertigo, dizziness, liver injury, fatigue, nausea, vomiting
Contraindications	Children <6 years, severe cardiovascular disease
Drug interactions	MAO inhibitors, antihypertensives

Atorvastatin

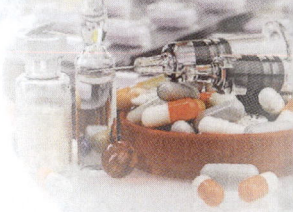

Drug name	Atorvastatin
Category	Lipid-lowering agent
Route	Oral
Strength	Tab (10 mg, 20 mg, 40 mg)
Brands	Atorlip (Tab), Atorva (Tab), Lipitor (Tab)
Mechanism of action	Acts by inhibiting hMG-CoA reductase enzyme
Pharmacokinetics	Rapidly absorbed but poor bioavailability due to high first pass metabolism, *Half-life:* 14 hours, metabolized in liver extensively, excreted primarily via bile
Indications	Hypercholesterolemia
Dosage as per indications	*Children >10 years of age:* 10 mg/day
Maximum dosage	20 mg/day
Dose adjustments	Hepatic impairment
Adverse effects	Myopathy, rhabdomyolysis
Contraindications	Hypersensitivity, acute liver disease
Drug interactions	Cyclosporine, CYP3A4 inhibitors, digoxin

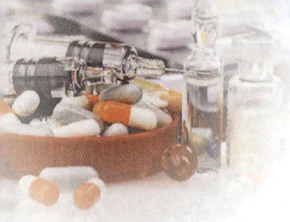

Atropine Sulfate

Drug name	Atropine sulfate
Category	Anticholinergic
Route	Oral, Intravenous, Intramuscular, Subcutaneous
Strength	Tab (0.4 mg, 0.6 mg); Inj (0.05 mg/mL, 0.1 mg/mL, 0.3 mg/mL, 0.4 mg/mL, 0.5 mg/mL, 0.8 mg/mL, 1 mg/mL)
Brands	Atro (Inj), Tropin (Inj), Tropine (Inj)
Mechanism of action	Inhibits the action of acetylcholine by binding to acetylcholine receptors
Pharmacokinetics	Effect on heart rate within 2–4 minutes of IV administration. Partly metabolized in the liver. *Elimination half-life:* 2–5 hours, increases in small children. Up to 50% protein bound
Indications	Cardiopulmonary resuscitation; Organophosphate poisoning
Dosage as per indications	• *Cardiac resuscitation:* 0.02 mg/kg/dose IV every 5 minutes × 2–3 doses • *Preanesthetic dose:* 0.01 mg/kg/dose SC/IV/IM, maximum: 0.4 mg/dose; minimum: 0.1 mg/dose, may repeat q 4–6 h • *Organophosphate poisoning:* 0.02 mg/kg body weight possibly repeated several times until signs and symptoms disappear
Maximum dosage	0.6 mg/dose; maximum dose in children: 1 mg, in adolescents: 2 mg
Dose adjustments	To use with caution in renal and hepatic derangement
Adverse effects	Blurred vision, dry mouth, tachycardia, constipation, urinary retention
Contraindications	Glaucoma, thyrotoxicosis, obstructive uropathy
Drug interactions	Drugs with anticholinergic activity
Remarks	Not used in neonates <3 kg

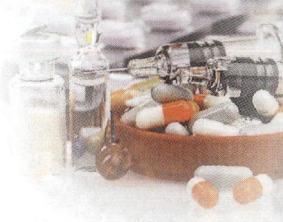

Azathioprine

Drug name	Azathioprine
Category	Immunosuppressant
Route	Oral, Intravenous
Strength	Tab (50 mg); Inj (100 mg/vial)
Brands	Azoran (Tab), Imuran (Tab)
Mechanism of action	Immunosuppressive, antimetabolite, suppresses delayed hypersensitivity and cellular cytotoxicity and to lesser extent antibody responses
Pharmacokinetics	Well-absorbed orally, *Half-life:* 5 hours, extensively metabolized in RBCs and liver
Indications	In transplants for immunosuppression; Autoimmune diseases like rheumatoid arthritis and systemic lupus erythematosus (SLE)

Dosage as per indications	Oral
	• *Transplant:*
	  – Initially start at 3–5 mg/kg/day given mostly as single dose and then decrease to maintenance dose of 1–3 mg/kg/day
	• Rheumatoid arthritis, SLE
	  – Start at 1 mg/kg/day till max of 2.5 mg/kg/day

Maximum dosage	2.5 mg/kg/day
Dose adjustments	Renal derangement
Adverse effects	Leukopenia, thrombocytopenia, hepatotoxic, increased risk of infections and malignancy
Contraindications	Hypersensitivity
Drug interactions	Allopurinol, ribavirin, drugs affecting myelopoiesis

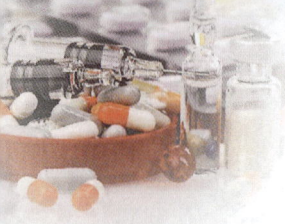

Azithromycin

Drug name	Azithromycin
Category	Antibiotic, Macrolide
Route	Oral, Intravenous
Strength	Tab (250 mg, 500 mg); Susp (100 mg/5 mL, 200 mg/5 mL); Inj (500 mg/vial)
Brands	Azithro (Inj, Tab, Syp), Azee (Tab, Syp), Aziwok (Tab, Syp)
Mechanism of action	Binds to the 50S-ribosomal subunit and prevents translocation of peptide chains from one side of the ribosome to the other, inhibiting RNA-dependent protein synthesis
Pharmacokinetics	Bioavailability around 35–40%. Peak plasma levels obtained in 2–3 hours. The terminal plasma-elimination half-life 2 to 4 days
Indications	Enteric fever; Acute respiratory infections; Otitis media; *Mycoplasma* infection
Dosage as per indications	• *Otitis media, community-acquired pneumonia, tonsillitis:* 10 mg/kg PO on day 1 followed by 5 mg/kg/day OD on days 2–5, maximum dose 500 mg on day 1 followed by 250 mg from days 2 to 5 • *Uncomplicated typhoid fever:* 20 mg/kg/day PO × 7 days • *Mycobacterium avium complex prophylaxis:* 20 mg/kg/dose PO once a week
Maximum dosage	1 g/day
Dose adjustments	Dose adjustment in severe hepatic/renal impairment
Adverse effects	Increased liver enzymes, cholestatic jaundice, GI disturbances
Contraindications	Hypersensitivity to azithromycin, erythromycin, any macrolide
Drug interactions	Antacids, digoxin, ergot derivatives
Remarks	Avoid use in infants <6 months of age

Aztreonam

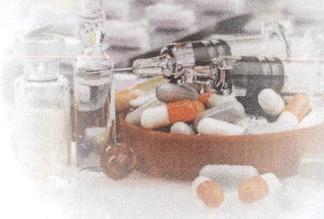

Drug name	Aztreonam
Category	Antibiotic, Monobactam
Route	Intravenous, Intramuscular
Strength	Inj (500 mg, 1 g, 2 g per vial)
Brands	Azactam (Inj), Aztreo (Inj), Aztrone (Inj)
Mechanism of action	Bactericidal. Acts by inhibiting bacterial cell wall synthesis
Pharmacokinetics	Around 50% bound to plasma proteins. The serum half-life 1.5–2 hours, mainly eliminated by kidney
Indications	Multidrug-resistant aerobic gram-negative infections; Enteric fever
Dosage as per indications	• *0–6 days:* 30 mg/kg/dose q 12 h • *>7 days:* 30 mg/kg/dose q 8 h *Children:* • *Mild to moderate infections:* 30 mg/kg/dose q 8 h • *Moderate to severe:* 30 mg/kg/dose q 6 h
Maximum dosage	2 g/dose
Dose adjustments	Dose reduction needed in renal and hepatic impairment
Adverse effects	Hypoglycemia, rash, fever, taste disturbance, increase in liver enzymes, eosinophilia
Contraindications	Hypersensitivity
Drug interactions	If aztreonam and metronidazole are to be used together, they should be administered separately
Remarks	Dilute to a final concentration of 20 mg/mL. Weekly monitoring of renal, hepatic and hematological functions

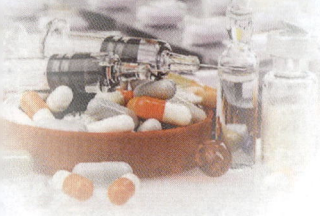

Baclofen

Drug name	Baclofen
Category	Central muscle relaxant
Route	Oral, Intrathecal
Strength	Tab (10 mg, 25 mg); Inj (0.5 mg/mL, 2 mg/mL)
Brands	Bacmax (Tab), Liofen (Inj, Tab)
Mechanism of action	Gamma-aminobutyric acid agonist, inhibits monosynaptic and polysynaptic reflexes at the spinal level by activating GABA receptors
Pharmacokinetics	Peak plasma concentration: 2 hours, elimination half-life: 5.5 hours, excreted primarily from kidney
Indications	Severe chronic spasticity as in cerebral palsy
Dosage as per indications	0.75–2 mg/kg/day oral q 8 h
Maximum dosage	<8 years: 60 mg/day; >8 years: 80 mg/day
Dose adjustments	Deranged renal function
Adverse effects	Drowsiness, fatigue, nausea, vertigo, psychiatric disturbances, urinary frequency, hypotonia, rash
Contraindications	Hypersensitivity
Drug interactions	Other muscle relaxant drugs
Remarks	Dosage is increased over 3 days to get the desired effect or till maximum dose achieved if needed. Stop slowly. Use cautiously in children with seizure disorder

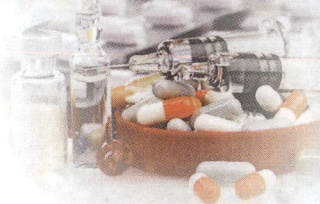

Beclomethasone Dipropionate (BDP)

Drug name	Beclomethasone dipropionate (BDP)
Category	Steroid, Antiasthmatic
Route	Oral, Nasal, Inhalational
Strength	Metered Dose Inhaler (MDI) (50 µg/puff, 100 µg/puff, 200 µg/puff); Rotacaps (100 µg, 200 µg, 400 µg), Nasal Spray (50 µg/spray)
Brands	Besone (Inhaler), Beclate (Inhaler, Rotacap, Nasal spray)
Mechanism of action	Has glucocorticoid receptor binding activity. When converted to becometasone-17-monopropionate (B-17-MP) via esterase enzyme, has anti-inflammatory activity
Pharmacokinetics	Has extensive first pass metabolism. Highly plasma protein bound. Half-life BDP and B-17-MP are 30 minutes and 2.5 hours respectively
Indications	Asthma; Allergic rhinitis

Dosage as per indications	• *Oral inhalation:*
	  – *6–11 years:* 100–200 µg (low dose), 200–400 µg (medium dose), >400 µg (high dose)
	  – *>11 years:* 200–500 µg (low dose), 500–1000 µg (medium dose), >1000 µg (high dose)
	• *Nasal inhalation:*
	  – *6–12 years:* 1 spray in each nostril TID
	  – *>12 years:* 1 spray in each nostril TID or 2 sprays in each nostril BID

Maximum dosage	• *6–11 years:* 400 µg (oral inhalational MDI) • *>11 years:* 1000 µg (oral inhalational MDI)
Dose adjustments	Not needed in renal and hepatic derangement
Adverse effects	• *Short-term:* Hoarseness, oral candidiasis. • *Long-term (with high doses):* Cushingoid features, adrenal suppression, growth retardation, decreased bone mineral density, cataract, psychological illnesses
Contraindications	Hypersensitivity. Not recommended in children <6 years
Drug interactions	Other drugs with steroidal activity
Remarks	Rinse mouth after each use of MDI. Avoid using in doses exceeding the recommended doses

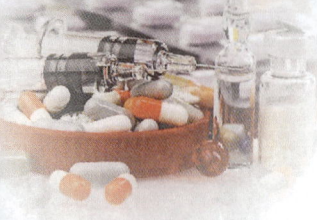

Bedaquiline

Drug name	Bedaquiline
Category	Antitubercular
Route	Oral
Strength	Tab (100 mg)
Brands	Sirturo (Tab)
Mechanism of action	Diarylquinoline antimycobacterial, inhibits mycobacterial enzyme adenosine 5'-triphosphate synthase
Pharmacokinetics	Highly protein bound, metabolized via CYP3A4 enzymatic pathway, half-life around 5–6 months, mainly eliminated in feces
Indications	Multidrug-resistant tuberculosis (MDR-TB)
Dosage as per indications	400 mg once daily for week 1 and 2 followed by 200 mg 3 times per week from 3rd week to 24th week
Maximum dosage	Not known
Dose adjustments	In liver derangement, end-stage renal disease
Adverse effects	Nausea, headache, QT prolongation, liver dysfunction
Contraindications	Hypersensitivity
Drug interactions	Drugs affecting QT interval, CYP3A4 inducers and inhibitors
Remarks	To be given with food

Benzathine Penicillin

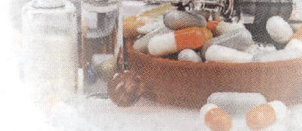

Drug name	Benzathine penicillin
Category	Antibiotic, Penicillin
Route	Intramuscular
Strength	Inj (1.2 MU, 2.4 MU, 4.8 MU vials)
Brands	Longacillin (Inj), Pencom LA (Inj), Penidure LA (Inj)
Mechanism of action	Bactericidal. Inhibits bacterial cell wall synthesis by blocking penicillin-binding proteins
Pharmacokinetics	Is converted to benzylpenicillin by hydrolysis. Peak plasma levels noted in 24 hours. Nearly 50% plasma protein bound. Plasma protein binding is approximately 55%. Eliminated mainly by kidneys
Indications	Rheumatic heart disease for secondary prophylaxis
Dosage as per indications	• <6 years: 0.6 MU IM every 21 days • >6 years: 1.2 MU IM every 21 days
Maximum dosage	1.2 MU/dose
Dose adjustments	Dose adjustments needed in deranged renal functions
Adverse effects	Candidiasis, diarrhea, nausea, hypersensitivity, rash, fever, urticaria, impact on renal hepatic and hematopoietic system in chronic use
Contraindications	Hypersensitivity to penicillin, cephalosporin or other beta-lactam agents
Drug interactions	Probenecid, methotrexate, anticoagulants
Remarks	To be given only after test dose; can cause severe anaphylaxis. Never give IV as it may result in cardiac arrest and death. The injection must not be administered into tissue with reduced perfusion. The injection should be administered as slowly as possible. Children should be observed for at least half hour after injection for anaphylaxis

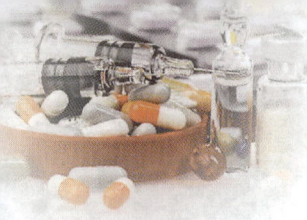

Benzyl Penicillin

Drug name	Benzyl penicillin
Category	Antibiotic, Penicillin
Route	Oral, Intravenous
Strength	Tab (2 lakh, 4 lakh, 8 lakh units); Inj (5 lakh, 10 lakh units vials)
Brands	Benzyl Pen (Inj), Pentids (Tab)
Mechanism of action	Bactericidal; inhibiting bacterial cell wall biosynthesis
Pharmacokinetics	Maximum concentration achieved in 15–30 minutes. *Plasma half-life:* 30 minutes. Most of the drug is eliminated by renal route mainly tubular secretion
Indications	Rheumatic fever; Streptococcal infection
Dosage as per indications	• *For penicillin-sensitive infections*: 1–2 lakh units/kg/day IV infusion q 4–6 h • *For meningitis and endocarditis*: 2–3 lakh units/kg/day IM q 4 h (maximum dose 24 million U/day) • *For rheumatic fever prophylaxis*: 2 lakh units (125 mg) BD
Maximum dosage	24 million U/day
Dose adjustments	The dose and frequency of administration should be decreased in both renal and hepatic impairment
Adverse effects	Hypersensitivity, pseudomembranous colitis, hypokalemia, hypernatremia
Contraindications	Hypersensitivity
Drug interactions	Probenecid acid decreases tubular secretion and increases the levels
Remarks	Only freshly prepared solutions should be used. Administer 30 minutes before or 2 hours after meals

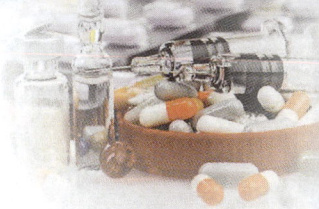

Bevacizumab

Drug name	Bevacizumab
Category	Antiangiogenic
Route	Intravenous, Intravitreal
Strength	Inj 400 mg/vial
Brands	Avastin (Inj), Bevatas (Inj), Bevacirel (Inj)
Mechanism of action	It binds to VEGF, prevents the interaction of VEGF to its receptors leading to inhibition of endothelial cell proliferation and new blood vessel formation
Pharmacokinetics	*Half-life:* 20 days, limited studies available
Indications	Malignancy (solid tumors); Retinopathy of prematurity (ROP)
Dosage as per indications	• *Recurrent/poor-prognosis solid cancers:* 5–10 mg/kg IV every 2–4 weeks • *Retinopathy of prematurity (ROP):* Intravitreal bevacizumab is also being used to treat severe ROP. Doses used have varied from 0.031 mg to 0.625 mg with varying success
Maximum dosage	Not known
Dose adjustments	Not known
Adverse effects	Lymphopenia, reversible posterior leukoencephalopathy syndrome, hypertension, intravitreal injection may lead to retinal detachment, recurrence, refractive errors, nystagmus, and strabismus during follow-up
Contraindications	Hypersensitivity
Drug interactions	No known drug interaction; studies limited

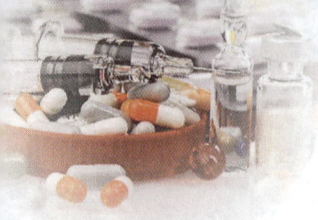

Bisacodyl

Drug name	Bisacodyl
Category	Laxative and purgative (Diphenylmethane derivatives group)
Route	Oral, Rectal
Strength	Tab (5 mg); Suppository (5 mg, 10 mg); Enema (10 mg/30 mL)
Brands	Dulcolax (Tab, Suppository)
Mechanism of action	It acts locally by 2 mechanisms. It exerts hydragogue effect as a contact laxative. It stimulates the mucosa of large intestine and rectum leading to peristalsis and promotion of accumulation of water and electrolytes
Pharmacokinetics	Poorly absorbed orally. Rapidly hydrolyzed to its active form bis-(p-hydroxyphenyl)-pyridyl-2-methane (BHPM), by esterases of the enteric mucosa. Maximum laxative effect is noted 6–12 hours after oral intake and 20–60 minutes after suppository. Majorly eliminated in feces. *Half-life:* 7–10 hours
Indications	Laxative
Dosage as per indications	• *Oral:* 0.3 mg/kg/day or 5–10 mg administered 6 hours before the desired effect • *Rectal:* >11 years: 10 mg
Maximum dosage	*Oral:* 30 mg/24 h
Dose adjustments	Not known
Adverse effects	Abdominal cramps, vomiting, nausea, rectal irritation
Contraindications	Ileus, intestinal obstruction, acute abdomen, severe dehydration, galactose intolerance, known hypersensitivity
Drug interactions	Intestinal motility agents
Remarks	Do not chew or crush tablets, do not give within 1 hour of antacids. Should not be used in children and adolescents under the age of 12 years

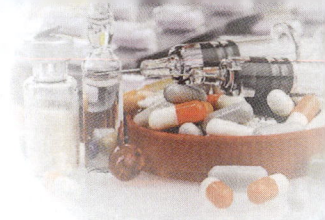

Bleomycin

Drug name	Bleomycin
Category	Chemotherapeutic drug, Glycopeptide antibiotic
Route	Intravenous, Intramuscular, Subcutaneous
Strength	Inj (15 IU)
Brands	Bleocel (Inj), Bleotex (Inj), Bleo (Inj)
Mechanism of action	Acts by inhibition of DNA synthesis
Pharmacokinetics	50% systemically absorbed, *Half-life:* Around 2 hours, metabolized in liver, around two-thirds eliminated in urine in active form
Indications	Non-Hodgkin lymphoma; Hodgkin lymphoma; Testicular cancer; Squamous cell carcinoma
Dosage as per indications	0.25–0.50 units/kg (10–20 units/m^2) IV/IM/SC weekly or twice weekly
Maximum dosage	Not known
Dose adjustments	Cautious use in patients with renal impairment
Adverse effects	Fever, thrombocytopenia, anaphylaxis, rash, pulmonary toxicity (fibrosis, interstitial pneumonitis)
Contraindications	Hypersensitivity, severe pulmonary disease
Drug interactions	Nephrotoxic drugs, digoxin

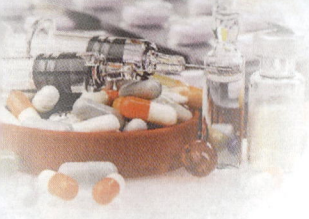

Budesonide

Drug name	Budesonide
Category	Steroid
Route	Inhalation
Strength	MDI (100 µg, 200 µg/puff); Rotacap (200 µg, 400 µg/puff); Respule (0.25 mg, 0.5 mg, 1 mg per 2 mL)
Brands	Budecort, Derinide, Pulmicort
Mechanism of action	Acts by its anti-inflammatory effect
Pharmacokinetics	*Half-life:* 2–2.5 hours after nebulization, absorbed drug metabolized via CYP3A4 enzymatic pathway
Indications	Bronchial asthma

Dosage as per indications	*As inhaler (MDI):*
	• *6–11 years:* Low dose: 100–200 µg/day, medium dose: 200–400 µg/day, high dose: >400 µg/day
	• *12 years and above:*
	  – *Low dose:* 200–400 µg/day
	  – *Medium dose:* 400–800 µg/day
	  – *High dose:* >800 µg/day
	As nebulization:
	• *3 months–12 years:* 250–500 µg twice daily
	• *12–18 years:* 500–1,000 µg twice daily

Maximum dosage	1 mg/day, higher doses up to 2 mg have been tried in adolescents
Dose adjustments	Not known for inhalational route
Adverse effects	Infections, immunosuppression, growth delay, low bone mineral density
Contraindications	Hypersensitivity
Drug interactions	Drugs affecting CYP3A4 pathway
Remarks	Not to be used alone in acute severe attack of asthma

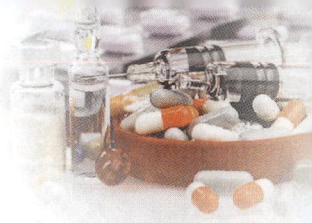

Budesonide with Formoterol

Drug name	Budesonide with formoterol
Category	Inhaled corticosteroid with inhaled long-acting beta-2 agonist
Route	Inhalational
Strength	MDI (100 μg + 6 μg, 200 μg + 6 μg, 400 μg + 6 μg, 400 μg + 12 μg per puff); Rotacap (100 μg + 6 μg, 200 μg + 6 μg, 400 μg + 6 μg, 400 μg + 12 μg per puff); Respules (0.5 mg + 20 μg, 1 mg + 20 μg per 2 mL). • Delivered dose for 200/6 combination is 160/4.5 μg and 100/6 combination is 80/4.5 μg
Brands	Budamate, Foracort, Formonide, Symbicort
Mechanism of action	Budesonide acts as anti-inflammatory drug whereas formoterol fumarate acts locally in the lung. It stimulates intracellular adenyl cyclase leading relaxation of bronchial smooth muscle and hence bronchodilation. It also inhibits release of mast cell mediators
Pharmacokinetics	Inhaled formoterol acts locally in lung, absorbed drug is metabolized by glucuronidation and O-demethylation followed by conjugation to inactive metabolites. Around 50–60% of both drugs are excreted in urine
Indications	Bronchial asthma
Dosage as per indications	*Children:* 1–2 puffs per day of 100/6 combination, adolescents: 1–4 puff divided twice daily of 200/6 combination
Maximum dosage	• It is based on the total dose of formoterol per day • *Adolescents:* 72 μg of formoterol (54 μg delivered dose) • *Children 6–11 years:* 48 μg (36 μg delivered dose)
Dose adjustments	To be used with caution in liver derangement

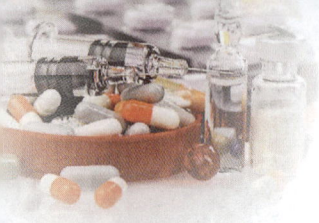

Adverse effects	Infections, immunosuppression, growth delay, low bone mineral density, tachycardia, hypokalemia
Contraindications	Hypersensitivity
Drug interactions	Drugs affecting CYP3A4 pathway, beta blockers, diuretics
Remarks	For children >6 years

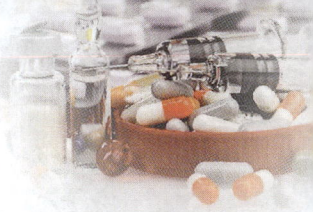

Bumetanide

Drug name	Bumetanide
Category	Loop diuretic
Route	Oral, Intravenous
Strength	Tab (1 mg); Inj (0.25 mg/mL)
Brands	Bumex (Tab, Inj)
Mechanism of action	Has diuretic/natriuretic action, acts on the ascending limb of the loop of Henle by inhibiting electrolyte reabsorption. Diuretic effect begins in 30 minutes and peaks in 1–2 hours
Pharmacokinetics	Almost completely absorbed from GI tract, high bioavailability after oral intake. Highly protein bound. Elimination half-life 45–150 minutes
Indications	Diuresis
Dosage as per indications	Oral/IV • *Till 6 months of age:* 0.01–0.05 mg/kg/dose once a day • *Above 6 months:* 0.015–0.1 mg/kg/dose once daily-QID
Maximum dosage	10 mg/24 hours
Dose adjustments	Required in hepatic derangement
Adverse effects	Cramps, dizziness, hypotension, headache, electrolyte losses (hypokalemia, hypocalcemia, hyponatremia, hypochloremia), encephalopathy, metabolic acidosis
Contraindications	Hypersensitivity, anuria, oliguria, hepatic coma, electrolyte imbalance
Drug interactions	Lithium, cardiac glycosides, NSAIDs
Remarks	• Cross-allergenicity may occur in patients allergic to sulfonamides • Not recommended for <12 years

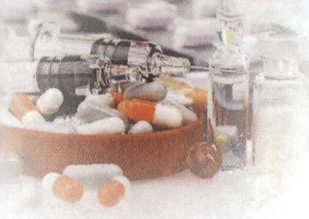

Busulfan

Drug name	Busulfan
Category	Cytotoxic chemotherapy, Alkylating drug
Route	Oral, Intravenous
Strength	Tab (2 mg); Inj (60 mg)
Brands	Bucelon (Inj, Tab), Mylefan (Tab), Myleran (Tab)
Mechanism of action	It is a bifunctional alkylating agent. It hydrolyses and subsequently forms reactive carbonium ions which damage DNA through alkylating
Pharmacokinetics	Limited data available. Around one-third of the drug is bound to albumin. It is metabolized in the liver, where it is conjugated with glutathione and then undergoes extensive oxidative metabolism
Indications	Chronic myelogenous leukemia (CML); Marrow conditioning
Dosage as per indications	• *CML initial dose:* ≤12 kg: 1.1 mg/kg (based on actual body weight); >12 kg: 0.8 mg/kg (based on actual body weight) • Doses are administered every 6 hours as 2 hours infusions over 4 days for a total of 16 doses • *Marrow-ablative conditioning regimen:* 0.5 mg/kg to 1 mg/kg orally q 6 h for 4 days. • *Hematopoietic stem cell transplant program:* ≤6 years: 40 mg/m^2/dose q 6 h for 4 days
Maximum dosage	Not known
Dose adjustments	• No dose modification needed in renal impairment, but monitoring is needed • Dose adjustment needed in severe hepatic impairment
Adverse effects	Gastrointestinal symptoms, anorexia, weight loss, amenorrhea, cough, impaired fertility, interstitial lung fibrosis, bone marrow suppression, hepatic veno-occlusive disease
Contraindications	Hypersensitivity, resistance
Drug interactions	Immunosuppressive drugs
Remarks	Busulfan should be discontinued if lung toxicity develops

Caffeine Citrate

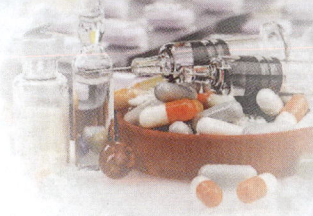

Drug name	Caffeine citrate
Category	Respiratory stimulant (Methylxanthine)
Route	Oral, Intravenous
Strength	Inj (20 mg/mL); Oral sol (20 mg/mL)
Brands	Capnea (Inj, Sol)
Mechanism of action	Has antagonistic effect on adenosine receptors. Increases respiratory drive thereby improving breathing pattern. It increases metabolic rate, heart rate, cardiac contractility and output, cerebral and splanchnic vasoconstriction, and vasodilator effect on other vascular smooth muscle
Pharmacokinetics	Rapid onset of action, within few minutes. Rapidly distributed into the brain
Indications	Neonatal apnea
Dosage as per indications	20 mg/kg intravenous infusion as loading followed by 10 mg/kg/day oral/intravenous maintenance after 24 hours
Maximum dosage	Not known
Dose adjustments	Dose adjustment needed in renal and hepatic impairment
Adverse effects	Tachycardia, neurologic and GI side effects
Contraindications	Hypersensitivity
Drug interactions	Adenosine, tizanidine, drugs affecting heart rate
Remarks	Do not use in cardiac arrhythmias, do not use caffeine benzoate as it increases the risk of kernicterus

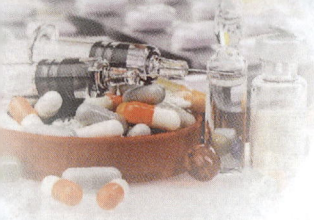

Calcium Carbonate

Drug name	Calcium carbonate
Category	Calcium supplement
Route	Oral
Strength	Chewable Tab (250 mg, 500 mg, 1,000 mg, 1,250 mg); Susp (250 mg/5 mL)
Brands	Shelcal (Tab, Syp), Os-cal (Tab, Syp), Tums (Tab)
Mechanism of action	Acts to revert negative calcium balance, also acts as antacid in stomach and phosphate binder in intestine
Pharmacokinetics	Once taken orally, breaks into soluble calcium salts absorbed in small intestine and distributed to bones. Calcium filtered via renal system is reabsorbed in ascending limb of the loop of Henle and the proximal and distal convoluted tubules. Eliminated mainly via feces
Indications	For prevention/treatment of hypocalcemia; As part of treatment of rickets
Dosage as per indications	• *Neonates:* 50–150 mg/kg/day in 1–4 divided doses • *Children:* 45–65 mg/kg/day in 1–4 divided doses
Maximum dosage	1 g/day
Dose adjustments	In renal derangement
Adverse effects	Constipation, hypophosphatemia, hypomagnesemia, nausea, vomiting, headache
Contraindications	Hypersensitivity
Drug interactions	Iron, inotropes
Remarks	Do not take iron and calcium together

Calcium Gluconate

Drug name	Calcium gluconate
Category	Injectable calcium (9% elemental calcium)
Route	Intravenous
Strength	Inj 10% containing 100 mg/mL of Calcium Gluconate equivalent to Elemental Calcium of 8.9 mg/mL or 0.45 mEq/mL of Ca^{++}
Brands	Betasone (Inj), Glucuriv (Inj), Glumig (Inj)
Mechanism of action	Mainly distributed in skeleton (99%). Ionized form, the biologically active form, contributes to 50% of total serum calcium. Rest around 50% is protein bound
Pharmacokinetics	Calcium gluconate injection is 100% bioavailable following intravenous injection. Not affected by first pass metabolism. Calcium itself does not undergo direct metabolism. Increased urinary calcium excretion is noted after intravenous administration of calcium gluconate
Indications	Hypocalcemia; Hyperkalemia
Dosage as per indications	• *Hypocalcemia:* 1–2 mL/kg/dose, to be given slow intravenous under cardiac monitoring • *Maintenance:* 2–4 mL/kg/day q 6 h • *Hyperkalemia:* 0.5 mL/kg over 5–10 minutes
Maximum dosage	10 mL/dose
Dose adjustments	• *Renal impairment:* Start at the lowest dose of the recommended dose range • *Hepatic impairment:* No modifications
Adverse effects	Hypotension, bradycardia, arrhythmias
Contraindications	Digitalized children
Drug interactions	Ceftriaxone (precipitate complexes in neonates), cardiac glycosides, drugs causing hypercalcemia (thiazides, calcipotriene, vitamin A/D)
Remarks	• Extravasation can cause tissue necrosis, calcinosis cutis • Dilute preferably in dextrose, do not exceed infusion rate >100 mg/min • Not compatible with drugs containing phosphates/bicarbonates

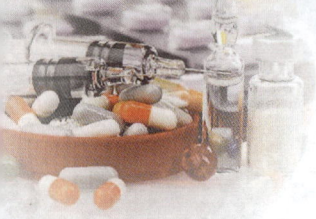

Capreomycin

Drug name	Capreomycin
Category	Antitubercular
Route	Intramuscular
Strength	Inj (500 mg, 750 mg, 1 g)
Brands	Capreo (Inj), Kapocin (Inj)
Mechanism of action	Acts similar as an aminoglycoside; inhibit protein synthesis by binding to the 70S ribosomal unit
Pharmacokinetics	Not known
Indications	Multidrug-resistant tuberculosis (MDR-TB)
Dosage as per indications	15–120 mg/kg/day
Maximum dosage	1 g/day
Dose adjustments	Renal dysfunction
Adverse effects	Nephrotoxic, hearing damage
Contraindications	Hypersensitivity, renal failure
Drug interactions	Nephrotoxic drugs, neuromuscular blocking agents

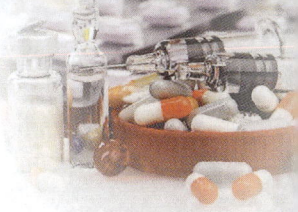

Captopril

Drug name	Captopril
Category	Antihypertensive, Angiotensin-converting enzyme inhibitor
Route	Oral
Strength	Tab (12.5 mg, 25 mg, 50 mg)
Brands	Aceten (Tab), Angiopril (Tab)
Mechanism of action	Inhibitor of angiotensin-I converting enzyme causing suppression of the plasma renin-angiotensin-aldosterone system
Pharmacokinetics	Nearly three-fourths of the oral intake is absorbed. Maximum effect noted 1–1.5 hours after oral administration. Nearly one-third bound to plasma protein. Elimination half-life: 2 hours. Most eliminated in urine over 24 hours
Indications	Hypertension
Dosage as per indications	• *Neonates:* 0.1–0.4 mg/kg/day PO q 6–24 h • *Children:* Initial dose: 0.3–0.5 mg/kg/dose q 8 h; titrate upward, if needed; maximum 6 mg/kg/day q 8–12 h
Maximum dosage	6 mg/kg/24 hours; max 450 mg/24 hours
Dose adjustments	Dose adjustment needed in renal impairment
Adverse effects	Rash, proteinuria, neutropenia, angioedema, dysgeusia, hypotension, and hyperkalemia
Contraindications	Hypersensitivity, bilateral renal artery stenosis
Drug interactions	Antihypertensives, diuretics
Remarks	Use with caution in collagen vascular disease

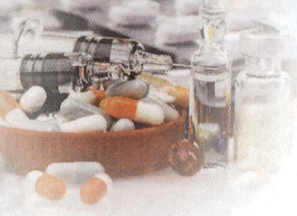

Carbamazepine

Drug name	Carbamazepine
Category	Anticonvulsant
Route	Oral
Strength	Tab (200 mg, 400 mg); Syp (100 mg/5 mL)
Brands	Acetol (Tab), Tegretol (Tab), Carbatol (Tab), Mazetol (Tab), Zeptol (Tab). (Syrup not available in India)
Mechanism of action	Causes voltage-dependent blockade of sodium channels thereby stabilizing hyperexcited nerve membranes, inhibiting repetitive neuronal discharges, and reducing synaptic propagation of excitatory impulses
Pharmacokinetics	Near complete absorption after oral intake, highly bound to plasma proteins (70–80%), metabolized in liver, elimination half-life: 36 hours
Indications	Partial seizures; Tonic-clonic seizures; Atonic seizures; Akinetic epilepsy; Mesial temporal lobe epilepsy syndrome; Trigeminal neuralgia; Postherpetic neuralgia
Dosage as per indications	• 10–30 mg/kg/day q 8 h, PO • Initiate therapy at 30–50% of initial dose and increase over 5–7 days
Maximum dosage	*Maximum initial dose:* • *6–12 years:* 100 mg/dose • *>12 years:* 200 mg/dose *Maximum maintenance dose:* • *6–15 years:* 1000 mg/day • *>15 years:* 1200 mg/day
Dose adjustments	Adjust dose in renal impairment
Adverse effects	Sedation, diplopia, Stevens–Johnson syndrome, urinary retention, aplastic anemia, liver dysfunction
Contraindications	Heart block, hypersensitivity, bone marrow depression, hepatic porphyria, on monoamine oxidase (MAO) inhibitor
Drug interactions	Phenytoin, benzodiazepines, valproate, ethosuximide
Remarks	Therapeutic blood levels 4–12 mg/L

Carbenicillin

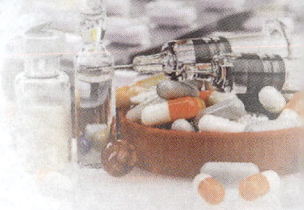

Drug name	Carbenicillin
Category	Antibiotic, Carboxypenicillin
Route	Intravenous, Intramuscular
Strength	Inj (1 g, 5 g)
Brands	Carbelin (Inj)
Mechanism of action	Inhibits cell wall synthesis in bacteria
Pharmacokinetics	Rapidly absorbed from small intestine, nearly 30% drug is excreted unchanged in urine, excreted via renal route, half-life around 1 hour
Indications	Effective against bacteria responsible for causing urinary tract infections including *Pseudomonas aeruginosa*; *Escherichia coli*; and some *Proteus* species
Dosage as per indications	400–600 mg/kg/day q 4 h IV or q 6 h IM
Maximum dosage	Not known
Dose adjustments	Required in renal and hepatic derangement
Adverse effects	Hypersensitivity, hypokalemia, bleeding
Contraindications	Hypersensitivity
Drug interactions	Probenecid acid
Remarks	It is not resistant to beta-lactamases

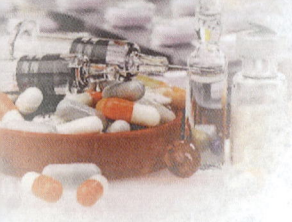

Carbimazole

Drug name	Carbimazole
Category	Antithyroid drug
Route	Oral
Strength	Tab (5 mg, 10 mg, 20 mg)
Brands	Anti-Thyrox (Tab), Neo-Mercazole (Tab), Thyrocab (Tab)
Mechanism of action	It inhibits thyroid peroxidase, organification of iodide and their uptake by tyrosyl radicals thus stopping thyroid hormonogenesis
Pharmacokinetics	Most is rapidly absorbed in gut within 15–30 minutes. It is hydrolyzed to methimazole, the active metabolite. It undergoes oxidative decomposition in the liver and in the thyroid. Carbimazole half-life is 5–5.5 hours. Methimazole average half-life is 6.5 hours but can be as long as 20 hours in thyroid gland. Carbimazole is mostly excreted in the urine as methimazole and metabolites
Indications	Hyperthyroidism
Dosage as per indications	• 1–2 mg/kg/day divided 8 hourly • *Adolescents and adults:* Initially 20 mg daily divided 8 hourly, gradually can increase up to maximum of 40–45 mg/day, maintenance 5–10 mg daily
Maximum dosage	Not known
Dose adjustments	In liver derangement
Adverse effects	Alopecia, bone marrow suppression, loss of taste, pancreatitis
Contraindications	Hypersensitivity, granulocytopenia, liver failure
Drug interactions	Theophylline, digitalis, chloroquine, steroids, beta blockers

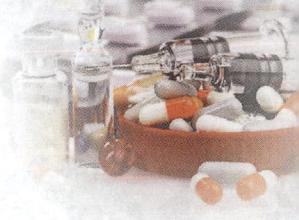

Carnitine

Drug name	Carnitine
Category	Supplement
Route	Oral, Intravenous
Strength	Tab (330 mg, 500 mg); Syp (50 mg/5 mL); Inj (500 mg/2.5 mL)
Brands	Carnitor (Inj, Syp, Cap), Carnivit (Tab), Nucarnit (Inj), Carnicare (Cap)
Mechanism of action	Required as co-factor in transport of long chain fatty acids and in krebs cycle
Pharmacokinetics	Absorbed in small intestine, poor systemic availability when taken orally, eliminated via urine
Indications	Primary carnitine deficiency (inborn error of metabolism); For cardioprotective action
Dosage as per indications	50–100 mg/kg/day q 8–12 h
Maximum dosage	*Oral:* 3 g/dose; *IV:* 300 mg/kg/24 hours
Dose adjustments	Not known
Adverse effects	Nausea, vomiting, diarrhea, pain abdomen, increased risk of seizures
Contraindications	Hypersensitivity
Drug interactions	Warfarin
Remarks	Caution in severe renal disease

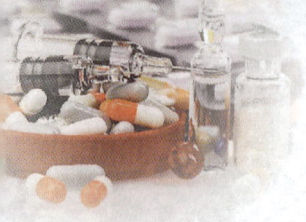

Carvedilol

Drug name	Carvedilol
Category	Beta blocker, Antihypertensive
Route	Oral
Strength	Tab (3.125 mg, 6.25 mg, 12.5 mg, 25 mg)
Brands	Caditone (Tab), Cardinome (Tab), Cardivas (Tab), Carloc (Tab)
Mechanism of action	Selective alpha-1 receptor and nonselective beta blocker with vasodilatory action by reducing peripheral vascular resistance and suppression of renin-angiotensin system
Pharmacokinetics	Rapidly absorbed after oral administration, peak concentration achieved after 1 hour; almost completely bound to plasma proteins. Elimination half-life around 6 hours
Indications	Hypertension
Dosage as per indications	0.05 mg/kg/dose BD, increase every 2 weeks by 0.05 mg/kg/dose for the first increment and then 0.1 mg/kg/dose over 3 months till max 0.35 mg/kg/dose BD
Maximum dosage	25 mg BD
Dose adjustments	Dose adjustment required in renal disease, contraindicated in liver dysfunction
Adverse effects	Hypotension, dizziness, AV block, arrhythmia
Contraindications	Hypersensitivity, heart failure, significant hepatic dysfunction, bronchial asthma, AV block
Drug interactions	Verapamil or diltiazem
Remarks	To be used with caution in hyperthyroidism, diabetes, heart disease

Caspofungin Acetate

Drug name	Caspofungin acetate
Category	Antifungal, Echinocandin
Route	Intravenous
Strength	Inj (50 mg, 70 mg vials)
Brands	Casfung (Inj), Cancidas (Inj)
Mechanism of action	Inhibits the synthesis of beta (1,3)-D-glucan, required for cell wall formation of filamentous fungi and yeast
Pharmacokinetics	Highly bound to plasma proteins, metabolized by hydrolysis and N-acetylation, eliminated slowly from kidneys. Average half-life: 10 hours
Indications	For treating fungal infections caused by *Aspergillus*; *Candida* species
Dosage as per indications	Loading dose 70 mg/m^2 IV once followed by 50 mg/m^2 IV once daily
Maximum dosage	70 mg/day
Dose adjustments	- No dose adjustment in renal disease and mild hepatic derangement - Dose adjustment needed in moderate to severe hepatic derangement
Adverse effects	Rash, fever, diarrhea, increased liver enzymes, hypotension, hypokalemia, hypersensitivity, nausea, vomiting
Contraindications	Hypersensitivity
Drug interactions	Drugs affecting liver enzymes
Remarks	Use with caution in hepatic impairment and in children <3 years

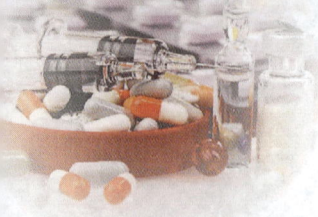

Cefaclor

Drug name	Cefaclor
Category	Antibiotic, Cephalosporin (Second generation)
Route	Oral
Strength	Tab (125 mg, 250 mg, 500 mg); Susp (125 mg/5 mL); Drops (50 mg/mL)
Brands	Distaclor (Cap/Tab, Susp, Drops), Keflor (Cap/Tab, Susp), Vercef (Cap/Tab, Susp)
Mechanism of action	Active against gram-positive bacteria, gram-negative bacteria, and anaerobes
Pharmacokinetics	Well absorbed orally, half-life 0.6–0.9 hours, mostly excreted unchanged in urine
Indications	Inhibition of cell wall synthesis
Dosage as per indications	20–40 mg/kg/day in three divided doses
Maximum dosage	1 g/day
Dose adjustments	In renal derangement
Adverse effects	Diarrhea, hepatitis, cholestatic jaundice, eosinophilia
Contraindications	Hypersensitivity
Drug interactions	Probenecid, anticoagulants

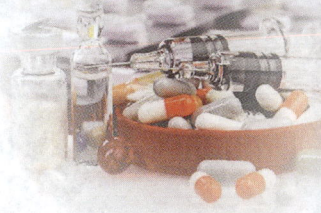

Cefadroxil

Drug name	Cefadroxil
Category	Cephalosporin antibiotic (First generation)
Route	Oral
Strength	Cap/Tab (1 g, 500 mg, 250 mg, 125 mg); Susp (125 mg/5 mL)
Brands	Cefadrox, Kefloxin, Cefadur, Droxyl
Mechanism of action	Inhibits cell wall synthesis
Pharmacokinetics	Rapidly absorbed after oral absorption, mostly excreted unchanged in urine, *Half-life:* 90 minutes
Indications	Active against both gram-positive; Gram-negative bacteria
Dosage as per indications	15 mg/kg/dose 12 hourly
Maximum dosage	2 g/day
Dose adjustments	In renal impairment
Adverse effects	Hepatic dysfunction, agranulocytosis, thrombocytopenia, arthralgia
Contraindications	Hypersensitivity
Drug interactions	Doxycycline, anticoagulants, certain vaccines (BCG, typhoid)

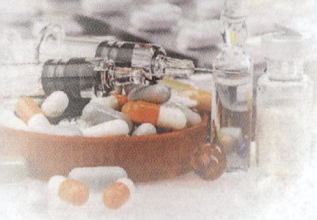

Cefazolin Sodium

Drug name	Cefazolin sodium
Category	Antibiotic, Cephalosporin (First generation)
Route	Intravenous, Intramuscular
Strength	Inj (250 mg, 500 mg, 1 g vials)
Brands	Cefadin (Inj), Ciprid (Inj), Reflin (Inj)
Mechanism of action	Bactericidal; inhibits cell wall synthesis blocking the penicillin-binding proteins
Pharmacokinetics	Maximum serum levels attained by an hour, almost three-fourths bound to plasma proteins. *Half-life:* 1.5–2 hours. Mostly excreted in urine. Does not undergo significant metabolism
Indications	Effective against gram-positive bacteria; Commonly used for streptococcal; Staphylococcal infections
Dosage as per indications	50–100 mg/kg/day q 6 h IV/IM
Maximum dosage	6 g/day
Dose adjustments	Required in renal derangement
Adverse effects	Increased liver enzymes, leukopenia, thrombocytopenia, false-positive Coombs test
Contraindications	Hypersensitivity
Drug interactions	Anticoagulants
Remarks	To use cautiously in renal disease/patients allergic to penicillin

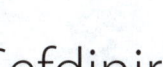

Cefdinir

Drug name	Cefdinir
Category	Antibiotic, Cephalosporin (Third generation)
Route	Oral
Strength	Inj (500 mg, 1 g); Tab/Cap (300 mg); Susp (125 mg/5 mL)
Brands	Adcef (Cap/Tab, Susp), Cefdiel (Cap, Inj, Susp), Zefdinir (Cap/Susp)
Mechanism of action	Inhibits cell wall synthesis
Pharmacokinetics	Variably absorbed, half-life around 90 minutes, poorly metabolized, mainly excreted via renal route
Indications	Acts on both gram-positive; Gram-negative bacteria
Dosage as per indications	14 mg/kg/day OD or two divided doses
Maximum dosage	600 mg/day
Dose adjustments	In renal derangement
Adverse effects	Seizures, cholestatic jaundice, hemolytic anemia, pseudomembranous colitis
Contraindications	Hypersensitivity
Drug interactions	Antacid, probenecid, iron

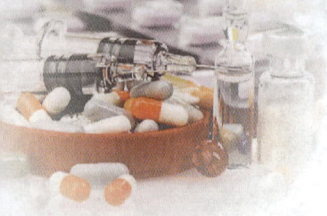

Cefepime

Drug name	Cefepime
Category	Antibiotic, Cephalosporin (Fourth generation)
Route	Intravenous, Intramuscular
Strength	Inj (250 mg, 500 mg, 1 g vials)
Brands	C-Pime (Inj), Adpime (Inj), Cefepime (Inj), Kefpime (Inj)
Mechanism of action	Bactericidal against gram-positive and gram-negative bacteria. Acts by inhibiting cell wall synthesis
Pharmacokinetics	• High absorption after parental administration • Mostly eliminated unchanged, with elimination half-life around 2 hours
Indications	Serious gram-positive; Gram-negative infections
Dosage as per indications	• 100 mg/kg/day q 8–12 h IV/IM • *Meningitis/serious infections:* 150 mg/kg/d q 8 h
Maximum dosage	2 g 8 hourly
Dose adjustments	Dose adjustment needed in renal dysfunction but not in hepatic dysfunction
Adverse effects	Nausea, vomiting, pain abdomen, deranged liver enzymes, false-positive Coombs test
Contraindications	Hypersensitivity
Drug interactions	Other bacteriostatic agents
Remarks	To use cautiously in patients allergic to penicillin

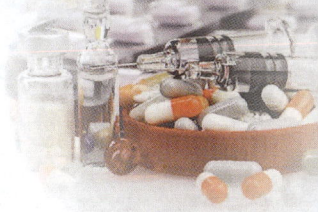

Cefixime

Drug name	Cefixime
Category	Antibiotic, Cephalosporin (Third generation)
Route	Oral
Strength	Syp (50 mg/5 mL); Tab (100 mg, 200 mg, 400 mg)
Brands	Cefex (Syp, Tab), Extacef (Syp, Tab), Omnatax O (Syp, Tab), Taxim-O (Syp, Tab), Zifi (Syp, Tab)
Mechanism of action	Bactericidal activity against gram-positive and gram-negative organisms
Pharmacokinetics	Oral bioavailability from 25 to 50%. More than 50% protein bound, some part metabolized in liver, rest eliminated unchanged in the urine by glomerular filtration, half-life: 3–4 hours
Indications	Dysentery; Enteric fever; UTI. Mainly active against gram-negative bacteria
Dosage as per indications	8–10 mg/kg/day q 12 h *Enteric fever:* 15–20 mg/kg/day q 12 h
Maximum dosage	1200 mg/day
Dose adjustments	Needed in renal derangement
Adverse effects	Nausea, vomiting, pain abdomen, false-positive Coombs test
Contraindications	Hypersensitivity
Drug interactions	Anticoagulants
Remarks	To use cautiously in renal disease/patients allergic to penicillin

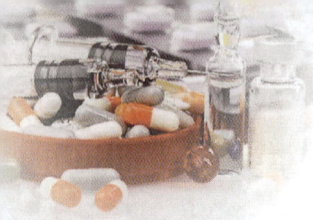

Cefoperazone-sulbactam

Drug name	Cefoperazone-sulbactam
Category	Antibiotic, Cephalosporin (Third generation)
Route	Intravenous, Intramuscular
Strength	Inj (available as 1:1 or 1:2 ratio of Sulbactam and Cefoperazone; for 1:1 preparation—500 mg:500 mg, 1 g:1 g; for 1:2 preparation—500 mg:1 g, 1 g:2 g vials)
Brands	Cefobid (Inj), Magnex (Inj)
Mechanism of action	Interferes with cell wall synthesis by binding to penicillin-binding proteins. Sulbactam is an irreversible inhibitor of beta-lactamases produced by most beta-lactam antibiotic-resistant organisms
Pharmacokinetics	Highly protein bound, mainly excreted by kidney (mainly sulbactam) and bile (mainly cefoperazone). Serum half-life around 1 hour for sulbactam and 1.7 hours for cefoperazone. Not significantly metabolized
Indications	Active against gram-positive; Gram-negative; *Pseudomonas* infection
Dosage as per indications	For 1:1 ratio *Nonsevere infections:* 40–80 mg/kg/day (20–40 mg/kg/day cefoperazone) q 6–12 h *Severe infections:* Up to 160 mg/kg/day (80 mg/kg/day cefoperazone) q 6–12 h
Maximum dosage	*Sulbactam:* 80 mg/kg/day (4 g/day) *Cefoperazone:* 80 mg/kg/day. Doses up to 160 mg/kg/day can be given but as 1:2 ratio preparation
Dose adjustments	Dose modification in hepatic, renal dysfunction, and biliary obstruction
Adverse effects	Bleeding, hypersensitivity
Contraindications	Known allergy to penicillins, sulbactam, cefoperazone
Drug interactions	Anticoagulants
Remarks	Does not penetrate the CSF well

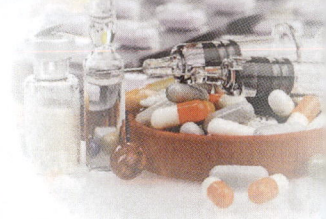

Cefotaxime

Drug name	Cefotaxime
Category	Cephalosporin (Third generation)
Route	Intravenous, Intramuscular
Strength	Inj (250 mg, 500 mg, 1 g)
Brands	Biotax (Inj), Taxim (Inj), Omnatax (Inj)
Mechanism of action	Acts by inhibiting cell wall synthesis by binding to PBPs
Pharmacokinetics	Well absorbed when administered intramuscular/intravenous. Eliminated via kidneys, nearly one-third remaining unchanged, rest as metabolites. *Half-life:* 1 hour
Indications	Bactericidal against gram-negative; Gram-positive bacteria

Dosage as per indications	• *Infections:* 100–150 mg/kg/day q 6–8 h; *Meningitis:* 200 mg/kg/day q 6 h IV
	• *Neonate:*
	  – *<7 days: >2 kg:* 100–150 mg/kg/day q 12 h, *<2 kg:* 100 mg/kg/day q 12h
	  – *>7 days: >2 kg:* 150–200 mg/kg/day q 6–8 h, 1.2–2 kg: 150 mg/kg/day q 12 h, <1.2 kg: 100 mg/kg/day q 12 h

Maximum dosage	12 g/day
Dose adjustments	In renal derangement
Adverse effects	Nausea, vomiting, pain abdomen, false-positive Coombs test
Contraindications	Hypersensitivity
Drug interactions	Probenecid acid

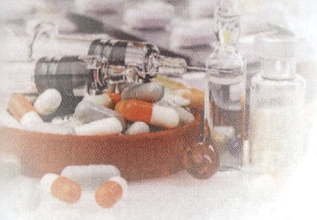

Cefoxitin

Drug name	Cefoxitin
Category	Antibiotic, Beta-lactam, Cephalosporin (Second generation)
Route	Intravenous
Strength	Inj (1 g, 2 g vials)
Brands	Mefoxin (Inj)
Mechanism of action	Acts by inhibiting cell wall synthesis by binding to penicillin binding proteins (PBP)
Pharmacokinetics	Poorly metabolized, mostly eliminated unchanged by the kidney. Elimination half-life: 45 minutes. Poor CSF penetration
Indications	Effective against gram-negative bacteria; Anaerobes
Dosage as per indications	80–160 mg/kg/day divided in q 4–6 h intervals
Maximum dosage	12 g/24 hours
Dose adjustments	Dose adjustment in renal dysfunction
Adverse effects	Hypoprothrombinemia, leukopenia, thrombocytopenia, diarrhea, interstitial nephritis
Contraindications	Hypersensitivity
Drug interactions	Aminoglycosides, probenecid
Remarks	May falsely elevate creatinine levels and can cause false-positive urine–reducing substance

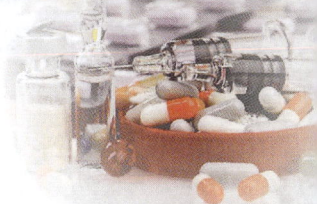

Cefpodoxime Proxetil

Drug name	Cefpodoxime proxetil
Category	Antibiotic, Cephalosporin (Second generation)
Route	Oral
Strength	Syp (50 mg, 100 mg); Tab (100 mg, 200 mg)
Brands	Cedon (Syp, Tab), Cefoprox (Syp, Tab), Cepodem (Syp, Tab)
Mechanism of action	Acts by inhibiting cell wall synthesis
Pharmacokinetics	Cefpodoxime proxetil is converted to its active metabolite, cefpodoxime. Around 50% absorbed when taken orally, *Half-life:* 2–3 hours, poorly bound to protein. Around 50% absorbed when taken orally
Indications	Active against gram-positive; Gram-negative bacteria
Dosage as per indications	10 mg/kg/day q 12 h
Maximum dosage	400 mg/24 hours
Dose adjustments	Dose adjustment in moderate to severe renal impairment; no dose adjustment in hepatic derangement
Adverse effects	Nausea, vomiting, diarrhea, vaginal candidiasis, false-positive Coombs test
Contraindications	Hypersensitivity
Drug interactions	H_2 blockers, antacids, probenecid
Remarks	Tablets should be taken with food, syrup can be taken anytime irrespective of food intake

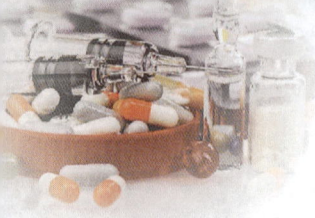

Cefprozil

Drug name	Cefprozil
Category	Antibiotic, Cephalosporin (Second generation)
Route	Oral
Strength	Tab (250 mg, 500 mg); Susp (125 mg/5 mL)
Brands	3Cef (Tab, Susp), Refzil O (Tab, Susp)
Mechanism of action	Inhibits cell wall synthesis
Pharmacokinetics	Well absorbed orally, *Half-life:* 90 minutes, excreted via renal route
Indications	Acts against gram-positive; Gram-negative bacteria
Dosage as per indications	15–30 mg/kg/day divided 12 hourly
Maximum dosage	<12 years: 1 g/day
Dose adjustments	In renal derangement
Adverse effects	Diarrhea, eosinophilia, direct Coombs test positive, hepatic dysfunction, decreased leukocyte count
Contraindications	Hypersensitivity
Drug interactions	Warfarin, furosemide, nephrotoxic drugs

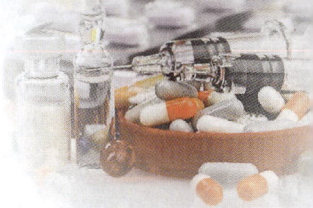

Ceftazidime

Drug name	Ceftazidime
Category	Antibiotic, Cephalosporin (Third generation)
Route	Intravenous, Intramuscular
Strength	Inj (250 mg, 500 mg, 1 g vials)
Brands	Cefopam S (Inj), Cefopar S (Inj), Ceftop (Inj), Magnex (Inj), Zostum (Inj)
Mechanism of action	Inhibits bacterial cell wall synthesis following attachment to penicillin binding proteins (PBPs)
Pharmacokinetics	Low-serum protein binding; not metabolized much, mainly excreted unchanged in urine, half-life of about 2 hours
Indications	Gram-negative sepsis; *Pseudomonas* in particular
Dosage as per indications	- 100–150 mg/kg/day q 8 h - *Neonate:* <7 days:100 mg/kg/day q 12 h; >7 days: >1.2 kg: 150 mg/kg/day q 8 h, <1.2 kg: 100 mg/kg/day q 12 h
Maximum dosage	6 g/24 hours
Dose adjustments	Dose adjustment needed in renal impairment and severe hepatic impairment
Adverse effects	Rash, deranged liver enzymes, false-positive Coombs test
Contraindications	Hypersensitivity
Drug interactions	Probenecid increases ceftazidime levels
Remarks	Good *Pseudomonas* coverage and CSF penetration

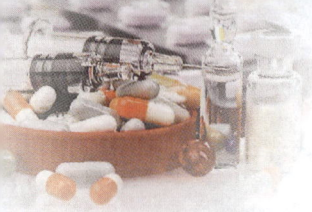

Ceftriaxone Sodium

Drug name	Ceftriaxone sodium
Category	Antibiotic, Cephalosporin (Third generation)
Route	Intravenous, Intramuscular
Strength	Inj (250 mg, 500 mg, 1 g vials)
Brands	Monocef (Inj), Mahacef (Inj), Gramocef (Inj), Oframax (Inj)
Mechanism of action	Inhibits bacterial cell wall synthesis by attaching to penicillin binding proteins and inhibiting cell wall (peptidoglycan) biosynthesis
Pharmacokinetics	Highly protein bound, poorly metabolized, significantly cleared in urine and bile. Highly plasma protein bound. Half-life 6–9 hours
Indications	Serious gram-negative infections including meningitis; Septicemia
Dosage as per indications	• *AOM:* 50–75 mg/kg/day q 12 h • *Meningitis:* 100 mg/kg/day q 12 h
Maximum dosage	4 g/24 hours
Dose adjustments	Required in renal derangement and hepatic dysfunction
Adverse effects	Deranged liver enzymes, diarrhea, cholelithiasis (reversible), gallbladder sludging false-positive Coombs test
Contraindications	Do not use simultaneously with calcium containing solutions in neonates
Drug interactions	Calcium injections, anticoagulant, probenecid
Remarks	Has good CNS penetration

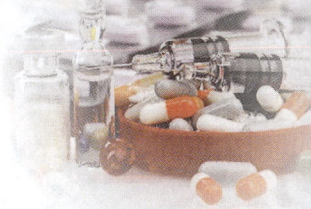

Cefuroxime Axetil

Drug name	Cefuroxime axetil
Category	Antibiotic, Cephalosporin (Second generation)
Route	Oral, Intravenous
Strength	Syp (125 mg/5 mL); Tab (125 mg, 250 mg, 500 mg); Inj (250 mg, 750 mg, 1.5 g vials)
Brands	Altacef (Inj, Syp, Tab), Bigcef (Tab, Inj), Cefakind (Tab, Syp), Cefasyn (Tab, Inj)
Mechanism of action	Attaches to penicillin binding proteins leading to interruption of cell wall (peptidoglycan) biosynthesis, causing bacterial cell lysis
Pharmacokinetics	Rapidly absorbed from the gut. Metabolized to acetic acid and acetaldehyde. Mainly excreted by renal route using glomerular filtration and tubular secretion. Serum half-life around 1 hour
Indications	Effective against both gram-positive; Gram-negative bacteria
Dosage as per indications	• *Intravenous:* 75–150 mg/kg/day q 6–8 h • *Oral:* 20–30 mg/kg/day q 12 h
Maximum dosage	• *IV:* 1,500 mg/dose • *Oral:* 1 g/24 h
Dose adjustments	Reduce dose in renal impairment
Adverse effects	GI disturbances, thrombophlebitis, false-positive Coombs test
Contraindications	Hypersensitivity
Drug interactions	Probenecid, anticoagulants
Remarks	To use cautiously in renal disease/patients allergic to penicillin

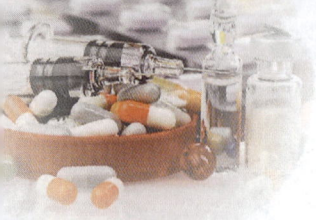

Cephalexin

Drug name	Cephalexin
Category	Antibiotic, Cephalosporin (First generation)
Route	Oral
Strength	Syp (125 mg/5 mL); Tab (125 mg DT, 250 mg DT); Cap (250 mg, 500 mg)
Brands	Bluecef (Syp, Cap, Tab), Cefanor (Cap, Tab), Phexin (Tab, Syp, Cap)
Mechanism of action	Bactericidal against both gram-positive and gram-negative organisms. Acts by inhibiting cell wall synthesis
Pharmacokinetics	Rapidly absorbed after oral administration from the gut, *Half-life:* 1 hour. Poorly metabolized, mostly excreted unchanged in the urine by glomerular filtration and tubular secretion
Indications	Gram-positive; Gram-negative infections including respiratory tract infection and UTI
Dosage as per indications	25–100 mg/kg/day q 6–8 h
Maximum dosage	4 g/24 hours
Dose adjustments	To use cautiously in renal disease with adjusted doses
Adverse effects	GI disturbances, false-positive Coombs test
Contraindications	Hypersensitivity
Drug interactions	Probenecid, cholestyramine, metformin
Remarks	Administer doses on an empty stomach 2 hours prior or 1 hour after meals

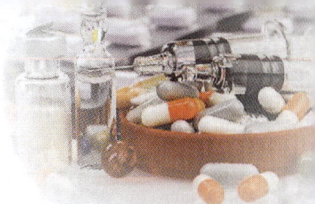

Cetirizine Dihydrochloride

Drug name	Cetirizine dihydrochloride
Category	Antihistamine
Route	Oral
Strength	Tab (5 mg, 10 mg); Syp (5 mg/5 mL)
Brands	Alercet (Syp, Tab), Cetlong (Syp, Tab), Cetrine (Syp, Tab), Zyrtec (Syp, Tab)
Mechanism of action	Potent and selective antagonist of peripheral H_1 receptors
Pharmacokinetics	Rapidly absorbed, peak levels in 1 hour, highly protein bound, metabolized by dealkylation, nearly 50% eliminated in urine, elimination half-life 8 hours
Indications	Allergic rhinitis
Dosage as per indications	• *2–6 years:* 2.5 mg BD or 5 mg OD • *>6 years:* 5–10 mg OD
Maximum dosage	• *2–6 years:* 5 mg/day • *6–12 years:* 10 mg/day
Dose adjustments	In renal impairment
Adverse effects	Sedation, dryness of mouth, GI upset, headache
Contraindications	Hypersensitivity, creatinine clearance <10 mL/min
Drug interactions	Sedatives
Remarks	Not recommended below 2 years

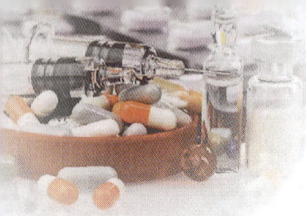

Chloral Hydrate

Drug name	Chloral hydrate
Category	Sedative, Hypnotic (Nonbarbiturate)
Route	Oral, Rectal
Strength	Syp (40 mg/mL)
Brands	Aquachloral Supprettes, PMS-Chloral Hydrate (CAN), Chloral Hydrate-Odan (CAN), Somnote *(No Indian brand available)*
Mechanism of action	Acts by potentiating the function of GABA receptors, inhibition of excitatory amino acid-activated currents
Pharmacokinetics	Rapidly absorbed from the gut after oral intake, effect noted within 30 minutes, lasts for 4–8 hours. Rapidly metabolized by the liver and erythrocytes to its active metabolite trichloroethanol
Indications	Sedation; Hypnosis
Dosage as per indications	• *Hypnotic:* 50 mg/kg/day PO up to 1 g per single dose; may be given in divided doses • *Sedative:* 25 mg/kg/day PO up to 500 mg per single dose; may be given in divided doses
Maximum dosage	• *2–12 years:* 1 g/dose • *>12 years:* 2 g/dose
Dose adjustments	Mild to moderate renal, hepatic derangement
Adverse effects	Sedation, respiratory depression
Contraindications	Severe hepatic renal or cardiac derangement, arrhythmias
Drug interactions	Drugs prolonging QT interval
Remarks	Use with caution in those with underlying respiratory illness

Chloramphenicol

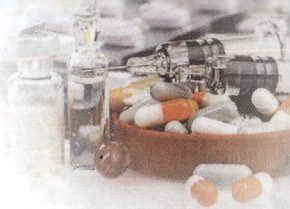

Drug name	Chloramphenicol
Category	Antibiotic
Route	Oral, Intravenous
Strength	Cap (250 mg, 500 mg); Susp (125 mg/5 mL); Inj (1 g)
Brands	Chlorocap (Cap), Chloromycetin (Cap, Syp), Paraxin (Inj, Cap, Syp)
Mechanism of action	By interfering with bacterial protein synthesis
Pharmacokinetics	Widely distributed in body tissues and fluids including cerebrospinal fluid. Well absorbed from gut, metabolized in liver, variable half-life from 3 to 12 hours, higher in younger age
Indications	Active against many gram-positive; Gram-negative organisms; *Spirilla*; *Rickettsia*
Dosage as per indications	• 50–75 mg/kg/day q 8 h PO; 100 mg/kg/day q 6 hourly IV • *Meningitis:* 75–100 mg/kg/day IV divided 6 hourly
Maximum dosage	4 g/24 hours
Dose adjustments	Hepatic and renal impairment
Adverse effects	Bone marrow suppression; gray baby syndrome (in newborns) at serum levels >50 mg/L
Contraindications	Hypersensitivity
Drug interactions	Anticoagulants, hypoglycemic agents, phenytoin
Remarks	Caution in renal/hepatic disease, G6PD deficiency, and in neonates

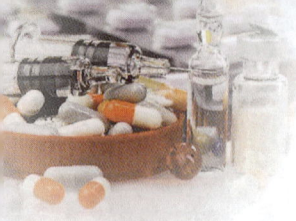

Chloroquine Phosphate

Drug name	Chloroquine phosphate
Category	Antimalarial
Route	Oral
Strength	Tab [250 mg (150 mg base)]; Syp (50 mg/5 mL)
Brands	Emquine (Syp, Tab), Jagquin (Syp, Tab), Lariago (Syp, Tab), Malaquin (Syp, Tab)
Mechanism of action	Alters the properties of DNA. Also binds to ferriprotoporphyrin IX causing lysis of plasmodial membrane. It inhibits the erythrocytic stage
Pharmacokinetics	Has high oral bioavailability. It is widely distributed in body tissues with a distribution half-life of 2–6 days and terminal elimination phase of 10–60 days. Nearly 50% is plasma protein bound
Indications	Uncomplicated malaria
Dosage as per indications	10 mg/kg (base) followed by 5 mg/kg (base) after 6 hours, 24 hours and 48 hours from first dose OR 10 mg/kg (base) followed by 10 mg/kg (base) after 24 hours followed by 5 mg/kg (base) after 48 hours from first dose
Maximum dosage	600 mg for 10 mg/kg, 300 mg for 5 mg/kg
Dose adjustments	In renal impairment
Adverse effects	Nausea, vomiting, prolonged QT interval, blurred vision, increased liver enzymes, headache, vision abnormalities
Contraindications	Hypersensitivity
Drug interactions	Antacids, ampicillin, kaolin, cimetidine
Remarks	To repeat dose, if vomiting within 30 minutes of intake; coadministration with mefloquine increases the risk of seizures

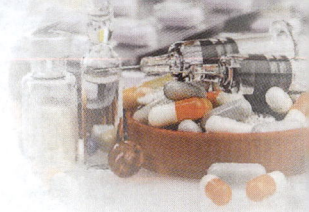

Chlorothiazide

Drug name	Chlorothiazide
Category	Diuretic
Route	Oral, Intravenous
Strength	Tab (12.5 mg); Inj (0.5 g, not available in India)
Brands	Available as a combination with other antihypertensives
Mechanism of action	Affects the distal renal tubules, increases excretion of sodium and chloride in nearly same amounts along with some loss of potassium and bicarbonate
Pharmacokinetics	Not metabolized much, eliminated by the kidney. Nearly 50% protein bound. Plasma half-life 1–2 hours
Indications	Hypertension
Dosage as per indications	• <6 months: 20–40 mg/kg/d q 12 h PO/IV • >6 months: 20 mg/kg/d q 12 h PO/IV
Maximum dosage	6 months–2 years: 375 mg/day, 2–12 years: 1 g/day, >12 years: 2 g/day
Dose adjustments	Caution in hepatic/renal disease
Adverse effects	Pancreatitis, hypokalemia, hypomagnesemia
Contraindications	Anuria, hypersensitivity
Drug interactions	NSAIDS, corticosteroids, antihypertensives, antidiabetics
Remarks	Available as a combination with other antihypertensives

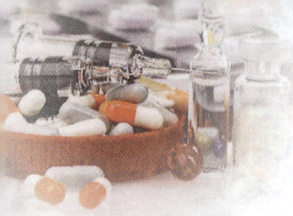

Chlorpheniramine Maleate

Drug name	Chlorpheniramine maleate
Category	Antihistamine
Route	Oral, Intravenous, Intramuscular, Subcutaneous
Strength	Tab (2 mg, 4 mg); Syp (2 mg/5 mL); Inj (10 mg/mL)
Brands	Anistamin (Inj), Cipium (Tab), Piriton (Tab)
Mechanism of action	Acts by competing with histamine for H_1 receptor sites on cells and tissues along with anticholinergic activity.
Pharmacokinetics	Nearly 70% bound to plasma proteins. Well absorbed from the gastrointestinal tract, following oral administration. Effects start within 30 minutes, peaks by 1–2 hours and lasts for 4–6 hours. Plasma half-life: 12–15 hours
Indications	Antihypertensive; Diuretic

Dosage as per indications	• *Oral:* 0.35 mg/kg/day PO q 4–6 h or dose based on age bands as
	  – *2–6 years:* 1 mg/dose PO q 4–6 h
	  – *6–12 years:* 2 mg/dose PO q 4–6 h
	  – *≥12 years:* 4 mg/dose q PO 4–6 h
	• IV/IM/SC: 5–20 mg once, max 40 mg/24 h

Maximum dosage	*Oral:* *2–6 years:* 6 mg/day *6–12 years:* 12 mg/day *>12 years:* 24 mg/day *IV/IM:* 40 mg/day
Dose adjustments	Required in renal and hepatic derangement
Adverse effects	Sedation, dryness of mouth, blurred vision, urinary retention
Contraindications	Hypersensitivity
Drug interactions	Other sedatives, anticholinergic agents
Remarks	To be used with caution in patients with asthma

Chlorpromazine

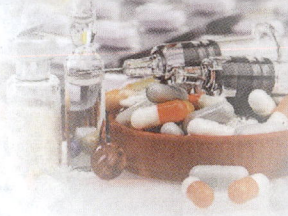

Drug name	Chlorpromazine
Category	Antiemetic, Phenothiazine derivative
Route	Oral, Injection
Strength	Tab (10 mg, 25 mg, 50 mg, 100 mg); extended release Caps (30 mg, 75 mg, 150 mg, 200 mg, 300 mg); Syp (10 mg/5 mL); Suppository (25 mg, 100 mg); Inj (25 mg/mL)
Brands	Chlorpromazine (Inj, Cap, Tab), Megatil (Inj, Cap, Tab), Sun Prazin (Cap, Tab)
Mechanism of action	Acts to exert antagonist effect on dopamine receptors, serotonergic receptors along with alpha adrenergic blocking effect
Pharmacokinetics	Rapidly absorbed and widely distributed in the body. It is metabolized in the liver and kidney, excreted in the urine and bile. Has a high affinity to plasma proteins. Half-life 30 hours
Indications	Psychosis; Emesis
Dosage as per indications	*Psychosis (>6 months)* • *IM or IV:* 2.5–4 mg/kg/day q 6–8 h • *PO:* 2.5–6 mg/kg/day q 4–6 h *Antiemetic (>6 months)* • IV/IM/PO: 0.5–1 mg/kg/dose 6–8 hourly
Maximum dosage	IM/IV: <5 years: 40 mg/24 hours, 5–12 years: 75 mg/24 hours; PO: 500 mg/24 hours
Dose adjustments	Use with caution in renal and hepatic derangement
Adverse effects	Drowsiness, jaundice, lowered seizure threshold, extrapyramidal or anticholinergic symptoms, hypotension, arrhythmias, neuroleptic malignant syndrome, bone marrow suppression
Contraindications	Hypersensitivity, bone marrow depression, urinary retention, agranulocytosis
Drug interactions	Sedatives, carbamazepine, drugs prolonging QT interval, fluoxetine, haloperidol
Remarks	Not to be used simultaneously with carbamazepine in oral form

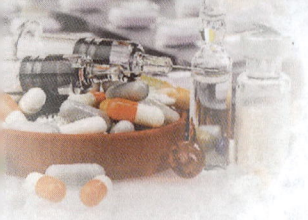

Cholecalciferol

Drug name	Cholecalciferol
Category	Vitamin D_3 supplement
Route	Oral
Strength	Tab (60,000 IU); Cap (60,000 IU); Sachet (60,000 IU); Syp (1000 IU/5 mL, 2000 IU/5 mL, 60,000 IU/5 mL); Drops (400 IU/mL, 800 IU/mL)
Brands	Calcirol (Sachet), Calcital (Sachet, Cap), D-Sol (Sachet, Tab, Drops), Wal-D3 (Cap, Syp, Drops)
Mechanism of action	Increases calcium and phosphorus absorption in small intestine and promotes renal reabsorption of calcium and phosphate. The vitamin helps in bone mineralization
Pharmacokinetics	Cholecalciferol is hydroxylated in liver 25-hydroxyvitamin D and further hydroxylated again in kidneys to form 1, 25-dihydroxyvitamin D, the active form. Cholecalciferol is easily absorbed from the small intestine. Excreted in bile and feces. Half-life 50 days
Indications	Rickets; Vitamin D deficiency
Dosage as per indications	*Term neonates and infants:* • *Prevention:* 400 IU/day (0–1 year) as routine • *Treatment:* 2,000 IU/day for minimum of 3 months *1–18 years:* • *Prevention:* 600 IU/day (only when indicated) • *Treatment:* 3,000–6,000 IU/day for minimum of 3 months
Maximum dosage	60,000 IU/week in infants >3 months
Dose adjustments	Renal and hepatic derangement
Adverse effects	Weakness, fatigue, loss of appetite, nausea, vomiting, dry mouth, metallic taste
Contraindications	Hypersensitivity
Drug interactions	Diuretics, phenytoin, steroids, barbiturates

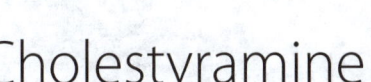

Cholestyramine

Drug name	Cholestyramine
Category	Oral
Route	Bile acid sequestrant
Strength	Sachet (4 g, 5 g, 9 g)
Brands	Choltran (Sachet), Clostran (Sachet)
Mechanism of action	It limits reabsorption of bile acids in gut by forming a resin which acts as bile acid sequestrant
Pharmacokinetics	Not absorbed from gut, half-life 6 minutes, metabolism by bile acids, excreted via feces
Indications	Hypercholesteremia; As antipruritic in partial bile duct obstruction
Dosage as per indications	250–500 mg/kg/day (anhydrous) divided 8 hourly
Maximum dosage	8 g/day
Dose adjustments	Not known
Adverse effects	Constipation, fat soluble vitamin deficiency
Contraindications	Hypersensitivity
Drug interactions	Anticoagulants, mycophenolate
Remarks	To be taken after meals, with juice or water. Not to be given in complete biliary obstruction

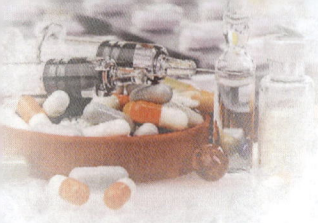

Ciprofloxacin

Drug name	Ciprofloxacin
Category	Antibiotic, Fluoroquinolone
Route	Oral, Intravenous
Strength	Syp (125 mg/5 mL); Tab (250 mg, 500 mg); Inj (200 mg/100 mL, 100 mg/50 mL)
Brands	Cifran (Tab/Cap, Inj), Ciplox (Tab/Cap, Inj), Cipflacin (Syp), Coflox (Tab/Cap), Alcipro (Tab/Cap, Inj)
Mechanism of action	Inhibition of both type II topoisomerase (DNA-gyrase) and topoisomerase IV, required for bacterial DNA replication, transcription, repair and recombination
Pharmacokinetics	Rapidly absorbed from small intestine after oral administration, maximum serum concentrations after 1–2 hours later. High bioavailability 70–80%. Metabolized via CYP1A2, half-life around 4 hours
Indications	Dysentery; UTI; Enteric infections
Dosage as per indications	• *Intravenous:* 10–20 mg/kg/day q 8–12 h • *Oral:* 20–30 mg/kg/day q 8–12 h
Maximum dosage	*Oral:* 1.5 g/24 hours, *IV:* 400 mg/dose
Dose adjustments	To use cautiously in renal disease/liver disease
Adverse effects	Rash, deranged liver enzymes, neutropenia, gynecomastia, diarrhea
Contraindications	Hypersensitivity
Drug interactions	Caffeine, methotrexate, theophylline, warfarin
Remarks	Do not give antacids within 1–2 hours of ciprofloxacin intake

Clarithromycin

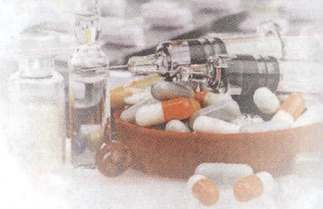

Drug name	Clarithromycin
Category	Antibiotic
Route	Oral
Strength	Tab (250 mg, 500 mg); Syp (125 mg/5 mL)
Brands	Claribid (Tab, Syp), Claricin (Tab, Syp), Clarimac (Tab), Synclar (Tab, Syp)
Mechanism of action	Acts by binding to the 50S ribosomal subunit of susceptible bacteria resulting in inhibition of protein synthesis
Pharmacokinetics	Rapidly absorbed after oral administration, peak levels attained after 2–3 hours, metabolized in liver (CYP3A4), eliminated in urine, half-life 3–5 hours
Indications	Active against gram-positive; Gram-negative bacteria; Mycobacteria; *Mycoplasma*; *Ureaplasma*; *Chlamydia*; *Toxoplasma*; *Borrelia*
Dosage as per indications	15 mg/kg/day q 12 h, PO *Mycobacterium avium* complex prophylaxis 15 mg/kg/dose PO once a week
Maximum dosage	500 mg/dose
Dose adjustments	Adjust dose in renal failure
Adverse effects	QT prolongation, arrhythmias, torsades de pointes
Contraindications	Hypersensitivity
Drug interactions	Cephalosporins, aminoglycosides, nephrotoxic drugs, drugs prolonging QT interval
Remarks	Not to be given in patients allergic to erythromycin and liver dysfunction. Avoid use in infants <6 months age, patients on cisapride

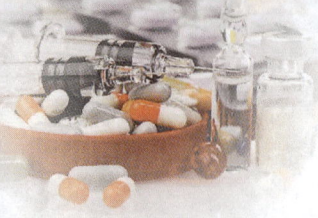

Clindamycin

Drug name	Clindamycin
Category	Antibiotic, Lincomycin
Route	Oral, Injection, Topical gel
Strength	Oral sol (75 mg/5 mL); Tab/Cap (150 mg, 300 mg); Inj (300 mg/2 mL); 1% Ointment for topical use in Acne
Brands	Clinbid (Inj, Cap), Dalacin C (Inj, Cap), Dalcinex (Inj, Cap, Susp)
Mechanism of action	Bacteriostatic against gram-positive aerobes and anaerobic bacteria. Bind to the 50S subunit of the bacterial ribosome and inhibit protein synthesis
Pharmacokinetics	Rapidly absorbed after oral intake; widely distributed in body fluids but not cerebrospinal fluid. Highly plasma protein bound. Metabolized in liver (CYP3A4/CYP3A5). *Half-life:* after oral: 2.5 hours
Indications	Gram-positive aerobic; Anaerobic infections; malaria; Toxoplasmosis; Pneumocystis pneumonia
Dosage as per indications	• *Neonates:* 5–7.5 g/kg/dose IV or PO, duration between 2 doses varying with gestational age and day of life • *Pediatric:* PO: 10–40 mg/kg/24 h q 6–8 h; max dose: 1.8 g/24 h IM/IV: 25–40 mg/kg/24 h in divided doses every 6–8 h; max dose: 2.7 g/24 h • *Malaria:* 10 mg/kg/dose q 12 h • *Toxoplasmosis:* 5–7.5 mg/kg/dose IV/PO q 6 h (max 600 mg/dose) • *Secondary prophylaxis:* 7–10 mg/kg/dose PO q 8 h • *PCP:* 10 mg/kg/dose IV/PO q 6 h (max 600 mg IV, max 450 mg PO)
Maximum dosage	Oral: 1.8 g/24 h, IV: 2.7 g/24 h
Dose adjustments	In severe hepatic or renal derangement
Adverse effects	Diarrhea, GI intolerance, nausea, vomiting, and anorexia
Contraindications	Hypersensitivity
Drug interactions	Tubocurarine, pancuronium, anticoagulants
Remarks	Do not exceed IV infusion rate of 30 mg/min, does not cross blood brain barrier

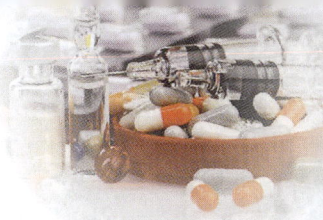

Clobazam

Drug name	Clobazam
Category	Antiepileptic, Benzodiazepine
Route	Oral
Strength	Tab (5 mg, 10 mg, 20 mg)
Brands	Aedon (Tab), Clobaday (Tab), Clobatar (Tab), Frisium (Tab)
Mechanism of action	It acts by increasing GABAergic transmission by acting on GABA receptors
Pharmacokinetics	After oral administration, rapidly and extensively absorbed. Peak plasma levels attained in 0.5–4.0 hours. It is rapidly and extensively metabolized in the liver. Mean half-life 1.5 days
Indications	• As an add-on drug in complex partial; Generalized tonic-clonic; Generalized tonic; Absence; Myoclonic; and Atonic seizures • Lennox–Gastaut syndrome; Febrile seizure prophylaxis
Dosage as per indications	• 0.3–1 mg/kg/day HS or divided in two doses • For febrile seizure prophylaxis 0.5 mg/kg/dose 12 hours for 48 hours
Maximum dosage	• *<30 kg:* 10 mg BD • *>30 kg:* 20 mg BD (To be started slowly and increased gradually till the given dose by end of 2 weeks)
Dose adjustments	Use with caution in hepatic impairment
Adverse effects	Drowsiness, ataxia, constipation, insomnia, aggressive behavior
Contraindications	Hypersensitivity
Drug interactions	Azelastine, olanzapine, proton pump inhibitors, azole antifungal agents, CNS depressants, cimetidine, and calcium channel blockers
Remarks	Avoid in children below 3 years; do not discontinue abruptly

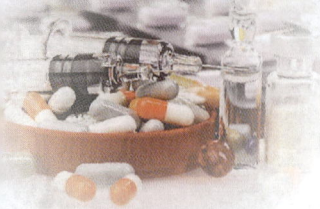

Clonazepam

Drug name	Clonazepam
Category	Antiepileptic, Benzodiazepine
Route	Oral
Strength	Tab (0.5 mg, 1 mg, 2 mg)
Brands	Clonotril (Tab), Rivotril (Tab)
Mechanism of action	Acts like other benzodiazepines to increase GABAergic transmission. Generalized EEG abnormalities are more readily suppressed than focal EEG abnormalities
Pharmacokinetics	Quickly and completely absorbed after oral administration. Peak plasma concentrations attained in 1–4 hours. Has high bioavailability. Metabolism primarily in liver. The elimination half-life is 24–36 hours. More than half the drug is excreted via urine
Indications	Myoclonic seizures; Status epilepticus; Absence seizures
Dosage as per indications	<30 kg—initial dose: 0.05 mg/kg/24 h q 8 h; increase by 0.25–0.5 mg/d to maximum of 0.1–0.2 mg/kg/24 h PO in three divided doses; For >30 kg—initial: 1.5 mg/24 h PO; increase by 0.5–1 mg/24 h
Maximum dosage	20 mg/24 h
Dose adjustments	Use with caution in hepatic and renal impairment
Adverse effects	Drowsiness, thrombocytopenia, leukopenia, increased bronchial secretions
Contraindications	Severe liver disease
Drug interactions	Carbamazepine, phenytoin, and phenobarbital
Remarks	Use with caution in patients with compromised respiratory function, porphyria and renal impairment. Do not discontinue abruptly

Clonidine Hydrochloride

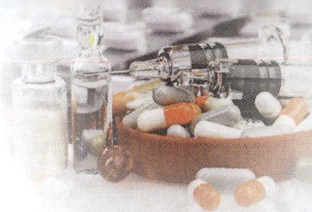

Drug name	Clonidine hydrochloride
Category	Antihypertensive, Central alpha-adrenergic agonist
Route	Oral, Injection, Transdermal
Strength	Tab (100 µg, 200 µg, 300 µg); Inj (100 µg/mL); Transdermal patch (0.1, 0.2, 0.3 mg/24 h × 7 days)
Brands	Arkamin (Tab), Clodict (Tab), Clonidine Hydrochloride (Inj), Clonidine (patch)
Mechanism of action	Acts centrally by stimulating alpha-2 adrenergic receptors and producing a reduction in sympathetic tone, prevents vascular changes in migraine by diminishing the responsiveness of peripheral vessels to constrictor and dilator stimuli
Pharmacokinetics	Highly absorbed after oral administration with peak effect within 1–3 hours. Around 40% bound to plasma proteins. Rapidly distributed and crosses the blood–brain barrier. Onset of action within 0.5–1 hour orally and 2–3 days when given transdermal
Indications	Hypertension; Especially in chronic kidney disease
Dosage as per indications	1–2 µg/kg/dose q 6 h
Maximum dosage	- *<12 years:* Max dose: 25 µg/kg/24 h up to 0.9 mg/24 h - *>12 years:* Max dose: 2.4 mg/24 h
Dose adjustments	Required in renal derangement
Adverse effects	Dry mouth, dizziness, drowsiness, constipation, fatigue
Contraindications	Severe bradyarrhythmia, sick sinus syndrome or AV block of 2nd or 3rd degree, or in patients with known hypersensitivity
Drug interactions	β-blockers may exacerbate rebound hypertension during and following the withdrawal of clonidine
Remarks	Do not discontinue abruptly, taper gradually over 1 week

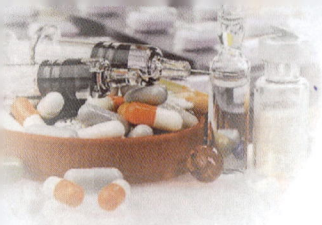

Cloxacillin

Drug name	Cloxacillin
Category	Antibiotic, Penicillinase-resistant penicillin
Route	Oral, Intravenous
Strength	Syp (125 mg/5 mL); Inj (500 mg vial); Cap (250 mg, 500 mg)
Brands	Aclox (Inj), Neoclox (Inj, Cap), Bioclox (Inj, Cap), Klox (Tab/Cap)
Mechanism of action	Acts by inhibiting synthesis of the bacterial wall
Pharmacokinetics	Not much data available; fairly absorbed from gut, highly protein bound, metabolized via breakdown of beta-lactam ring, around 40% excreted in urine, plasma half-life around half hour
Indications	Gram-positive infections; Especially *Staphylococcus*; *Streptococcus*; *Pneumococcus*
Dosage as per indications	50–100 mg/kg/day q 6 h IV or PO (1 h before or 2 h after meals) Meningitis: 200 mg/kg/day q 4 h (maximum up to 4 g/day has been tried)
Maximum dosage	2 g/24 hours
Dose adjustments	Dose adjustment in hepatic dysfunction
Adverse effects	Nausea, vomiting, diarrhea, hypersensitivity
Contraindications	Contraindicated in hypersensitivity to penicillin, flucloxacillin-associated jaundice/hepatic dysfunction
Drug interactions	Oral contraceptives and warfarin
Remarks	Administer 1 hour before meals or 2 hours after meals

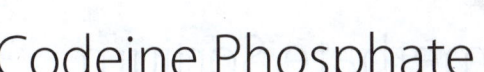

Codeine Phosphate

Drug name	Codeine phosphate
Category	Narcotic, Analgesic, Antitussive
Route	Oral
Strength	Tab (15 mg, 30 mg, 60 mg); Syp (Codeine 10 mg + Chlorpheniramine 4 mg/5 mL)
Brands	Ascoril C (Syp), Codeine Sulfate (Tab), Corex (Syp), Tossex (Syp)
Mechanism of action	Acts via μ opioid receptors, exerts analgesic effect by conversion to morphine
Pharmacokinetics	It is metabolized in the liver, mainly excreted in the urine
Indications	As cough suppressant; Severe pain (Postoperative; Chemo/Radiation therapy)
Dosage as per indications	• *Pain:* 0.5–1 mg/kg/dose q 4–6 h, maximum 60 mg/dose • *Cough:* 1–1.5 mg/kg/24 h q 4–6 h
Maximum dosage	240 mg/24 hours
Dose adjustments	In renal derangement
Adverse effects	Constipation, drowsiness, respiratory depression
Contraindications	Children <12 years, children between 12 and 18 years with compromised respiratory function
Drug interactions	Sedatives, MAOI, anticholinergics, anesthetics
Remarks	Do not use in postoperative pain after tonsillectomy/adenoidectomy

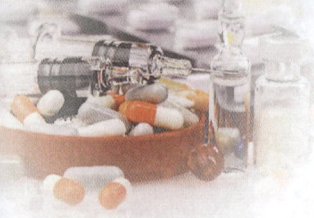

Colistimethate Sodium (Colistin)

Drug name	Colistimethate sodium (Colistin)
Category	Cyclic polypeptide antibacterial agent, Polymyxin group
Route	Intravenous, Intramuscular, Intrathecal, Intraventricular
Strength	Inj (1 MIU, 2 MIU, 3 MIU vials)
Brands	Colinem (Inj), Xylistin (Inj), Koolistin (Inj)
Mechanism of action	Damages the cell membrane of the bacterium. Selective acts on aerobic gram-negative bacteria having hydrophobic outer membrane
Pharmacokinetics	Has extensive renal tubular reabsorption, cleared by both renal and extrarenal routes; half-life 3 hours
Indications	Acts on gram-negative bacteria
Dosage as per indications	• 2.5–5 mg/kg/day q 6–12 h IV of colistin base (1 mg of colistin base = 2.67 mg colistimethate sodium = 33,333 IU of colistimethate sodium) • For treating ventriculitis in neonates, it may additionally be given intrathecally or intraventricularly as 10 mg/day
Maximum dosage	Not known
Dose adjustments	In renal impairment
Adverse effects	Nephrotoxicity, neurotoxicity
Contraindications	Hypersensitivity
Drug interactions	Quinolones, muscle relaxants
Remarks	Avoid coadministration with other nephrotoxic drugs

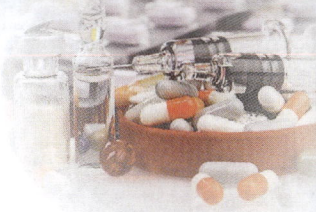

Cycloserine

Drug name	Cycloserine
Category	Antitubercular drug
Route	Oral
Strength	Cap/Tab (250 mg)
Brands	Coxerin (Cap), Cyclorin (Cap), Myser (Cap)
Mechanism of action	Inhibits L-alanine racemase and D-alanylalanine synthetase required for bacterial cell wall synthesis
Pharmacokinetics	Rapidly and completely absorbed, half-life 10 hours
Indications	MDR-TB
Dosage as per indications	10 mg/kg/day q 12 hourly
Maximum dosage	1 g/day
Dose adjustments	Renal dysfunction
Adverse effects	Headache, drowsiness, irritability, vertigo, seizures
Contraindications	Hypersensitivity
Drug interactions	Ethionamide, isoniazid, neurotoxic drugs

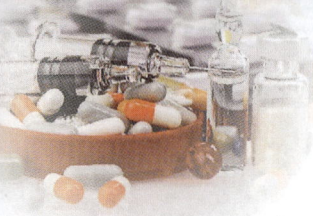

Cyclosporine

Drug name	Cyclosporine
Category	Immunosuppressant
Route	Oral, Intravenous
Strength	Cap (50 mg, 100 mg); Inj (50 mg/mL); Oral sol (100 mg/mL, 50 mL)
Brands	Neoral (Cap, Syp), Arpimune (Cap), Graftin (Cap), Cyclophil ME (Cap)
Mechanism of action	Cyclic polypeptide with immunosuppressive agent, acts specifically and reversibly on lymphocytes
Pharmacokinetics	Following oral administration, peak blood concentrations of cyclosporine obtained in 1–2 hours, bioavailability varies in different patients, metabolized mainly in liver, elimination is mainly by biliary route
Indications	Nephrotic syndrome; Aplastic anemia; In organ transplant recipients to decrease GVHD
Dosage as per indications	*Oral:* 15 mg/kg as single oral dose initially followed by maintenance doses of 5–8 mg/kg/day *Intravenous (IV):* 4–6 mg/kg/day IV infusion over 2–4 hours until patient can tolerate orally
Maximum dosage	Not known
Dose adjustments	Dose reduction in hepatic impairment, renal function monitoring needed
Adverse effects	Nephrotoxic, hypertension, hirsutism
Contraindications	Hypersensitivity
Drug interactions	Fluconazole, ketoconazole, erythromycin, carbamazepine, rifampicin, phenytoin and phenobarbitone

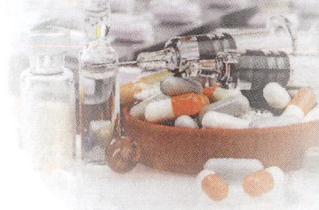

Cyproheptadine Hydrochloride

Drug name	Cyproheptadine hydrochloride
Category	Antihistaminic, Appetite stimulant
Route	Oral
Strength	Tab (2 mg, 4 mg); Syp (2 mg/5 mL)
Brands	Apetiz (Tab, Syp), Apitol (Tab, Syp), Ciplactin (Tab, Syp), Practin (Tab, Syp)
Mechanism of action	Antagonist/inverse agonist of H1 receptors, antagonist of 5-HT2 receptors. Also has anticholinergic, antiserotonergic, and antidopaminergic activities
Pharmacokinetics	Well absorbed after oral intake, peak levels after 1–3 hours, terminal half-life 8 hours
Indications	Allergic manifestations; Appetite stimulant
Dosage as per indications	- Children 0.25–0.5 mg/kg/day q 8–12 h - 2–6 years 2 mg q 8–12 h - >6 years 4 mg q 8–12 h
Maximum dosage	- *2–6 years:* 12 mg/day - *>6 years:* 16 mg/day
Dose adjustments	Dose adjustment needed in hepatic and renal impairment
Adverse effects	Sedation, dryness of mouth, blurred vision, urinary retention
Contraindications	Neonates and children suffering from asthma, glaucoma, or GI/GU obstruction, and therapy with MAO inhibitors
Drug interactions	MAO inhibitors

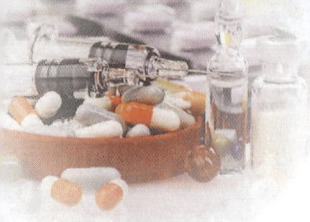

Daptomycin

Drug name	Daptomycin
Category	Antibiotic (Cyclic lipopeptide)
Route	Intravenous
Strength	Inj (350 mg)
Brands	Cubicin (Inj), Dapmicin (Inj), Daptocure (Inj)
Mechanism of action	Acts by binding to bacterial cell membranes. It inhibits DNA, RNA, and protein synthesis
Pharmacokinetics	Highly protein bound, poorly metabolized, eliminated mainly by kidneys
Indications	Reserved drug used for *Staphylococcus aureus*-induced bacteremia/right-sided infective endocarditis; Complicated skin and skin structure infections by gram-positive bacteria such as *Staphylococcus aureus*; *Streptococcus* and vancomycin-susceptible *Enterococcus faecalis*
Dosage as per indications	• *1–2 years:* 10 mg/kg • *2–6 years:* 9 mg/kg • *7–11 years:* 7 mg/kg • *12–17 years:* 5 mg/kg Given once in 24 hours, for younger children over 60 minutes, in older children over 30 minutes
Maximum dosage	Not known
Dose adjustments	In renal derangement
Adverse effects	Myopathy, peripheral neuropathy, eosinophilic pneumonia, rhabdomyolysis, bleeding diathesis due to deranged INR
Contraindications	Hypersensitivity
Drug interactions	HMG-CoA reductase inhibitors, drugs increasing INR

Darunavir (DRV)

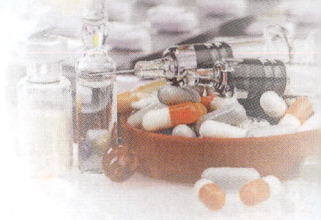

Drug name	Darunavir (DRV)
Category	Antiretroviral agent, Protease inhibitor
Route	Oral
Strength	Tab (300 mg, 600 mg, 800 mg); Susp (100 mg/mL)
Brands	Daruvir (Tab)
Mechanism of action	It inhibits HIV-1 protease enzyme thus inhibiting the cleavage of HIV-1 encoded Gag-Pol polyproteins in infected cells required for formation of mature virus particles. Primarily metabolized by CYP3A, 95% bound to plasma proteins, mostly eliminated in feces, terminal half-life around 15 hours
Pharmacokinetics	Antiretroviral agent; protease inhibitor
Indications	HIV/AIDS
Dosage as per indications	*Dosing according to weight band:* *10–11 kg:* DRV 200 mg + RTV 32 mg *11–12 kg:* DRV 220 mg + RTV 32 mg *12–13 kg:* DRV 240 mg + RTV 40 mg *13–14 kg:* DRV 260 mg + RTV 40 mg *14–15 kg:* DRV 280 mg + RTV 48 mg *15–30 kg:* DRV 375 mg + RTV 48 mg *30–40 kg:* DRV 450 mg + RTV 100 mg *≥40 kg:* DRV 600 mg + RTV 100 mg RTV—ritonavir
Maximum dosage	Not known
Dose adjustments	Not needed in mild to moderate hepatic and renal impairment
Adverse effects	Skin rash, hepatitis, fat maldistribution, diarrhea, nausea, headache, and hyperlipidemia
Contraindications	Hypersensitivity, not recommended in children <3 years or weight <10 kg because of risk of seizures
Drug interactions	Other antiretroviral drugs
Remarks	DRV should be administered with food

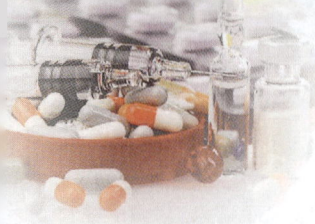

Deferasirox

Drug name	Deferasirox
Category	Chelating agent
Route	Oral
Strength	Tab (100 mg, 250 mg, 400 mg, 500 mg)
Brands	Asunra (Tab), Desirox (Tab), Defrijet (Tab)
Mechanism of action	It is a tridentate ligand that has high affinity for iron. It also promotes iron excretion
Pharmacokinetics	Maximum plasma levels attained in 1.5–4 hours. Highly bound to plasma protein. The main metabolic pathway is glucuronidation followed by biliary excretion
Indications	Thalassemia (as iron chelator in iron overload)
Dosage as per indications	20 mg/kg PO per day; dose may be titrated by increasing by 5–10 mg based on serum ferritin; if serum ferritin persistently >2,500 µg/L
Maximum dosage	40 mg/kg/day
Dose adjustments	Needed in both hepatic and renal impairment
Adverse effects	Increased risk of bleeding, kidney disease, GI upset, deranged liver enzymes
Contraindications	Hypersensitivity, with other iron chelators, renal failure
Drug interactions	Other iron chelators
Remarks	• Tablet should not be chewed or swallowed whole but dispersed in apple or orange juice or in water before consumption • Preferably taken empty stomach or 30 minutes prior to food

Deferiprone

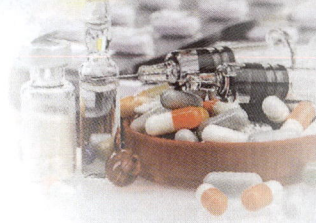

Drug name	Deferiprone
Category	Chelating agent
Route	Oral
Strength	Cap (250 mg, 500 mg)
Brands	Kelfer (Cap)
Mechanism of action	It is a bidentate ligand which binds iron strongly
Pharmacokinetics	Rapidly absorbed from gut. Peak serum levels in 45–60 minutes. It is eliminated mainly via renal route. The elimination half-life around 2–3 hours
Indications	Thalassemia (as iron chelator in iron overload)
Dosage as per indications	75–100 mg/kg/day divided 8–12 hourly
Maximum dosage	100 mg/kg/day
Dose adjustments	No dose adjustments in renal impairment and mild to moderate hepatic impairment
Adverse effects	Joint pain, agranulocytosis, zinc deficiency
Contraindications	Hypersensitivity, recurrent agranulocytosis, pregnancy and breastfeeding
Drug interactions	Drugs associated with neutropenia, those affecting UGT1A6
Remarks	Do not use in pregnancy, breastfeeding, in patients having low TLC. It can be used with desferrioxamine

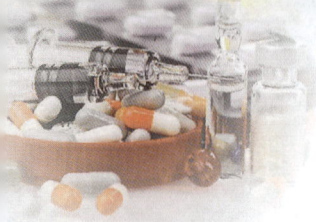

Deflazacort

Drug name	Deflazacort
Category	Glucocorticoid
Route	Oral
Strength	Tab (1 mg, 6 mg, 18 mg, 30 mg, 36 mg); Syp (6 mg/5 mL)
Brands	Cortimax (Tab), Defcort (Tab, Syp), Defnalone (Tab)
Mechanism of action	• Has anti-inflammatory action and immunosuppressant • Acts through the glucocorticoid receptor
Pharmacokinetics	Rapidly converted by esterases to 21-des deflazacort (active metabolite). Nearly 40% protein bound. Mainly eliminated in urine
Indications	As immunomodulator and anti-inflammatory; Especially in cases of muscular dystrophies
Dosage as per indications	0.25–1.5 mg/kg/day in 1–3 divided doses
Maximum dosage	Not known
Dose adjustments	Not needed
Adverse effects	As with other corticosteroids
Contraindications	Hypersensitivity
Drug interactions	CYP3A4 inducers and inhibitors
Remarks	Not preferred in children <5 years

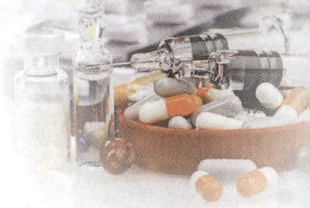

Desferrioxamine

Drug name	Desferrioxamine
Category	Chelating agent
Route	Intravenous, Subcutaneous
Strength	Inj (500 mg, 1,000 mg)
Brands	Desferal (Inj)
Mechanism of action	Chelates trivalent iron ions to produce stable and nontoxic compounds. Acts on both free or bound iron
Pharmacokinetics	Rapidly absorbed after intramuscular/subcutaneous administration. Metabolized by plasma proteins, eliminated from kidneys
Indications	For chelation in thalassemia; Acute iron poisoning
Dosage as per indications	• *Chronic iron overload:* 20–40 mg/kg/day SC over 8–12 hours using battery operated pump • *Acute iron poisoning:* 15 mg/kg/h OR 50 mg/kg/dose q 6 h IV
Maximum dosage	Maximum 40 mg/kg/day or 6 g over 24 hours IV
Dose adjustments	Dose adjustment needed in renal impairment
Adverse effects	Flushing, erythema, hypotension, tachycardia, leg cramps, fever, hearing loss, and cataracts
Contraindications	Anuria, primary hemochromatosis, severe renal disease
Drug interactions	Oral vitamin C
Remarks	Iron mobilization may be poor in children aged 3 years and less

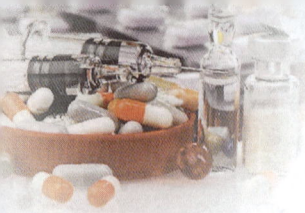

Desloratadine

Drug name	Desloratadine
Category	Antihistaminic
Route	Oral
Strength	Tab (5 mg)
Brands	Allerde (Tab), Clarinex (Tab), Neoloridin (Tab), Deslor (Tab)
Mechanism of action	Selectively blocks peripheral histamine H_1 receptors
Pharmacokinetics	Well absorbed, effect starts in 30 minutes with maximum concentration achieved in 3 hours, the terminal phase half-life around 27 hours
Indications	Antiallergic; Allergic rhinitis
Dosage as per indications	2–5 years: 1 mg OD; 6–12 years: 2.5 mg OD
Maximum dosage	Not known
Dose adjustments	Dose adjustment in renal insufficiency
Adverse effects	Dryness of mouth, tiredness, headache, tachycardia, sore throat
Contraindications	Hypersensitivity
Drug interactions	Ketoconazole, macrolides like erythromycin/azithromycin
Remarks	To be used with caution in children with history of seizures

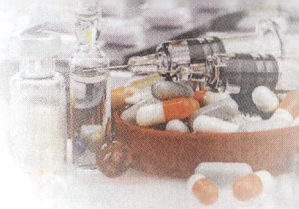

Desmopressin

Drug name	Desmopressin
Category	Vasopressin analog
Route	Oral, Inhalational
Strength	Inj (4 µg/mL); Tab (0.1 mg, 0.2 mg); Nasal spray (10 µg/mL)
Brands	Minrin (Spray, Tab, Inj), Desmospray (Nasal spray)
Mechanism of action	Reduces urine production by stimulating vasopressin (V2) receptors and hence increasing water reabsorption in the kidney
Pharmacokinetics	Oral bioavailability is much lesser than nasal and intravenous route. Half-life when given intravenously is around 3 hours. The drug in mainly eliminated by kidneys
Indications	Diabetes insipidus; Primary nocturnal enuresis
Dosage as per indications	• *Diabetes Insipidus:* 0.05 mg once to twice a day oral; can be gradually increased till desired response or maximum 0.6 mg once at bedtime • *Primary nocturnal enuresis:* Nasal spray 10 µg once daily up to maximum of 30 µg in single or 2 divided doses (as nasal spray) for 28 days
Maximum dosage	As mentioned above
Dose adjustments	In renal derangement
Adverse effects	Hyponatremia, hypertension, water intoxication, convulsions
Contraindications	Hypersensitivity, renal impairment, hyponatremia
Drug interactions	Tricyclic antidepressants (TCAs), selective serotonin reuptake inhibitors (SSRIs), opioids, NSAIDs, antiepileptics, vasoconstrictors

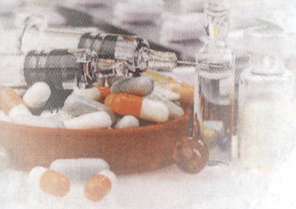

Dexamethasone

Drug name	Dexamethasone
Category	Glucocorticoid
Route	Oral, Intravenous, Intramuscular
Strength	Tab (0.5 mg, 1 mg, 1.5 mg, 2 mg, 4 mg); Inj (4 mg/mL)
Brands	Decadron (Inj, Tab), Dexona (Inj, Tab)
Mechanism of action	Synthetic glucocorticoid, high anti-inflammatory effect along with antiallergic and immunosuppressive actions
Pharmacokinetics	Well absorbed from the gut and sites of local application. Rapidly distributed, highly bound to plasma proteins, half-life: 36–54 hours, metabolized mainly in the liver but also in the kidney
Indications	Asthma; Croup; Airway edema; Cerebral edema; Antiemetic
Dosage as per indications	• *Airway edema:* 0.5–2 mg/kg/24 h IV/IM ÷ q 6 h (begin 24 hours before extubation and continue for 4–6 doses after extubation) • *Asthma exacerbation:* 0.6 mg/kg/dose (max 16 mg/dose) PO/IV/IM Q 24 h × 1 or 2 doses • *Croup:* 0.6 mg/kg/dose single dose • *Antiemetic (chemotherapy induced):* Initial: 10 mg/m^2/dose IV; max dose: 20 mg; subsequent: 5 mg/m^2/dose Q 6 h IV • *Anti-inflammatory:* Child: 0.08–0.3 mg/kg/24 h PO, IV, IM ÷ q 6–12 h • *Brain tumor-associated cerebral edema:* Loading dose: 1–2 mg/kg/dose IV/IM × 1 maintenance: 1–1.5 mg/kg/24 h ÷ q 4–6 h
Maximum dosage	16 mg/24 h
Dose adjustments	Not needed
Adverse effects	Gastritis, increased risk of infections, side effects similar to other steroids
Contraindications	Active untreated infections; and fungal, viral, and mycobacterial ocular infections
Drug interactions	Rifampicin, rifabutin, carbamazepine, phenobarbitone, phenytoin, primidone enhance the metabolism of corticosteroids
Remarks	Slow withdrawal should be done in patients receiving systemic steroids for more than 2–3 weeks

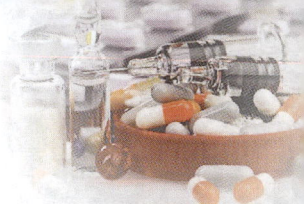

Dextromethorphan

Drug name	Dextromethorphan
Category	Antitussive
Route	Oral
Strength	Syp (30 mg/5 mL)
Brands	Lastuss LA (Syp), Suppressa (Syp)
Mechanism of action	Synthetic morphine derivative (pharmacologically nonopioid), acts on the cough center in the medulla, raising the threshold for the cough reflex
Pharmacokinetics	Rapidly absorbed from the gastrointestinal tract, peak plasma concentrations in 2–2.5 hours. Has low oral bioavailability due to extensive first-pass in the liver. The onset of action: 15–30 minutes, total duration of action: 3–6 hours
Indications	Dry cough
Dosage as per indications	1–2 mg/kg/day q 8 h
Maximum dosage	120 mg/day
Dose adjustments	Dose adjustment in hepatic impairment
Adverse effects	Nausea, vomiting, dizziness
Contraindications	Hypersensitivity, patients taking monoamine oxidase inhibitors (MAOIs), or within 14 days of stopping MAOI treatment, those on SSRIs, respiratory failure
Drug interactions	MAO inhibitors
Remarks	Avoid in children less than 4 years

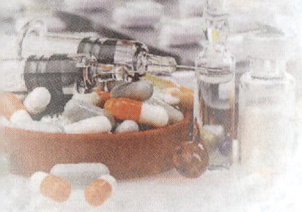

Diaminodiphenyl Sulfone (DDS)

Drug name	Diaminodiphenyl sulfone (DDS)
Category	Antibacterial (Sulfone group)
Route	Oral
Strength	Tab (50 mg, 100 mg)
Brands	Dapsone (Tab)
Mechanism of action	Inhibits bacterial synthesis of dihydrofolic acid. Active against *Mycobacterium leprae*, *Pneumocystis jirovecii*
Pharmacokinetics	Highly absorbed, good bioavailability, has half-life of 10–80 hours, metabolized in liver, mostly eliminated in urine after glucuronidation
Indications	Leprosy; Pneumocystis prophylaxis
Dosage as per indications	1–2 mg/kg/day as single or two divided doses
Maximum dosage	100 mg/day
Dose adjustments	Liver derangement
Adverse effects	Hemolysis, methemoglobinemia, peripheral neuropathy, rash, hepatitis, anorexia, vomiting
Contraindications	Hypersensitivity to dapsone or sulfonamides. Avoid in patients with severe anemia, severe glucose-6-phosphate dehydrogenase (G-6PD) deficiency
Drug interactions	Probenecid, rifampicin, saquinavir, trimethoprim
Remarks	Not used in children <12 years

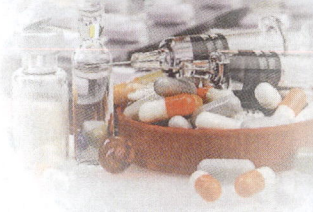

Diazepam

Drug name	Diazepam
Category	Benzodiazepine
Route	Oral, Intravenous, Rectal
Strength	Tab (2.5 mg, 5 mg); Syp (2 mg/5 mL); Inj (5 mg/mL ampoule); Suppository
Brands	Alzepam (Inj, Tab), Calmpose (Inj, Tab, Syp), Dizep (Inj, Tab), Valium (Inj, Tab), Zepose (Inj, Tab)
Mechanism of action	Has anticonvulsant, sedative and muscle relaxant effect. It acts on various receptors in brain and spinal cord to increase the inhibitory effect of GABA
Pharmacokinetics	*Onset of action:* 1–3 minutes (IV route); 2–10 minutes (rectal route). It is metabolized in liver and excreted via the kidney. Metabolized to two active metabolites, one of which, desmethyldiazepam, has an extended half-life
Indications	Sedation; Anxiety; Neonatal tetanus; Status Epilepticus; Termination of seizure
Dosage as per indications	• *Status epilepticus:* Intravenous: 0.2–0.5 mg/kg/dose, repeat at 3–5 minutes, if needed (for 2–3 doses); per-rectal: 0.3–0.5 mg/kg/dose • *Antianxiety, sedation, and muscle relaxation:* Oral 0.1–0.3 mg/kg/day q 4–8 h adjusted according to clinical response • *Neonatal tetanus:* 0.5–5 mg/kg/dose IV q 2–4 h
Maximum dosage	*<5 years:* 5 mg *>5 years:* 10 mg Max dose for sedation in child: 0.6 mg/kg for an 8-hour duration
Dose adjustments	Dose adjustment in renal and hepatic derangement
Adverse effects	Hypotension, respiratory depression
Contraindications	Myasthenia gravis, severe respiratory insufficiency, severe hepatic failure, and sleep apnea syndrome
Drug interactions	Protease inhibitors
Remarks	• Administer not >2 mg/min • *Antidote flumazenil:* Reverts sedation; not effective against respiratory depression. 0.01 mg/kg IV (maximum 0.2 mg), then 0.005–0.01 mg/kg/min; maximum cumulative dose: 1 mg; may repeat after 20 minutes; maximum 3 mg/h

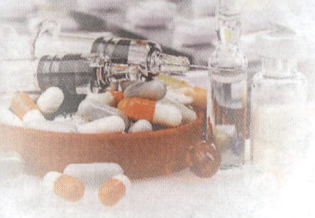

Diazoxide

Drug name	Diazoxide
Category	Antihypoglycemic agent, Antihypertensive
Route	Oral, Intravenous
Strength	Syp (50 mg/mL); Cap (50 mg); Inj (15 mg/mL ampoule)
Brands	Proglycem (Cap, Syp), Balila (Cap, Syp), DBL Diazoxide (Inj)
Mechanism of action	Not available
Pharmacokinetics	Not available
Indications	Hypoglycemia (hyperinsulinemic); Hypertensive crisis
Dosage as per indications	• *Hypertensive crisis:* 1–3 mg/kg/dose IV up to maximum of 150 mg/dose, repeat q 5–15 min, then q 4–24 h • *Hyperinsulinemic hypoglycemia:* 1 year: 3–8 mg/kg/day q 8–12 h
Maximum dosage	150 mg/dose
Dose adjustments	Renal impairment
Adverse effects	Hyponatremia, salt and water retention, GI disturbances, rash, ketoacidosis, hypertrichosis, arrhythmias, pulmonary hypertension (reversible)
Contraindications	Hypersensitivity to thiazides
Drug interactions	Antihypertensives, warfarin, enoxaparin, phenytoin
Remarks	Hyperglycemic effect noted within 1 hour of administration, watch for hypotension

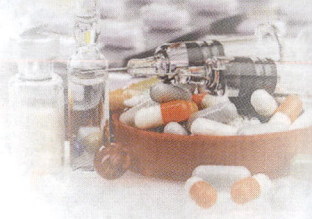

Diclofenac

Drug name	Diclofenac
Category	Nonsteroidal anti-inflammatory drug (NSAID)
Route	Oral, Intramuscular
Strength	Tab (50 mg, 75 mg, 100 mg); Inj (75 mg/3 mL)
Brands	Diclonac (Inj, Tab), Diclostar (Inj, Tab), Voveran (Inj, Tab)
Mechanism of action	Potent inhibitor of prostaglandin biosynthesis and a modulator of arachidonic acid release and uptake
Pharmacokinetics	Highly bound to plasma proteins, extensive first pass metabolism. The terminal half-life in plasma is 1–2 hours
Indications	Painkiller; Antipyretic
Dosage as per indications	1–3 mg/kg/day in 2–4 divided doses
Maximum dosage	150 mg/day
Dose adjustments	Renal and hepatic impairment
Adverse effects	Dizziness, headache, fluid retention, gastric bleeding or ulcer
Contraindications	Renal and hepatic failure, perforation, established heart failure, ischemic heart disease
Drug interactions	Anticoagulants
Remarks	Increases risk of bleeding

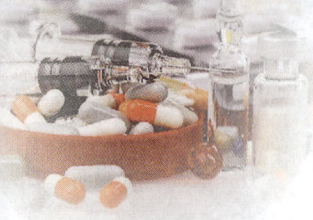

Dicyclomine

Drug name	Dicyclomine
Category	Antispasmodic
Route	Oral
Strength	Tab (10 mg, 20 mg); Drops (10 mg/mL); Syp (10 mg/5 mL)
Brands	Colispas (Tab, Syp, Drops), Meftal-Spas (Tab, Syp, Drops), Spasmo-Proxyvon (Tab, Syp, Drops)
Mechanism of action	Relieves gut smooth muscle spasm by anticholinergic effect (antimuscarinic) and direct effect upon smooth muscle (musculotropic)
Pharmacokinetics	Rapidly absorbed after oral administration, peak levels attained in 60–90 minutes. Predominantly excreted via urine
Indications	Infantile colic; Abdominal colic
Dosage as per indications	• *<6 months:* 5–10 drops 15 minutes before feeds • *6 months to 2 years:* 10–20 drops 15 minutes before feeds • *>2 years:* 1 mL every 6 hours
Maximum dosage	Not known
Dose adjustments	Hepatic and renal disease
Adverse effects	Tachycardia, dryness of mouth, GI disturbances
Contraindications	Bowel obstruction, hypersensitivity, children <6 months
Drug interactions	Anticholinergics, antiarrhythmics, antipsychotics

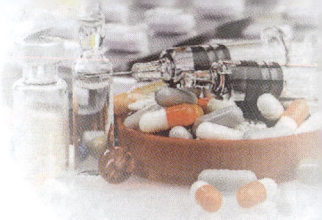

Didanosine

Drug name	Didanosine
Category	Antiretroviral agent, Reverse transcriptase inhibitor
Route	Oral
Strength	Tab, Cap (100 mg, 250 mg, 400 mg)
Brands	Dinosin (Tab), Virosine-DR (Tab), Dinex EC (Tab), DD-Retro (Tab)
Mechanism of action	It inhibits the activity of HIV-1 reverse transcriptase through its active metabolite dideoxyadenosine 5'-triphosphate
Pharmacokinetics	Not much known, rapidly absorbed, peak levels found between 15 and 90 minutes
Indications	HIV/AIDS
Dosage as per indications	180 mg/m^2/day divided into two doses
Maximum dosage	400 mg/day
Dose adjustments	In renal and hepatic insufficiency
Adverse effects	Headache, diarrhea, abdominal pain, pancreatitis, nausea, vomiting, peripheral neuropathy, dyselectrolytemia, hyperuricemia, increased liver enzymes, lactic acidosis, retinal pigmentation, CNS depression, rash/pruritus, myalgia, pancreatitis
Contraindications	Hypersensitivity
Drug interactions	Ciprofloxacin, ganciclovir, indinavir, methadone, nelfinavir, ribavirin, azole antifungals
Remarks	Administer empty stomach

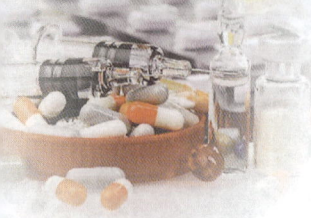

Diethylcarbamazine (DEC)

Drug name	Diethylcarbamazine (DEC)
Category	Antihelminthic
Route	Oral
Strength	Tab (50 mg, 100 mg); Syp (120 mg/5 mL)
Brands	Banocide (Tab, Syp), Hetrazan (Tab, Syp)
Mechanism of action	Acts by platelet-mediated triggering of the release of excretory antigen from microfilariae, with killing involving free radicals, drug-induced alteration of prostaglandin metabolism in microfilariae and/or in host endothelial cells, leading to immobilization of microfilariae on endothelial surfaces and adherence and killing by host platelets and granulocytes and inhibition of microtubule polymerization
Pharmacokinetics	Well absorbed orally, peak plasma levels: 1–2 hours, elimination half-life 10–12 hours. Elimination via renal excretion, elimination decreased in alkaline urine
Indications	Filariasis; Tropical pulmonary eosinophilia; Loeffler pneumonia
Dosage as per indications	- *Filariasis:* 6 mg/kg/day q 8 h, oral, for 3–4 weeks; repeat course after 6 months - *Tropical pulmonary eosinophilia and visceral larva migrans:* 10 mg/kg/day, 8 hours, oral for 4 weeks - *Loeffler pneumonia:* 15 mg/kg/day, single daily dose, for 4 days
Maximum dosage	Not known
Dose adjustments	In renal derangement
Adverse effects	Fever, chills, nausea, joint pain, muscle ache, visual disturbances, itching, facial swelling, headaches
Contraindications	Previous history of heart problems, gastrointestinal problems, and allergy
Drug interactions	None

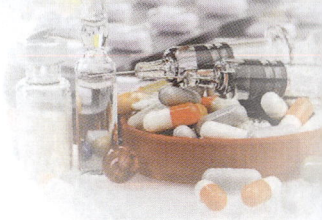

Digoxin

Drug name	Digoxin
Category	Antiarrhythmic
Route	Oral, Intravenous
Strength	Tab (0.25 mg, 0.5 mg); Elixir (0.5 mg/mL); Inj (0.5 mg/2 mL)
Brands	Cardioxin (Inj, Tab, Elixir), Dixin (Inj, Tab, Elixir), Lanoxin (Inj, Tab, Elixir)
Mechanism of action	Inhibits adenosine triphosphatase, affecting sodium-potassium (Na^+-K^+) exchange activity, this results in increased calcium ion influx availability at the time of excitation-contraction coupling
Pharmacokinetics	Well absorbed when taken orally. Around one-fourth of the drug is protein bound. Metabolized via hydrolysis, oxidation and conjugation. Excreted mainly through the kidney. *Half-life:* Full-term neonates and children 35 hours; infants 18–25 hours
Indications	Heart failure
Dosage as per indications	*Digitalizing dose (oral)* • *Preterm neonates:* 0.04 mg/kg/day • *Term neonates:* 0.06 mg/kg/day • *<2 years:* 0.04–0.05 mg/kg/day • *>2 years:* 0.04 mg/kg/day *Digitalizing dose (parenteral)* • *Two-thirds of oral dose:* ½ of digitalizing dose given stat, one-fourth after 8 hours and one-fourth after 16 hours • *Daily maintenance dose:* One-fourth of digitalizing dose
Maximum dosage	Not known
Dose adjustments	Doses to be adjusted in renal derangement
Adverse effects	AV block, cardiac dysrhythmias
Contraindications	Ventricular dysrhythmia
Drug interactions	Calcium channel blockers, adenosine
Remarks	Calcium infusion in patients on digoxin can precipitate ventricular fibrillation; inappropriate serum potassium and magnesium increase risk for digoxin toxicity. Digoxin levels appear falsely elevated in neonates or those with renal, hepatic, or heart failure

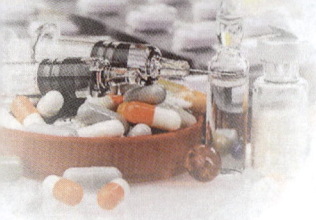

Dimenhydrinate

Drug name	Dimenhydrinate
Category	Antihistaminic
Route	Oral, Intravenous, Intramuscular
Strength	Tab (50 mg); Inj (50 mg/mL); Syp (15 mg/5 mL)
Brands	Dramamine (Inj, Syp, Tab), Draminate (Inj, Syp, Tab)
Mechanism of action	Effect seen after 20–30 minutes after oral and intramuscular administration; whereas immediate effect seen after IV administration
Pharmacokinetics	Well absorbed orally and parenteral. It is metabolized in liver and excreted in urine
Indications	Antiallergic; Motion sickness prevention
Dosage as per indications	*Up to 12 years:* 5 mg/kg/day q 6–8 h PO/IV/IM
Maximum dosage	• *2–6 years:* 75 mg/day • *6–12 years:* 150 mg/day
Dose adjustments	No renal and hepatic adjustments needed
Adverse effects	Drowsiness and anticholinergic side effects
Contraindications	Hypersensitivity
Drug interactions	CNS depressants, MAO inhibitors
Remarks	Not recommended in children <2 years. Use with caution in patients with seizures

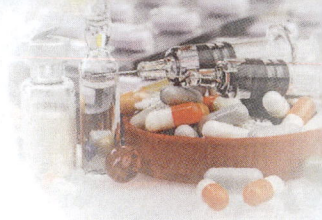

Dimercaprol

Drug name	Dimercaprol
Category	Chelating agent
Route	Intramuscular (deep)
Strength	Inj (100 mg/2 mL)
Brands	BAL (Inj)
Mechanism of action	It has sulfhydryl group which competes with the sulfhydryl groups on proteins/enzymes. As a result, the sulfhydryl group of dimercaprol instead of the enzyme/protein combines with the metals to form dimercaprol-metal complex
Pharmacokinetics	Rapidly absorbed, peak levels in 1-hour, maximum concentration found in liver and kidney. Rapidly metabolized, excreted mainly by kidneys, to some extent in bile
Indications	Useful in arsenic; Mercury; Gold poisoning; Also found effective in lead poisoning when used with sodium calcium edetate
Dosage as per indications	Varies with the metal involved • *Arsenic/gold poisoning:* – *Mild:* 2.5 mg/kg QID for 2 days, BD for 1 day, OD for next 10 days – *Severe:* 3 mg/kg 4 hourly for 2 days, QID for next 1 day, BD for next 10 days • *Mercury poisoning:* 5 mg/kg on day 1 followed by 2.5 mg/kg/dose 12–24 hourly for 10 days • *Acute lead poisoning:* 3–4 mg/kg alone as first dose, then 4-hourly with edetate calcium disodium injection (separate site) for 2–7 days
Maximum dosage	*Preferred maximum single dose:* 3 mg/kg, though in severe poisoning dose up to 5 mg/kg given
Dose adjustments	In renal and hepatic derangement
Adverse effects	Hemolysis in G6PD deficiency, fever, transient reduction of polymorphonuclear leukocytes, hypertension, tachycardia, nausea, headache
Contraindications	Hypersensitivity, allergy to peanuts/soya, iron poisoning, liver failure by causes other than arsenic poisoning
Drug interactions	Iron

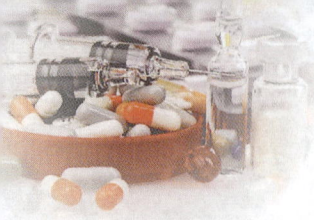

Diphenhydramine

Drug name	Diphenhydramine
Category	Antihistaminic
Route	Oral, Intravenous
Strength	Tab (25 mg, 50 mg); Syp (12.5 mg/5 mL); Inj (50 mg/mL, 10 mg/mL)
Brands	Benadryl (Inj, Cap, Syp), Kuffdryl (Cap)
Mechanism of action	Has anticholinergic and marked sedative effects by inhibiting the effects on H_1-receptors
Pharmacokinetics	Has rapid absorption after oral intake. Nearly 50% of the drug reaches systemic circulation. It is rapidly distributed and levels peak in 1–4 hours
Indications	Cough suppressant; Antiallergic, in phenothiazine toxicity
Dosage as per indications	1 mg/kg/dose PO q 6 h *Phenothiazine toxicity:* 1 mg/kg intravenous
Maximum dosage	300 mg/day
Dose adjustments	Required in hepatic impairment
Adverse effects	Nausea, vomiting, drowsiness, blurred vision
Contraindications	Neonates
Drug interactions	Sedatives, benzodiazepines, antidepressant
Remarks	Avoid in infants and young children

Disopyramide

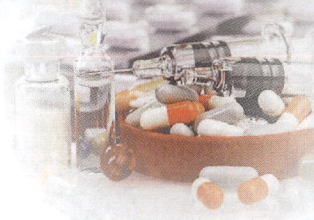

Drug name	Disopyramide
Category	Antiarrhythmic
Route	Intravenous, Oral
Strength	Inj (10 mg/mL); Tab (50 mg, 100 mg, 150 mg)
Brands	Norpace (Cap), Regubeat (Cap), Rythmodan (Inj)
Mechanism of action	Acts as a myocardial depressant to decrease membrane responsiveness and prolong the effective refractory period (ERP). The drug also has anticholinergic effects
Pharmacokinetics	Nearly 50% protein bound, only one-fourth drug is metabolized, rest excreted unchanged in urine. Has a half-life of 5–8 hours
Indications	Arrhythmia
Dosage as per indications	• 5–10 mg/kg/dose 12 hourly (slow release) in children; 5–7.5 mg/kg/dose 6 hourly in infants • *IV*: 5 mg/kg loading followed by oral maintenance
Maximum dosage	800 mg/day
Dose adjustments	In renal and hepatic insufficiency
Adverse effects	Hypoglycemia, arrhythmia
Contraindications	Hypersensitivity, second- or third-degree atrioventricular block, atrioventricular block, long QT syndrome
Drug interactions	Antiarrhythmic drugs, drugs at risk for torsades de pointes

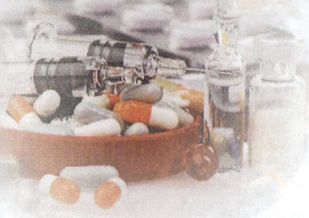

Dobutamine

Drug name	Dobutamine
Category	Inotrope
Route	Intravenous
Strength	Inj (1 mL/50 mg vial)
Brands	Cardiject (Inj), Dobucard (Inj), Dobustat (Inj), Cardiforce (Inj)
Mechanism of action	Selective β_1-adrenergic agonist leading to cardiac stimulation. It does not release endogenous norepinephrine
Pharmacokinetics	*Onset of action:* 2 minutes after IV administration. Peak levels attained in noted in 10 minutes. The effects reverse rapidly on stopping the drug. *Half-life:* 2 minutes. Mainly metabolized in liver
Indications	Shock
Dosage as per indications	5–20 µg/kg/min IV infusion
Maximum dosage	40 µg/kg/min
Dose adjustments	Adjustment done based on clinical response
Adverse effects	Arrhythmias, hypertension, tachycardia
Contraindications	Contraindicated in IHSS
Drug interactions	β-blockers, ionotropic agents
Remarks	Do not mix with sodium bicarbonate

Dolutegravir (DTG)

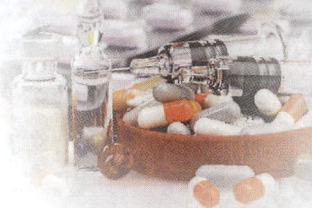

Drug name	Dolutegravir (DTG)
Category	Antiretroviral, Integrase inhibitor
Route	Oral
Strength	Tab (50 mg)
Brands	Doluvir (Tab), Instgra (Tab), Tivicay (Tab)
Mechanism of action	It inhibits HIV integrase required for HIV replication cycle
Pharmacokinetics	Rapidly absorbed following oral administration, half-life: 2–3 hours, highly bound plasma proteins, undergoes glucuronidation via UGT1A1, terminal half-life 14 hours
Indications	HIV/AIDS
Dosage as per indications	Used in children and adolescents with HIV infection whose body weight is >20 kg and age >6 years as 50 mg once a day
Maximum dosage	Not known
Dose adjustments	Needed in severe renal impairment, not needed in hepatic derangement
Adverse effects	Increased cholesterol and triglycerides, increased lipase, increased bilirubin, transaminitis, raised creatinine, hyperglycemia, insomnia, nausea, risk of neural tube defects in offspring if taken during pregnancy
Contraindications	Hypersensitivity
Drug interactions	Dofetilide, NRTIs, NNRTIs, protease inhibitor, metformin, rifampicin
Remarks	If coinfected with tuberculosis and on concomitant ATT, an additional tablet of DTG is given after 12 hours for the duration of TB treatment

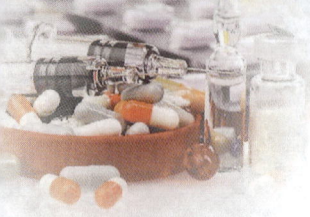

Domperidone

Drug name	Domperidone
Category	Antiemetic, Prokinetic
Route	Oral
Strength	Tab (10 mg); Syp (5 mg/5 mL)
Brands	Domped (Tab, Syp), Domstal (Tab, Syp), Vomistal (Tab, Syp)
Mechanism of action	It is a dopamine antagonist. It also has gastrokinetic effect producing antiemetic action. It also releases prolactin helping mothers with milk production
Pharmacokinetics	Rapidly absorbed after oral administration, peak levels noted in 60 minutes. Metabolized in liver
Indications	Vomiting
Dosage as per indications	0.2–0.4 mg/kg/dose 6–8 hourly
Maximum dosage	40 mg/day
Dose adjustments	Dose adjustment in renal impairment, contraindicated in hepatic impairment
Adverse effects	Gynecomastia in males, galactorrhea in females
Contraindications	Prolactinoma, intestinal obstruction, prolonged QT interval, moderate to severe hepatic impairment
Drug interactions	Drugs causing prolonged QT interval
Remarks	Does not cross blood–brain barrier

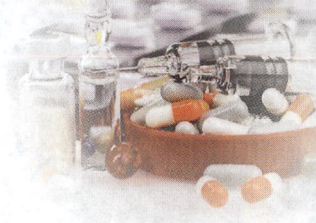

Dopamine

Drug name	Dopamine
Category	Inotrope
Route	Intravenous
Strength	Inj (40 mg/mL ampoule)
Brands	Dopacard (Inj)
Mechanism of action	• Stimulates β_1-adrenergic receptors, releases norepinephrine from its storage sites and causes vasodilatation of renal, mesenteric, coronary, and intracerebral vessels due to its dopaminergic action • At low doses (<2 µg/kg per minute) it has dopaminergic actions, most prominent effect noted as renal vasodilatation • At doses between 2 and 10 µg/kg per minute, it stimulates β_1-adrenergic receptors leading to cardiac stimulation • At doses above 10 µg/kg/min, vasoconstrictor action occurs due to additional stimulation of α-adrenergic receptors
Pharmacokinetics	• *Onset of action:* 5 minutes • *Duration of action:* 10 minutes. Nearly one-fourth of the drug is converted to norepinephrine during metabolism. The drug is mainly excreted in urine. Does not cross blood–brain barrier
Indications	Shock
Dosage as per indications	5–20 µg/kg/min
Maximum dosage	Preferred dose not >20 µg/kg/min Doses up to 50 µg/kg/min have been tried
Dose adjustments	Not known
Adverse effects	Arrhythmias, hypertension, vasoconstriction
Contraindications	Hyperthyroidism, pheochromocytoma, halogenated hydrocarbon anesthetics
Drug interactions	MAO inhibitors
Remarks	Do not mix with sodium bicarbonate

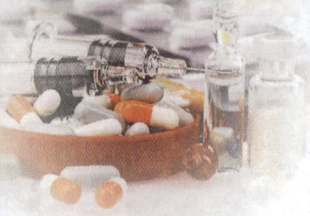

Doripenem

Drug name	Doripenem
Category	Antibiotic (Carbapenem)
Route	Intravenous
Strength	Inj (250 mg, 500 mg vials)
Brands	Doribax (Inj), Dorimed (Inj)
Mechanism of action	Acts as bactericidal drug by inhibiting bacterial cell wall biosynthesis by inactivating penicillin-binding proteins (PBPs)
Pharmacokinetics	Metabolized via dehydropeptidase to inactive form. Eliminated mainly by the kidneys. Terminal half-life 1 hour
Indications	Reserved antibiotic used for complicated urinary tract infections; Pyelonephritis mostly active against gram-negative bacteria including *Pseudomonas*
Dosage as per indications	500 mg IV 8 hourly
Maximum dosage	500 mg/dose
Dose adjustments	In renal derangement
Adverse effects	Seizures
Contraindications	Hypersensitivity
Drug interactions	Valproate, probenecid
Remarks	Not enough studies available for pediatric patients

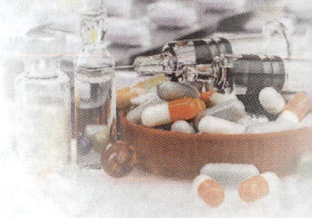

Doxapram

Drug name	Doxapram
Category	Respiratory stimulant
Route	Intravenous
Strength	Inj (20 mg/mL)
Brands	Dopram (Inj)
Mechanism of action	Acts via peripheral carotid chemoreceptors to stimulate respiration. With rising doses, it also acts as stimulant on respiratory centers in the medulla and brain
Pharmacokinetics	Not much known. Onset: 20–40 seconds after injection, peak effect: 1–2 minutes. Total duration of action: 5–12 minutes. The drug acts by increasing tidal volume and respiratory rate
Indications	Apnea of prematurity
Dosage as per indications	Begin at 0.5 mg/kg/h, increase gradually by 0.5 mg/kg/h till maximum of 2.5 mg/kg/h or early if control of apnea occurs
Maximum dosage	2.5 mg/kg/h
Dose adjustments	In both hepatic and renal derangement
Adverse effects	Hypotension, seizures
Contraindications	Hypersensitivity, head injury, seizures, asthma, hypertension
Drug interactions	Sodium bicarbonate, aminophylline, sympathomimetics, MAO inhibitors

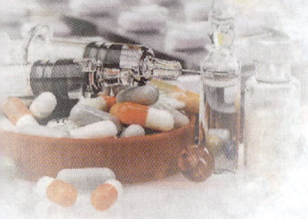

Doxycycline

Drug name	Doxycycline
Category	Bacteriostatic antibiotic, Tetracycline derivative
Route	Oral
Strength	Tab (100 mg, 200 mg); Syp (25 mg, 50 mg/5 mL)
Brands	Doxy-1 (Tab), Minicycline (Tab, Syp), Tetradox (Tab)
Mechanism of action	It inhibits protein synthesis by binding to 30S ribosomes after entering through the lipid bilayer and energy-dependent active transport pump
Pharmacokinetics	Rapidly absorbed with a very high bioavailability of around 93%, with high concentration in bile. Peak serum levels in 2–4 hours. Elimination by renal and biliary route
Indications	Active against many gram-positive; Gram-negative bacteria; And Parasites. Actively used in cholera; Scrub typhus; Malaria management
Dosage as per indications	5 mg/kg/day q 12 h; given as single dose in cholera
Maximum dosage	300 mg/day
Dose adjustments	Not needed in renal impairment
Adverse effects	GI symptoms, photosensitivity, hemolytic anemia, rash, skin manifestation, increased ICT
Contraindications	Hypersensitivity, pregnancy and lactation, sucrose intolerance
Drug interactions	Cyclosporine, antiepileptics
Remarks	Not recommended for children <8 years (risk of tooth enamel hypoplasia)

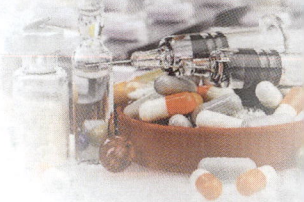

D-penicillamine

Drug name	D-penicillamine
Category	Chelating agent
Route	Oral
Strength	Tab (125 mg, 250 mg)
Brands	Artamine (Tab), Cuprimine (Tab), Distamine (Tab)
Mechanism of action	It chelates copper, reduces excess cystine excretion and interferes with the formation of cross-links between tropocollagen molecules, besides having an immunosuppressive action in rheumatoid arthritis
Pharmacokinetics	Rapidly but incompletely absorbed when taken orally, highly protein bound, peak levels in 1–3 hours. Mainly excreted via kidneys
Indications	Lead/copper poisoning; Wilson disease; cystinuria; Juvenile idiopathic arthritis (JIA)
Dosage as per indications	*Poisoning/Wilson/cystinuria:* • 20–40 mg/kg/day oral 8–12 hourly • *JIA:* 5–10 mg/kg/day as single dose
Maximum dosage	• *<10 years:* 0.5–0.75 g/day q 12 h • *>10 years:* 1 g/day q 12 h
Dose adjustments	In renal derangement, not needed in hepatic derangement
Adverse effects	Dermatitis, nausea, vomiting, hemolysis, drug eruptions, lupus-like syndrome, thyroiditis, marrow suppression, neuropathies, tinnitus
Contraindications	Hypersensitivity
Drug interactions	Sucralfate, antacids, iron, zinc
Remarks	Give vitamin B_6 and zinc as supplement. Penicillamine should preferably be given on an empty stomach

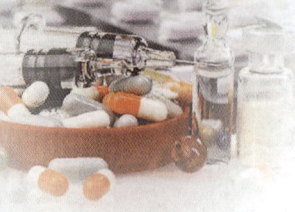

Drotaverine

Drug name	Drotaverine
Category	Antispasmodic
Route	Intravenous, Oral
Strength	Inj (20 mg/mL); Tab (40 mg, 80 mg); Susp (20 mg/5mL)
Brands	Baralgan (Inj, Tab), Drotin (Inj, Tab), Drovet (Inj, Tab)
Mechanism of action	Inhibiting phosphodiesterase-4 (PDE4), thereby increasing cAMP concentration, which causes smooth muscle relaxation
Pharmacokinetics	Incomplete absorption after oral intake with variable bioavailability. Mainly metabolized and eliminated in liver along with some amount undergoing biliary excretion. Half-life 10 hours
Indications	Functional bowel disorders; Pain abdomen due to renal/gallstones
Dosage as per indications	*Oral:* *1–6 years:* 20 mg 8 hourly *>6 years:* 40 mg 8 hourly
Maximum dosage	80 mg/day oral
Dose adjustments	Liver and kidney disease, acute/subacute intestinal obstruction
Adverse effects	Nausea, vomiting, dry mouth
Contraindications	Hypersensitivity
Drug interactions	Antimuscarinic drugs, benzodiazepines

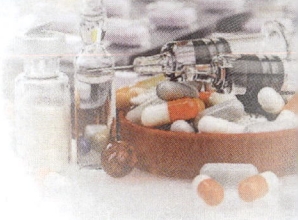

Edrophonium

Drug name	Edrophonium
Category	Cholinergic/Antimyasthenic
Route	Intravenous, Intramuscular
Strength	Inj (10 mg/mL)
Brands	Tensilon (Inj), Enlon (Inj). No Indian brand available
Mechanism of action	Inhibits acetylcholinesterase enzymes thereby prolonging the action of acetylcholine
Pharmacokinetics	*Rapidly absorbed, onset of action:* 30–60 seconds, duration of action: 10 minutes, primarily excreted from kidneys, half-life 0.5–1.5 hours
Indications	Myasthenia gravis
Dosage as per indications	*Initial dose:* 0.04 mg/kg/dose intravenous or intramuscular; if no response after 1 minute, give 0.16 mg/kg/dose to a total dose of 0.2 mg/kg
Maximum dosage	Initial maximum dose 1 mg; total maximum dose 5 mg
Dose adjustments	Not known
Adverse effects	Cholinergic crisis, arrhythmia, bronchospasm
Contraindications	Hypersensitivity, GI obstruction, arrhythmia
Drug interactions	Drugs with cholinergic or anticholinergic action

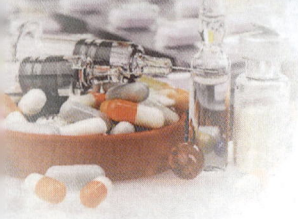

Efavirenz (EFV)

Drug name	Efavirenz (EFV)
Category	Antiretroviral, Non-nucleoside reverse transcriptase inhibitor (NNRTI)
Route	Oral
Strength	Caps (50 mg, 100 mg, 200 mg)
Brands	Efavir (Cap), Evirenz (Cap), Revenz (Cap)
Mechanism of action	It is a noncompetitive inhibitor of HIV-1 reverse transcriptase (RT)
Pharmacokinetics	Highly protein bound terminal half-life 50 hours
Indications	HIV/AIDS
Dosage as per indications	15 mg/kg once a day
Maximum dosage	600 mg/day
Dose adjustments	No or minimal adjustment in renal impairment, no adjustment needed for mild hepatic impairment, not to be given in severe hepatic derangement
Adverse effects	Rash, granulocytopenia, hepatotoxicity and psychosis
Contraindications	Not recommended in children <3 years age/weight <10 kg
Drug interactions	Terfenadine, astemizole, cisapride, midazolam

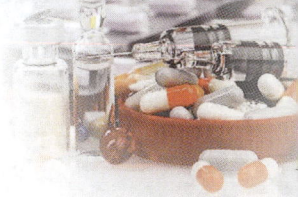

Emtricitabine (FTC)

Drug name	Emtricitabine (FTC)
Category	Antiretroviral, Nucleoside reverse transcriptase inhibitor (NRTI)
Route	Oral
Strength	Sol (10 mg/mL); Cap (200 mg)
Brands	Emtriva (Cap, Syp), Mebryl (Cap), Coviracil (Cap)
Mechanism of action	It is converted to 5-triphosphate which competitively inhibits HIV-1 reverse transcriptase thus terminating the DNA chain
Pharmacokinetics	Highly absorbed, peak plasma levels in 1–2 hours. Eliminated mainly by the kidneys
Indications	HIV/AIDS
Dosage as per indications	• *0–3 months:* 3 mg/kg OD • *3 months–17 years:* 6 mg/kg OD
Maximum dosage	240 mg/day
Dose adjustments	Dose adjustment needed in renal insufficiency
Adverse effects	• Headache, nausea, rash, hyperpigmentation of palms and soles, lactic acidosis, hepatotoxicity • Severe hepatitis in children with hepatitis B coinfected persons
Contraindications	Hypersensitivity
Drug interactions	Adefovir, orlistat, aminoglycosides

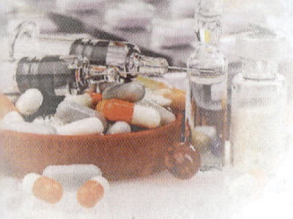

Enalapril Maleate

Drug name	Enalapril maleate
Category	Antihypertensive, Angiotensin-converting enzyme inhibitor
Route	Oral, Intravenous
Strength	Tab (2.5 mg, 5 mg); Inj (1.25 mg/mL) (not available in India)
Brands	Canapril (Tab), Dilvas (Tab), Envas (Tab), Enlacard (Tab)
Mechanism of action	Inhibits angiotensin-converting enzyme (ACE) leading to decreased plasma angiotensin II, increased plasma renin activity, and decreased aldosterone secretion
Pharmacokinetics	Rapidly absorbed when taken orally, peak serum levels in 1 hour. *Half-life:* 11 hours. Excretion is primarily renal
Indications	Hypertension
Dosage as per indications	• *Oral:* 0.1–0.5 mg/kg/day q 12–24 h • *Intravenous:* 0.005–0.01 mg/kg/dose q 8–24 h
Maximum dosage	*Oral:* 40 mg/24 hours, *IV:* 1.25 mg/dose
Dose adjustments	Dose adjustment in renal impairment
Adverse effects	Nausea, diarrhea, headache, dizziness, hyperkalemia, hypoglycemia, hypersensitivity, cough and hypotension
Contraindications	Bilateral renal artery stenosis
Drug interactions	Drugs affecting renin-angiotensin system, diuretics

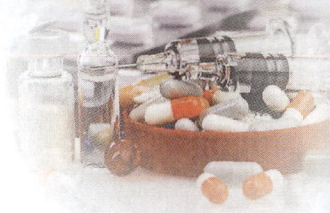

Enoxaparin

Drug name	Enoxaparin
Category	Anticoagulant
Route	Subcutaneous
Strength	Inj (20 mg, 40 mg, 60 mg, 80 mg)
Brands	Clexane (Inj), Enoxarin (Inj), Zaparin (Inj)
Mechanism of action	Inactivates factor Xa with a high anti-Xa activity and low anti-IIa or antithrombin activity mediated through antithrombin III (ATIII)
Pharmacokinetics	Very high bioavailability after subcutaneous injection. Metabolized in liver. *Half-life:* 5–7 hours
Indications	Deep vein thrombosis
Dosage as per indications	• *DVT treatment:* <2 months: 1.5 mg/kg/dose q 12 hourly; 2 months to 18 years: 1 mg/kg/dose q 12 hourly • *DVT prophylaxis:* <2 months: 1.5 mg/kg/dose q 24 hourly; 2 months to 18 years: 1 mg/kg/dose q 24 hourly
Maximum dosage	*Prophylaxis:* 30 mg/dose in children >2 months of age
Dose adjustments	Dose adjustment needed in hepatic and renal impairment
Adverse effects	Bleeding, confusion, edema thrombocytopenia, hypochromic anemia, and pain/erythema at injection site. Allergic reactions, headache, eosinophilia, alopecia, hepatocellular and cholestatic liver injury
Contraindications	Major bleed and drug-induced thrombocytopenia; prophylactic use is not recommended in patients with prosthetic heart valves
Drug interactions	Concurrent use with spinal or epidural anesthesia, or spinal puncture has resulted in long-term or permanent paralysis
Remarks	*Approximate anti-factor Xa activity:* 100 IU per 1 mg; target antifactor Xa levels of 0.1–0.3 units/mL. Protamine sulfate is the antidote; 1 mg protamine sulfate neutralizes 1 mg enoxaparin. Use with caution in uncontrolled arterial hypertension, bleeding diathesis, history of recurrent GI ulcers

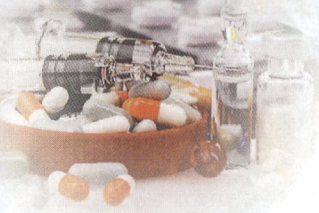

Ergotamine Tartrate

Drug name	Ergotamine tartrate
Category	Antimigraine
Route	Oral, Sublingual
Strength	Tab (2 mg)
Brands	Ergomar (Tab)
Mechanism of action	Specific and selective 5-hydroxytryptamine$_1$ (5HT$_{1D}$) receptor agonist responsible for cranial blood vessels vasoconstriction
Pharmacokinetics	Rapidly absorbed, nearly 70% concentration in 45 minutes. Eliminated by oxidative metabolism (via monoamine oxidase A) and excreted in the urine
Indications	Cluster headache
Dosage as per indications	Take one tablet sublingually soon after onset of headache. May take maximum of 10 mg/week
Maximum dosage	3 mg/24 h; 5 mg/week
Dose adjustments	Use with caution in renal or hepatic disease
Adverse effects	Nausea, vomiting, dizziness, paresthesia, muscle cramps. May cause rebound headache (withdrawal) if stopped abruptly after prolonged usage
Contraindications	Concurrent administration with protease inhibitors, macrolides like clarithromycin, azole antifungals, nitroglycerin, CYP450 3A4 inhibitors should not be used simultaneoulsy to avoid risk of ergotism
Drug interactions	Protease inhibitors, clarithromycin, erythromycin, CYP450 3A4 inhibitors, and nitroglycerin
Remarks	Do not crush tablet

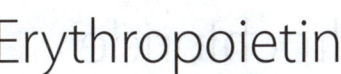

Erythropoietin

Drug name	Erythropoietin
Category	Glycoprotein hormone for erythropoiesis
Route	Intravenous, Subcutaneous
Strength	Inj (2,000 IU, 4,000 IU)
Brands	Epofer (Inj), Epomine (Inj), Eprex (Inj)
Mechanism of action	Glycoprotein hormone produced by kidney to regulate red blood cell (RBC) production, mainly acting at erythroid precursor level, though active at all stages. Acts by interfering with apoptosis and stimulating erythroid cell proliferation
Pharmacokinetics	• *Peak serum levels:* 12–18 hours after SC injection • *Half-life:* 4 and 24 hours after IV and SC injection, respectively
Indications	Chronic renal failure; Anemia of prematurity
Dosage as per indications	• *Chronic renal failure:* 50–100 IU/kg SC two to three times/week • *Anemia of prematurity:* 25–100 IU/kg/dose SC three times per week for 8–12 weeks
Maximum dosage	40,000–60,000 U/week
Dose adjustments	Dose adjustment needed in renal impairment
Adverse effects	Increased risk of thrombosis/stroke/cardiovascular event/death in those with Hb >11/CKD
Contraindications	Hypersensitivity, uncontrolled hypertension, severe coronary, peripheral arterial, carotid or cerebral vascular disease
Drug interactions	Captopril, carboplatin
Remarks	• Provide oral iron supplementation 2–3 mg/kg/d • SC route preferred to IV route • Monitor for hypertension, blood urea, serum creatinine, hematocrit and clotting time. Peak effect in 2–3 weeks • Reduce dose when target attained or when hematocrit increases >4 points in any 2 weeks period

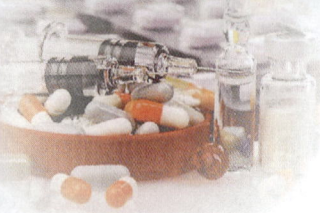

Esmolol Hydrochloride

Drug name	Esmolol hydrochloride
Category	Antihypertensive, Beta-1 selective adrenergic blocker
Route	Intravenous
Strength	Inj (10 mg/mL, 250 mg/mL)
Brands	Esocard (Inj), Miniblock (inj)
Mechanism of action	It is a cardioselective adrenergic receptor blocking agent. Steady state blood levels are obtained within 5 minutes
Pharmacokinetics	• Rapid onset of action, around 1–2 minutes, peak levels: 5 minutes, distribution half-life 2 minutes, elimination half-life: 9 minutes • Well absorbed when taken orally, 50% protein bound, metabolized in red blood cells, eliminated via kidneys
Indications	Hypertension
Dosage as per indications	• *Loading:* 100–500 µg/kg IV over 1 minute • *Maintenance dose:* 25–100 µg/kg/min infusion, may increase rate every 10 minutes by 25–50 µg/kg/min up to 500 µg/kg/min
Maximum dosage	700 µg/kg/min. Doses up to 1000 µg/kg/min have been tried
Dose adjustments	Dose adjustment needed in renal impairment
Adverse effects	Congestive heart failure, hypotension, nausea, vomiting, bronchospasm
Contraindications	Heart block (first degree), heart failure, cardiogenic shock, sinus bradycardia
Drug interactions	Acebutolol, acetaminophen, digoxin

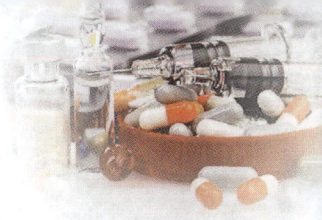

Etanercept

Drug name	Etanercept
Category	Tumor necrosis factor-α (TNF-α) receptor blocker
Route	Subcutaneous
Strength	Inj (25 mg/vial)
Brands	Enbrel (Inj), Enbrol (Inj)
Mechanism of action	Competitive inhibition of TNF binding to cell surface TNF receptors, leading to prevention of TNF actions including TNF-mediated cellular responses
Pharmacokinetics	Onset of action is 1–4 weeks, with peak effect: 3 months. *Half-life:* 70 hours
Indications	Juvenile Idiopathic Arthritis (JIA)
Dosage as per indications	*2–17 years:* 0.4 mg/kg/dose twice weekly given 72–96 hours apart
Maximum dosage	*Oral:* 50 mg/week and max single injection site dose of 25 mg
Dose adjustments	Not needed in renal and hepatic impairment
Adverse effects	GI discomfort, rash, infections, dizziness, lymphoma
Contraindications	Sepsis/severe infection
Drug interactions	Other immunosuppressants like cyclophosphamide, cyclosporine, anakinra and azathioprine, certain live vaccines
Remarks	Do not administer live vaccines concurrently with this drug

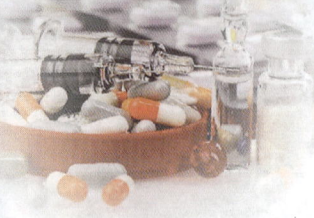

Ethambutol

Drug name	Ethambutol
Category	Antitubercular drug
Route	Oral
Strength	Tab (200 mg, 400 mg, 600 mg, 800 mg)
Brands	Combutol (Tab), Albutol (Tab), Ebutol (Tab)
Mechanism of action	Bacteriostatic against *Mycobacterium tuberculosis* and *M. bovis* by inhibiting arabinosyl transferase required for formation of arabinogalactan, a constituent of mycobacterium cell wall
Pharmacokinetics	Well absorbed, absorption not impaired by food. Mostly excreted in urine over 48 hours
Indications	Tuberculosis
Dosage as per indications	15–25 mg/kg/day
Maximum dosage	2.5 g/24 hours
Dose adjustments	Adjust dose in renal impairment
Adverse effects	Rash, peripheral neuropathy, hyperuricemia, GI disturbances
Contraindications	Do not use in optic neuritis
Drug interactions	Aluminum hydroxide
Remarks	Avoid use in children where visual acuity cannot be assessed. Drug should be immediately discontinued if any child develops visual deterioration on ethambutol

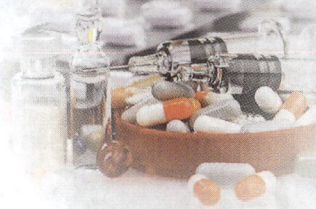

Ethionamide

Drug name	Ethionamide
Category	Antitubercular drug
Route	Oral
Strength	Tab (250 mg)
Brands	Ethiocid (Tab), Myobid (Tab)
Mechanism of action	Acts as both bacteriostatic or bactericidal, inhibit peptide synthesis in the organism
Pharmacokinetics	Highly absorbed and widely distributed after oral administration. Extensively metabolized in liver, half-life around 2 hours
Indications	Tuberculosis
Dosage as per indications	15–20 mg/kg/day
Maximum dosage	1 g/day
Dose adjustments	In hepatic derangement
Adverse effects	Hepatotoxicity, vitamin B_6 deficiency, optic neuritis
Contraindications	Hypersensitivity, severe hepatic derangement
Drug interactions	Cycloserine (Isoniazid)
Remarks	To be given in two divided doses

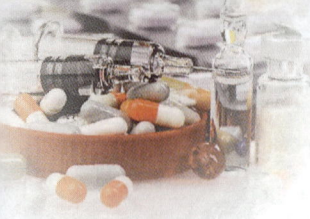

Ethosuximide

Drug name	Ethosuximide
Category	Anticonvulsant
Route	Oral
Strength	Tab (250 mg); Syp (250 mg/5 mL)
Brands	Ethosuximide (Tab, Syp), Zarontin (Tab, Syp)
Mechanism of action	Depression of the motor cortex and elevation of the threshold to convulsive stimuli
Pharmacokinetics	Well absorbed when taken orally but highly metabolized in liver, peak levels in 5–7 hours. Elimination half-life: 30 hours. Excreted mainly in the urine
Indications	Absence seizures
Dosage as per indications	• *Absence attacks:* 15 mg/kg/day q 12 h. Increase the dose every week till control of seizures • *Maintenance dose:* 20–40 mg/kg/day q 12 h
Maximum dosage	• *≤6 years:* 500 mg/day • *>6 years:* 1,500 mg/day
Dose adjustments	Dose adjustment required in renal and hepatic impairment
Adverse effects	Lupus-like syndrome, Stevens-Johnson syndrome (SJS), ataxia, blood dyscrasias
Contraindications	Use cautiously in renal and hepatic diseases
Drug interactions	Acetaminophen, acetazolamide, other antiepileptic drugs
Remarks	Do not withdraw the drug abruptly as it may precipitate absence seizures. Therapeutic levels are between 40 and 100 µg/mL

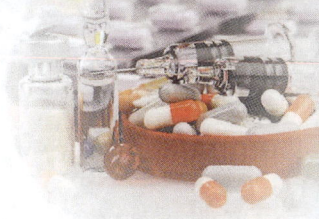

Famotidine

Drug name	Famotidine
Category	H_2 receptor antagonist
Route	Oral
Strength	Tab (10 mg, 20 mg, 40 mg)
Brands	Advantac (Tab), Facid (Tab), Famocid (Tab)
Mechanism of action	Inhibit gastric acid secretion (basal, nocturnal, postmeal, caffeine induced) by competitively blocking histamine-2 (H_2) receptor
Pharmacokinetics	When taken orally, onset of action: 1 hour, peak effect: 1–3 hours, total duration of action: 10–12 hours, has a dose-dependent therapeutic action. Has minimal first-pass metabolism. Eliminated via renal (around 70%) and hepatic (around 30%) route. Half-life 2–4 hours
Indications	Peptic ulcer disease; Gastritis
Dosage as per indications	0.5 mg/kg/dose once or twice a day
Maximum dosage	40 mg/day
Dose adjustments	In renal and hepatic derangement
Adverse effects	Altered bowel habits, headache, dizziness, pancytopenia, Stevens–Johnson syndrome, QT prolongation
Contraindications	Hypersensitivity
Drug interactions	Ketoconazole, itraconazole, triamterene, cefpodoxime

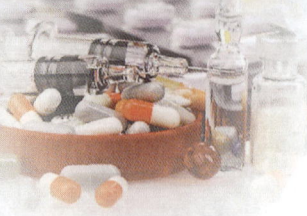

Faropenem

Drug name	Faropenem
Category	Antibiotic
Route	Oral
Strength	Tab (150 mg, 200 mg)
Brands	Duonem (Tab), Farobact (Tab), Faronem (Tab)
Mechanism of action	It is a beta-lactam antibiotic. The drug acts by inhibiting the synthesis of bacterial cell walls by competitively inhibiting the transpeptidase enzyme used for cross-linking peptides for peptidoglycan synthesis
Pharmacokinetics	Easily absorbed with bioavailability of around 70%. Half-life 1 hour, metabolized and excreted by kidney through enzyme dehydropeptidase
Indications	Broad-spectrum antibacterial activity against many gram-positive; Gram-negative aerobes; Anaerobes
Dosage as per indications	Not fully established; 15 mg/kg/day in three divided doses (in trials)
Maximum dosage	200–300 mg/dose 8 hourly
Dose adjustments	Renal impairment
Adverse effects	Nausea, vomiting, pain abdomen, diarrhea
Contraindications	Hypersensitivity
Drug interactions	Sodium valproate, imipenem, cilastatin, furosemide

Fentanyl

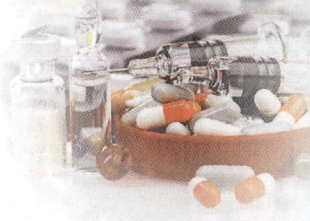

Drug name	Fentanyl
Category	Narcotic, Synthetic opiate
Route	Intravenous, Oral
Strength	Inj (50 µg/mL ampoule); Transdermal patch (25 µg/h, 50 µg/h); Tab (50 µg, 100 µg)
Brands	Durogesic (Tab, Patch), Fenstud (Inj, Patch), Verfen (Inj)
Mechanism of action	50–100 times more potent than morphine. Onset of action 1–2 minutes, peak effects: 10 minutes, total duration of action: 30–60 minutes, when given intravenously. Give IV dose over 3–5 minutes. Deposits in fat tissue
Pharmacokinetics	Acts almost immediately after IV administration, effect lasts for 30–60 minutes; variably bound in plasma, metabolized in liver, eliminated mainly in urine
Indications	Sedation; Pain reliever
Dosage as per indications	• *Infants:* 1–4 µg/kg/dose q 1–4 h IV; continuous infusion 0.5–5 µg/kg/h • *Children:* 1–3 µg/kg/dose q 1–4 h IV; continuous infusion 1–5 µg/kg/h PO 10–15 µg/kg/dose
Maximum dosage	400 µg/dose
Dose adjustments	Adjust dose in renal impairment
Adverse effects	Hypotension, bradycardia, GI upset, respiratory depression, chest wall rigidity, biliary tract spasm
Contraindications	Hypersensitivity Use with caution in bradycardia, respiratory depression, and increased intracranial pressure
Drug interactions	Not to be used with MAO inhibitors
Remarks	Rapid administration may cause respiratory depression, which may persist when analgesia effect lowers down

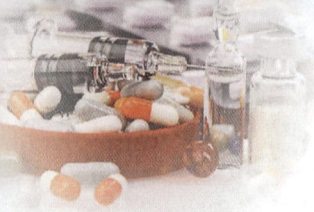

Ferrous Sulfate/Fumarate/Gluconate/Ascorbate

Drug name	Ferrous sulfate/Fumarate/Gluconate/Ascorbate
Category	Iron
Route	Oral
Strength	Tab (20 mg, 60 mg, 100 mg); Syp (30 mg/5 mL)
Brands	Tonoferon (Tab, Syp), Feronia-XT (Tab, Syp), Autrin (Tab), Trufer XT (Tab, Syp)
Mechanism of action	Has no intrinsic therapeutic activity except as a nutrient source
Pharmacokinetics	Incompletely absorbed from GI tract. Ferrous form has high absorption. Food decreases absorption
Indications	Iron deficiency anemia
Dosage as per indications	*Treatment:* • Elemental iron premature infant: 2–4 mg/kg/24 h in 1–2 divided doses • Child: 3–6 mg/kg/24 h divided once-TID *Prophylaxis:* • Elemental iron premature infant: 2 mg/kg/24 h (max: 15 mg) • Term infant: 1–2 mg/kg/24 h (max: 15 mg) • Child 2–12 years: 2 mg/kg/24 h (max: 30 mg) • Adolescent: 60 mg PO OD
Maximum dosage	Elemental iron PO OD *Premature infant:* 15 mg *Term infant:* 15 mg *Child:* 2–12 years: 30 mg *Adolescent:* 60 mg
Dose adjustments	None
Adverse effects	Gastritis, pain abdomen, nausea, constipation, black discoloration of teeth/tongue
Contraindications	Hypersensitivity, hemolytic anemia, hemosiderosis
Drug interactions	Antibiotics (penicillin, ciprofloxacin), antacids
Remarks	Antacids may decrease iron absorption. Avoid intake of iron with tea or coffee

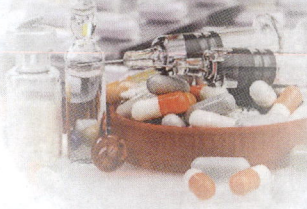

Fexofenadine Hydrochloride

Drug name	Fexofenadine hydrochloride
Category	Antihistaminic
Route	Oral
Strength	Tab (30 mg, 120 mg, 180 mg); Syp (30 mg/5 mL)
Brands	Allegra (Tab, Syp), Altiva (Tab, Syp), Fexidine (Tab, Syp)
Mechanism of action	It is a nonsedating antihistaminic which acts on H_1 receptors to block histamine action
Pharmacokinetics	It is rapidly absorbed orally with peak levels obtained 1–3 hours later. The drug is 60–70% plasma protein bound. Terfenadine is the active metabolite of this drug
Indications	Antiallergic
Dosage as per indications	• *6 months to 2 years:* 15 mg BD • *2–12 years:* 30 mg BD • *>12 years:* 60 mg BD or 120 mg OD
Maximum dosage	180 mg/day
Dose adjustments	Avoid use in renal impairment
Adverse effects	GI disturbances, drowsiness, fatigue
Contraindications	Hypersensitivity
Drug interactions	Co-administration of fexofenadine hydrochloride with erythromycin or ketoconazole increases the risk of cardiac arrhythmias

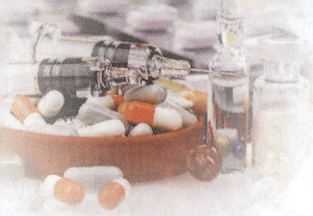

Fluconazole

Drug name	Fluconazole
Category	Antifungal, Azole
Route	Oral, Intravenous
Strength	Syp (200 mg/100 mL); Tab (50 mg, 150 mg); Inj (2 mg/mL)
Brands	Flucon (Tab, Syp), Forcan (Inj, Tab, Syp), Zocon (Inj, Tab, Syp)
Mechanism of action	It inhibits fungal cytochrome P-450-mediated 14 alpha-lanosterol demethylation, required for synthesis of fungal ergosterol for fungal cell membrane
Pharmacokinetics	Well absorbed orally. High bioavailability after oral and intravenous administration. Peak levels 30–90 minutes later; elimination half-life 15–20 hours. Mainly eliminated through renal route
Indications	Fungal infection
Dosage as per indications	Intravenous/oral • *Children:* 3–6 mg/kg/day OD • *Neonates:* Loading dose 12 mg/kg followed by 3–5 mg/kg/day OD
Maximum dosage	12 mg/kg/24 h
Dose adjustments	Dose adjustment needed in hepatic and renal disease
Adverse effects	Nausea, vomiting, abdominal pain, hepatitis, cholestasis, blood dyscrasias
Contraindications	Hypersensitivity; avoid in patients prone to arrhythmias
Drug interactions	Use with other medications that are known to prolong the QT interval and are metabolized via the CYP450 3A4 enzyme (e.g., erythromycin) is contraindicated

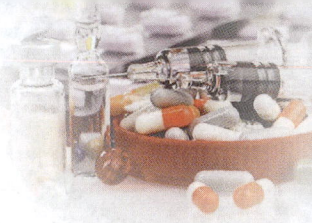

Flucytosine

Drug name	Flucytosine
Category	Antifungal, Antimetabolite
Route	Oral
Strength	Tab (250 mg, 500 mg); Syp (10 mg/mL, 50 mg/mL, not available in India)
Brands	Cytoflu (Tab): only Indian brand, Ancobon (Cap)
Mechanism of action	Flucytosine converts to 5-fluorouracil inside the fungal cell. Once converted, it incorporates into fungal RNA and inhibits synthesis of both DNA and RNA
Pharmacokinetics	Rapidly and almost completely absorbed from GI tract and widely distributed in body tissue and body fluids; has high bioavailability; main route of elimination is renal via glomerular filtration
Indications	Fungal infections
Dosage as per indications	• *Newborn:* 12.5–37.5 mg/kg per dose q 6 h PO • *Pediatric:* 50–150 mg/kg/24 h, q 6 h PO
Maximum dosage	150 mg/kg/day
Dose adjustments	Avoid in renal and hepatic dysfunction
Adverse effects	Bone marrow suppression, diarrhea, hepatitis, rash
Contraindications	Hypersensitivity, first trimester of pregnancy, avoid in hematological disorder
Drug interactions	Cytarabine, NSAIDs, nephrotoxic drugs
Remarks	*Therapeutic levels:* 25–100 mg/L. Monitor blood counts, kidney function tests, alkaline phosphatase and liver enzymes (SGOT, SGPT)

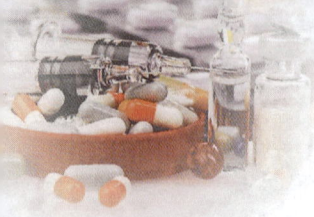

Fludrocortisone Acetate

Drug name	Fludrocortisone acetate
Category	Mineralocorticoid
Route	Oral
Strength	Tab (0.1 mg)
Brands	Florinef (Tab), Floricot (Tab)
Mechanism of action	It is a synthetic mineralocorticoid use along with hydrocortisone, acts similar to aldosterone and structurally similar to cortisol.
Pharmacokinetics	It increases sodium reabsorption and potassium excretion in kidneys. Has rapid and complete absorption after oral administration. It is highly protein bound, mostly eliminated in urine, with a half-life of 1–3.5 hours
Indications	Congenital adrenal hyperplasia (CAH)
Dosage as per indications	0.05–0.2 mg/24 h
Maximum dosage	Not known
Dose adjustments	In renal derangement
Adverse effects	Hypertension, hypokalemia, acne, rash, bruising, headaches, GI ulcers, and growth suppression. Monitor BP and serum electrolytes
Contraindications	Heart failure, systemic infections, hypertension, renal dysfunction
Drug interactions	Digoxin, phenytoin, and rifampin
Remarks	Gradually increase or decrease dose

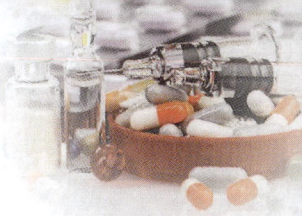

Flumazenil

Drug name	Flumazenil
Category	Antidote for benzodiazepine
Route	Intravenous
Strength	Inj (0.5 mg)
Brands	Fludot (Inj)
Mechanism of action	It competitively blocks activity at GABA/benzodiazepine receptor complex
Pharmacokinetics	*Onset of action:* 1–3 minutes. *Half-life:* 1 hour, completely metabolized in liver, mostly eliminated in urine in next 3 days
Indications	Benzodiazepine overdose; Reversal of benzodiazepine sedation
Dosage as per indications	• *Benzodiazepine overdose:* 0.01 mg/kg (max dose: 0.2 mg) IV every 1 minute to a maximum dose of 1 mg • *Reversal of benzodiazepine sedation:* Initial dose: 0.01 mg/kg (max dose: 0.2 mg) given over 15 seconds, can be repeated after 45 seconds (total maximum dose of 0.05 mg/kg or 1 mg, whichever is lesser)
Maximum dosage	As mentioned above
Dose adjustments	In liver dysfunction
Adverse effects	Seizures, panic attacks
Contraindications	Hypersensitivity
Drug interactions	Tricyclic antidepressants (TCAs)
Remarks	Does not reverse narcotic effects

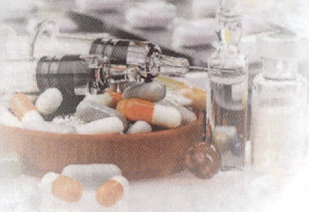

Flunarizine

Drug name	Flunarizine
Category	Calcium channel blocker
Route	Oral
Strength	Tab (5 mg, 10 mg)
Brands	Flunarin (Tab), Sibelium (Tab)
Mechanism of action	It is a calcium antagonist. It also inhibits sodium channel in brain only
Pharmacokinetics	Well absorbed after oral administration, highly protein bound, peak levels in 2–4 hours mainly metabolized in liver and excreted in feces. Terminal half-life: 18 days
Indications	Migraine prophylaxis; Treatment of vestibular vertigo
Dosage as per indications	*5–12 years:* 5 mg; *>12 years:* 10 mg
Maximum dosage	Not known
Dose adjustments	In liver dysfunction
Adverse effects	Depression, extrapyramidal symptoms galactorrhea, fatigue, weight gain
Contraindications	Hypersensitivity, depressive disorder
Drug interactions	Hepatic enzyme inducers

Fluoxetine

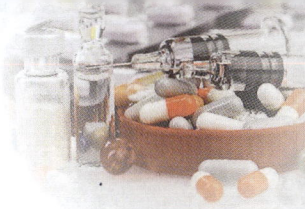

Drug name	Fluoxetine
Category	Antidepressant
Route	Oral
Strength	Tab (10 mg, 20 mg); Susp (20 mg/5 mL)
Brands	Flunil (Tab), Fluxel (Tab), Prodep (Tab, Susp)
Mechanism of action	Inhibits CNS neuronal uptake of serotonin
Pharmacokinetics	Highly protein bound, extensively metabolized in liver, elimination half-life: 1–3 days (short duration), 6–8 days (long duration)
Indications	Depression; Obsessive-compulsive disorder
Dosage as per indications	• Used in children >7 years • *Depression/obsessive-compulsive disorder:* Start at 5–10 mg once a day oral. May increase gradually to 20 mg over next few weeks as required
Maximum dosage	Not known
Dose adjustments	In renal and hepatic derangement
Adverse effects	Headache, drowsiness, insomnia, weight loss, depression
Contraindications	Monoamine oxidase (MAO) inhibitors
Drug interactions	TCAs, diuretics, selective serotonin reuptake inhibitors (SSRIs)

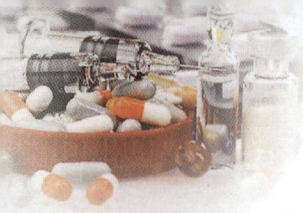

Fluticasone Propionate

Drug name	Fluticasone propionate
Category	Corticosteroid
Route	Inhalation, Nasal
Strength	MDI (25 µg/puff, 50 µg/puff, 125 µg/puff); Rotacap (50 µg, 100 µg)
Brands	Flohale (MDI, Rotacap), Flomale (MDI, Rotacap), Flutiflo (MDI, Rotacap)
Mechanism of action	It shows corticosteroid action by inhibiting various inflammatory cells like mast cells, eosinophils, basophils, lymphocytes, macrophages, neutrophils) and thereby decreasing inflammatory mediators such as histamine, leukotrienes, and cytokines
Pharmacokinetics	Not much available; Acts locally on lung
Indications	Asthma
Dosage as per indications	MDI 50–500 µg/day in two divided doses
Maximum dosage	500 µg/dose
Dose adjustments	Use cautiously in liver disease
Adverse effects	Oral thrush, dysphonia, dermatitis
Contraindications	Hypersensitivity
Drug interactions	CYP3A4 inhibitors
Remarks	Rinse mouth every time after use

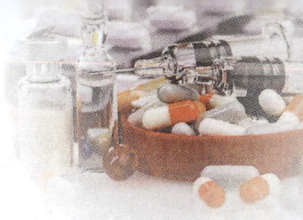

Folic Acid

Drug name	Folic acid
Category	Vitamin
Route	Oral
Strength	Tab (5 mg)
Brands	Folvite (Tab), Folacin (Tab)
Mechanism of action	Folic acid is converted to tetrahydrofolate in plasma and liver, which then acts as a coenzyme in several metabolic processes including hematopoiesis
Pharmacokinetics	Well absorbed orally from proximal small intestine. Bioavailability of drug is almost double of the natural sources. Mostly eliminated from urine
Indications	Anemia; Nutritional supplement; Severe malnutrition
Dosage as per indications	*Initial dose* • *Infant:* 15 µg/kg/dose • *Child:* 1 mg/dose *Maintenance* • *Infant:* 30–45 µg/24 h once daily • *Child:* 0.1–0.4 mg/24 h once daily
Maximum dosage	Not known
Dose adjustments	Not known
Adverse effects	Bloating, nausea, diarrhea, irritability, confusion, behavior changes or skin reactions on high doses
Contraindications	Hypersensitivity, untreated cobalamin deficiency
Drug interactions	Phenytoin, fosphenytoin, primidone, phenobarbitone
Remarks	Masks neurological abnormalities due to vitamin B_{12} deficiency

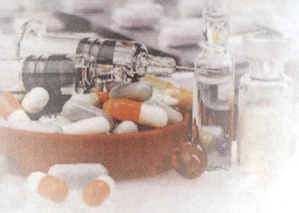

Formoterol Fumarate

Drug name	Formoterol fumarate
Category	Long-acting beta-2 adrenergic agonist (LABA)
Route	Inhalation
Strength	MDI (12 µg/puff); Rotacaps (6 µg)
Brands	Foratec (MDI, Rotacap), Deriform (MDI, Rotacap)
Mechanism of action	Stimulation of intracellular adenyl cyclase, which helps to increase cyclic AMP levels. This helps to relax bronchial smooth muscle and inhibits ion release of mediators from mast cells
Pharmacokinetics	Fast onset of action (1–3 minutes) with peak effects in 0.5–1 hour lasting over long duration (up to 12 hours)
Indications	Asthma
Dosage as per indications	Used in children >5 years of age as: MDI 12 BD
Maximum dosage	24 µg/24 h (12 µg spaced 12 hours apart)
Dose adjustments	Not known
Adverse effects	Increased risk of asthma-related deaths, nausea, pain abdomen
Contraindications	Avoid in patients with hyperthyroidism, diabetes, seizures, pheochromocytoma
Drug interactions	MAO inhibitors, xanthines, beta blockers
Remarks	Should be used with inhaled corticosteroid for asthma/bronchodilation

Foscarnet

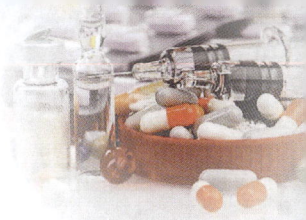

Drug name	Foscarnet
Category	Antiviral agent
Route	Intravenous
Strength	Inj (500 mg, 1 g)
Brands	Foscavir (Inj)
Mechanism of action	Directly inhibits viral specific DNA polymerase
Pharmacokinetics	Mainly eliminated by the kidneys mainly through glomerular filtration. Half-life: 2–4 hours
Indications	CMV retinitis
Dosage as per indications	60 mg/kg/dose q 8 h as slow IV infusion during induction phase followed by 90 mg/kg/dose OD IV infusion during maintenance phase
Maximum dosage	Not known
Dose adjustments	Avoid in patients with renal diseases
Adverse effects	Seizures, hallucinations, peripheral neuropathy, renal failure, dyspnea, chest pain, fever, nausea, diarrhea
Contraindications	Hypersensitivity
Drug interactions	Amphotericin, aminoglycosides, cidofovir
Remarks	Adequate hydration decreases risk of nephrotoxicity, do not give IV infusion rapidly, use with ciprofloxacin can precipitate seizures

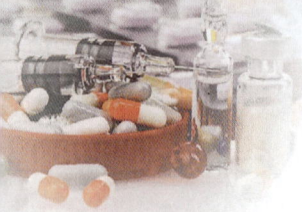

Fosphenytoin

Drug name	Fosphenytoin
Category	Anticonvulsant
Route	Intravenous
Strength	Inj (50 mg PE/mL per vial)
Brands	Fosolin (Inj), Fosophen (Inj), Milorgen (Inj)
Mechanism of action	Acts on voltage-dependent sodium channels and calcium channels of neurons, inhibits calcium flux across neuronal membranes, and increases sodium-potassium ATPase activity of neurons
Pharmacokinetics	Peak levels 30 minutes after intravenous medication. Highly bound to plasma proteins
Indications	Antiepileptic
Dosage as per indications	• *Loading:* 15–20 mg/kg phenytoin equivalent, PE (not to exceed 3 mg PE/kg/min) • *Maintenance dose:* 4–6 mg PE/kg/d IV/IM 1.5 mg fosphenytoin = 1 mg phenytoin = 1 mg phenytoin equivalent (PE)
Maximum dosage	Not known
Dose adjustments	Dose reduction needed in renal and hepatic impairment
Adverse effects	Ataxia, rash, nystagmus, slurring of speech, tinnitus
Contraindications	Sinus bradycardia, sinoatrial block, second- and third-degree A-V block and Adams–Stokes syndrome, acute intermittent porphyria
Drug interactions	Chlordiazepoxide, chloramphenicol, chlorambucil
Remarks	Indicated as substitute for oral phenytoin where intravenous phenytoin is not available/possible

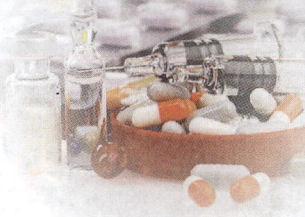

Furosemide

Drug name	Furosemide
Category	Loop diuretic
Route	Oral, Intravenous
Strength	Tab (40 mg); Inj (20 mg/2 mL); Drops (10 mg/mL)
Brands	Furoped (Drops), Lasix (Inj, Tab), Frusenex (Tab)
Mechanism of action	Inhibits active chloride transport in the thick ascending limb thereby decreasing reabsorption of sodium and chloride from the nephron
Pharmacokinetics	Around 60–65% absorption after oral intake. Terminal half-life 1½ hours
Indications	Edema; Hypertension; Fluid overload
Dosage as per indications	• *Neonates:* 0.5–1 mg/kg/dose q 8–24 h • *Maximum PO dose in newborn:* 6 mg/kg/dose. • *Children:* 0.5–2 mg/kg/dose q 6–12 h; or continuous IV infusion 0.05–1 mg/kg/h
Maximum dosage	*Intravenous:* 2 mg/kg/dose
Dose adjustments	Renal impairment
Adverse effects	Hypokalemia, alkalosis, dehydration, hyperuricemia, hypercalciuria
Contraindications	Shock, hypersensitivity
Drug interactions	Aminoglycosides
Remarks	Prolonged use in preterm neonates can cause nephrocalcinosis. In the presence of renal disease, it can cause ototoxicity when used with aminoglycosides

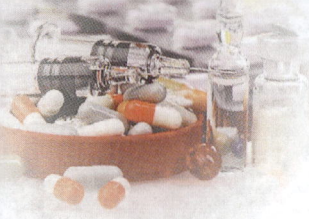

Gabapentin

Drug name	Gabapentin
Category	Anticonvulsant
Route	Oral
Strength	Caps (100 mg, 250 mg, 300 mg, 400 mg, 450 mg, 600 mg, 800 mg)
Brands	Gabapin (Cap), Neurontin (Cap), Progaba (Cap)
Mechanism of action	It acts by binding to α2δ (alpha-2-delta) subunit of voltage-gated calcium channels in brain
Pharmacokinetics	Following oral administration, peak plasma levels attained in 2–3 hours
Indications	Partial seizures; Refractory seizures
Dosage as per indications	Add on therapy for partial seizures. 15–35 mg/kg/day q 8 h. Can increase over several days to 50 mg/kg/day
Maximum dosage	2,400–3,600 mg/day
Dose adjustments	Adjust dose in renal impairment
Adverse effects	Somnolence, dizziness, ataxia, fatigue, nystagmus
Contraindications	Hypersensitivity
Drug interactions	Increased sedation with opioids
Remarks	Do not stop the drug abruptly

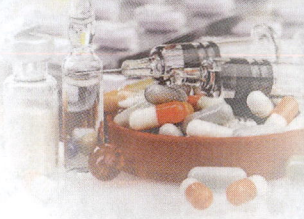

Ganciclovir

Drug name	Ganciclovir
Category	Antiviral, Synthetic analog of 2′-deoxyguanosine
Route	Oral, Intravenous
Strength	Cap (250 mg, 500 mg); Inj (500 mg)
Brands	Ganguard (Cap, Inj), Cymevene (Cap, Inj)
Mechanism of action	It has a virustatic effect. It inhibits viral DNA synthesis by preventing attachment of deoxyguanosine triphosphate into DNA by attaching ganciclovir triphosphate into viral DNA
Pharmacokinetics	Poor oral absorption. Mainly eliminated by renal route via glomerular filtration and active tubular secretion
Indications	CMV retinitis
Dosage as per indications	• 5 mg/kg/dose 12 hourly IV infusion during induction phase followed by 5 mg/kg/dose IV infusion OD during maintenance phase of treatment of CMV retinitis in immunocompromised hosts. • *For severe infections:* 10 mg/kg/dose q 8 h IV for 14 days
Maximum dosage	1000 mg/day
Dose adjustments	Dose adjustment needed in renal impairment
Adverse effects	Nephrotoxicity, neutropenia, thrombocytopenia, retinal detachment, confusion
Contraindications	Hypersensitivity
Drug interactions	Probenecid, didanosine, zidovudine, imipenem-cilastatin
Remarks	Minimum dilution is 10 mg/mL. Do not use subcutaneous and intramuscular routes

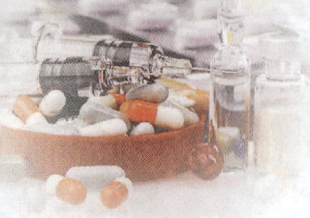

Gatifloxacin

Drug name	Gatifloxacin
Category	Antibiotic, Fluoroquinolone
Route	Oral
Strength	Tab (200 mg, 400 mg)
Brands	Aristogaticin (Tab), G-flox (Tab), Gabact (Tab)
Mechanism of action	Inhibition of DNA gyrase and topoisomerase 4
Pharmacokinetics	Well absorbed after oral administration with high bioavailability. Peak levels seen 1–2 hours after oral administration, poorly protein bound, mainly excreted by kidney in unchanged form
Indications	Active against gram-positive; Gram-negative bacteria
Dosage as per indications	10 mg/kg/dose OD
Maximum dosage	400 mg/day
Dose adjustments	Needed in renal derangement, not needed in mild to moderate hepatic derangement. Not known in patients with severe hepatic derangement
Adverse effects	Dysglycemia
Contraindications	Hypersensitivity
Drug interactions	10 mg/kg/dose OD
Remarks	400 mg/day

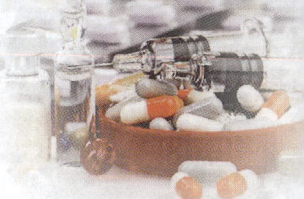

Gentamicin Sulfate

Drug name	Gentamicin sulfate
Category	Antibiotic, Aminoglycoside
Route	Intravenous, Intramuscular
Strength	Inj (10 mg/mL, 40 mg/mL ampoules)
Brands	Biogaracin (Inj), Gentacip (Inj), Gentapar (Inj)
Mechanism of action	Bactericidal. Binds with the proteins of the 30S subunits of the bacterial ribosomes, acts in proliferation and resting phase
Pharmacokinetics	• Mainly eliminated in the urine by glomerular filtration • *Half-life:* 2–3 hours
Indications	Gram-negative infections; UTI
Dosage as per indications	• 5.0–7.5 mg/kg/day q 8–12 h • *Intrathecal/intraventricular:* >3 months: 1–2 mg OD, adults: 4–8 mg OD
Maximum dosage	• *<10 years:* 320 mg/day • *>10 years:* 640 mg/day
Dose adjustments	Adjust dose in renal failure
Adverse effects	Nephrotoxicity, ototoxicity
Contraindications	Hypersensitivity
Drug interactions	Concurrent administration with other nephrotoxic/ototoxic drugs like aminoglycosides, NM blocking drugs, diuretics
Remarks	Use cautiously in patients receiving loop diuretics. It is eliminated faster in patients with burns

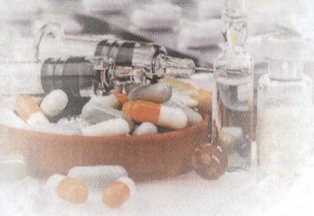

Glucagon Hydrochloride

Drug name	Glucagon hydrochloride
Category	Antihypoglycemic agent
Route	Intramuscular, Subcutaneous, Intravenous
Strength	Inj (1 mg/vial)
Brands	GlucaGen (Inj), HypoKit (Inj)
Mechanism of action	Converts liver glycogen to blood glucose
Pharmacokinetics	Half-life after IV administration: 8–18 minutes, degraded in liver, kidney and plasma
Indications	Refractory/resistant hypoglycemia
Dosage as per indications	*<25 kg:* 0.5 mg *>25 kg:* 1 mg
Maximum dosage	Not known
Dose adjustments	Preferable to start at low dose in renal and hepatic derangement
Adverse effects	Nausea, vomiting, urticaria, respiratory distress
Contraindications	Hypersensitivity, pheochromocytoma
Drug interactions	Beta blockers
Remarks	Always also administer glucose IV for hypoglycemia

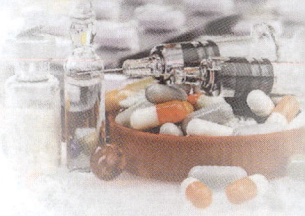

Granisetron

Drug name	Granisetron
Category	Antiemetic, 5HT3 antagonist
Route	Intravenous, Oral
Strength	Tab (1 mg); Inj (1 mg/mL)
Brands	Grandem (Inj, Tab), Granicip (Inj, Tab)
Mechanism of action	Antagonizes 5-hydroxytryptamine type 3 (5-HT3) receptors located peripherally on vagal nerve terminals and centrally in the chemoreceptor trigger zone of the area postrema
Pharmacokinetics	65% bound to plasma proteins, has hepatic metabolism via cytochrome P-450
Indications	Chemotherapy-induced nausea and vomiting (CINV)
Dosage as per indications	*Children ≥2 years and adults:* 10–20 µg/kg/dose IV over 15–60 minutes before chemotherapy; may repeat two three times after chemotherapy. Alternately, single dose of 40 µg/kg/dose PO 15–60 minutes before starting chemotherapy In adults 1 mg BD or 2 mg OD, started 1 hour prior to chemotherapy
Maximum dosage	Not known
Dose adjustments	Use cautiously in patients with liver disease, no renal adjustment needed
Adverse effects	Hypertension, hypotension, arrhythmia, agitation, insomnia
Contraindications	Hypersensitivity
Drug interactions	With drugs known to prolong QT interval

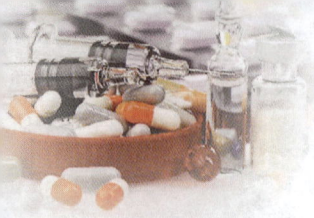

Granulocyte Colony-Stimulating Factor (G-CSF)

Drug name	Granulocyte colony-stimulating factor (G-CSF)
Category	Growth factor
Route	Subcutaneous
Strength	Inj (300 μg vial)
Brands	Filgrastim (Inj), Neupogen (Inj), Neukine (Inj)
Mechanism of action	Regulates neutrophil progenitor proliferation within the bone marrow and selected end-cell functional activation
Pharmacokinetics	Not much known elimination half-life 3.5 hours
Indications	Severe neutropenia
Dosage as per indications	5–10 μg/kg/day SC
Maximum dosage	Not known
Dose adjustments	Not known
Adverse effects	Bone pain, local tenderness, nausea
Contraindications	Avoid in myeloid malignancies
Drug interactions	Lithium
Remarks	To mobilize peripheral blood progenitor cells for hematopoietic stem cell transplantation and granulocytes for apheresis collection, and to decrease the duration of neutropenia after chemotherapy and to offset the neutropenia due to myelodysplasia, acquired immunodeficiency syndrome, and genetic disorders of granulocyte production

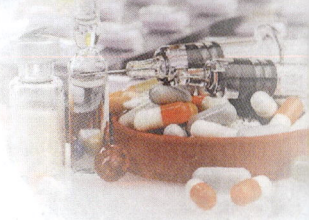

Griseofulvin

Drug name	Griseofulvin
Category	Antifungal
Route	Oral
Strength	Tab (125 mg, 250 mg, 500 mg)
Brands	Dermonorm (Tab), Grisovin FP (Tab)
Mechanism of action	Binds to tubulin, and interferes in microtubule function. This leads to inhibition of meiosis and cell division
Pharmacokinetics	Less than 50% of the oral dose is absorbed. The terminal plasma half-life lies between 10 and 20 hours, mostly excreted in the urine
Indications	Tinea capitis; Tinea unguium
Dosage as per indications	10 mg/kg/day q 6–12 h. The treatment duration is 4–6 weeks for tinea capitis and 4–6 months for tinea unguium
Maximum dosage	500 mg/day
Dose adjustments	No renal adjustment
Adverse effects	Leukopenia, allergy, photosensitivity
Contraindications	Contraindicated in porphyria and hepatic disease
Drug interactions	Phenobarbitone, cyclosporine, coumarin anticoagulants
Remarks	Absorption increases with fatty food

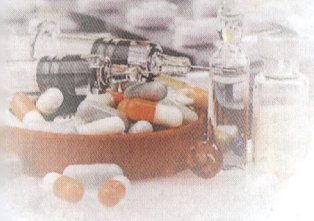

Haloperidol

Drug name	Haloperidol
Category	Antipsychotic, Butyrophenones group
Route	Oral, Intramuscular
Strength	Tab (0.25 mg, 1.5 mg, 5 mg, 10 mg); Syp (2 mg/mL); Inj (5 mg/mL)
Brands	Depidol (Tab, Inj), Halo (Tab, Inj), Serenace (Tab, Syp)
Mechanism of action	Central dopamine type 2 receptor antagonist, with low alpha-1 antiadrenergic activity and no antihistaminergic or anticholinergic activity
Pharmacokinetics	The average bioavailability after oral administration is 60–70%. Peak plasma levels attained within 2–6 hours of oral dosing. Average half-life is 24 hours
Indications	Psychosis; Autism; Tourette syndrome
Dosage as per indications	3–13 years: • *Antipsychotic:* 0.05–0.15 mg/kg/day q 8–12 h PO • *Acute agitation:* 0.01–0.03 mg/kg/day q 8–12 h PO • *Infantile autism:* 0.025–0.05 mg/kg/day q 8–12 h PO • *Tourette syndrome:* 0.05–0.075 mg/kg/day q 8–12 hourly • Initial dose not >0.5 mg/day, can be increased by 0.25–0.5 mg/day every 5–7 days >13 years: • *Acute agitation/psychosis:* 1–15 mg/dose PO • *Tourette syndrome:* 0.5–2 mg/dose BID–TID PO
Maximum dosage	<18 years: 5 mg/day, >18 years: 10–20 mg/day depending upon the condition for which treatment is being received
Dose adjustments	Dose adjustment in hepatic and severe renal impairment
Adverse effects	Extrapyramidal effects, drowsiness, headache, tachycardia, nausea, vomiting, ECG changes, acute oculogyric effects

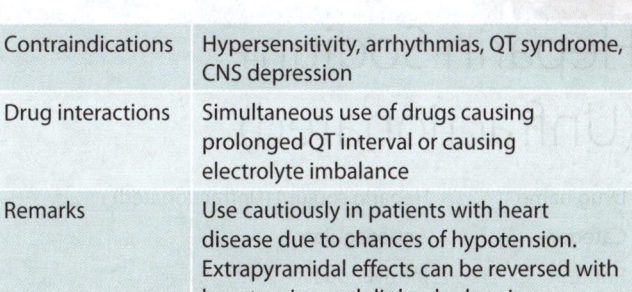

Contraindications	Hypersensitivity, arrhythmias, QT syndrome, CNS depression
Drug interactions	Simultaneous use of drugs causing prolonged QT interval or causing electrolyte imbalance
Remarks	Use cautiously in patients with heart disease due to chances of hypotension. Extrapyramidal effects can be reversed with benztropine and diphenhydramine

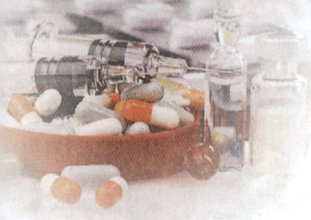

Heparin Sodium (Unfractionated)

Drug name	Heparin sodium (Unfractionated)
Category	Anticoagulant
Route	Intravenous
Strength	Inj (5,000 U/5 mL; 120 U = approximately 1 mg)
Brands	Hibor (Inj), Declot (Inj), Keparin (Inj)
Mechanism of action	Inhibits activated coagulation factors, including thrombin and factor X
Pharmacokinetics	Heparin is not absorbed from the gastrointestinal tract. Heparin and its metabolites are excreted in the urine. The half-life of heparin depends on the dose administered
Indications	As anticoagulant in thrombosis treatment; Extracorporeal membrane oxygenation (ECMO); Maintaining patency of central/arterial line
Dosage as per indications	*Dose for anticoagulation in infants and children:* • *Initial:* 50 U/kg bolus • *Maintenance:* 10–25 U/kg/h as IV infusion or 50–100 U/kg/dose q 4 h IV • *ECMO:* 50 U/kg intravenous bolus loading; 15–35 U/kg/h intravenous infusion • *Heparin flush:* Peripheral IV: 1–2 mL of 10 U/mL solution q 4 h; central line: 2–3 mL of 100 U/mL solution q 24 h; TPN (central line) and arterial line: Add heparin to make final concentration of 0.5–1 U/mL
Maximum dosage	>1 year: 7,700 U/day
Dose adjustments	Patients with increased risk of bleeding complications, elderly, hypertension, renal or hepatic insufficiency
Adverse effects	Bleeding, allergy, thrombocytopenia
Contraindications	Hypersensitivity
Drug interactions	Dicoumarol or warfarin sodium, angiotensin-converting enzyme (ACE) inhibitors, nitrates

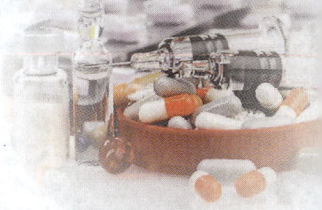

Remarks	• Monitoring based on APTT, therapeutic range 1.5–2.5 times normal. APPT is best measured 6–8 hours after initiation of changes in solution • *Antidote for heparin overdose/toxicity:* Protamine sulfate (1 mg per 100 U heparin in previous 4 hours) • Use preservative-free heparin in neonates

Heparin Sodium (Unfractionated)

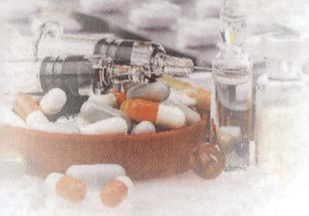

Heparin, Low Molecular Weight (Enoxaparin)

Drug name	Heparin, low molecular weight (Enoxaparin)
Category	Anticoagulant
Route	Subcutaneous
Strength	Inj (40 mg/0.4 mL, 30 mg/0.3 mL)
Brands	Clexane (Inj), Enoxarin (Inj), Thrombiflo (Inj)
Mechanism of action	Inhibits thrombosis by inactivating factor Xa. It does not affect bleeding time, platelet function, PT, or aPTT at recommended doses
Pharmacokinetics	Bioavailability is nearly 100% after SC Inj, based on anti-Xa activity. Mainly metabolized in the liver. Elimination half-life: 5–7 hours after SC Inj
Indications	Deep vein thrombosis (DVT)
Dosage as per indications	*DVT treatment:* • *Infants:* 1.5 mg/kg q 12 h SC • *Children and adults:* 1 mg/kg q 12 h SC
Maximum dosage	100 mg/dose
Dose adjustments	Renal and hepatic dysfunction
Adverse effects	Fever, confusion, edema, nausea, hemorrhage, thrombocytopenia
Contraindications	• Major bleeding and drug-induced thrombocytopenia • Use with caution in uncontrolled arterial hypertension, bleeding diathesis, history of recurrent GI ulcers, diabetic retinopathy, and severe renal dysfunction
Drug interactions	NSAIDS, other anticoagulants
Remarks	• Concurrent use with spinal or epidural anesthesia, or spinal puncture has resulted in long-term or permanent paralysis; potential benefits must be weighed against the risks • Monitoring based on antifactor Xa assay, therapeutic range 0.3–0.7 U/mL • Protamine sulfate is the antidote; 1 mg protamine sulfate neutralizes 1 mg enoxaparin

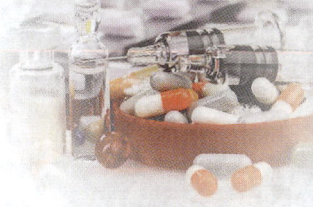

Hepatitis B Immunoglobulin (HBIG)

Drug name	Hepatitis B immunoglobulin (HBIG)
Category	Immunoglobulin (Human)
Route	Intramuscular, Intravenous
Strength	Inj (160 mg/mL, 200 IU/mL vials)
Brands	Bayhep B (Inj), HepaGam B (Inj), HyperHEP B (Inj), Nabi-HB (Inj)
Mechanism of action	Contains immunoglobulin G (IgG) with specifically high content of antibodies against hepatitis B virus surface antigen (HBs)
Pharmacokinetics	After an intramuscular dose, the drug is available in body's circulation after 2–3 days with a maximum half-life of 3–4 weeks
Indications	Prevention of hepatitis B following exposure
Dosage as per indications	• Newborn 0.5 mL IM up to 72 hours of birth, preferably within 12 hours of birth • Children 0.06 mL/kg single dose IM
Maximum dosage	500 IU/dose
Dose adjustments	None
Adverse effects	Flu-like symptoms, cold, nausea, vomiting, diarrhea, tremors, sore throat, rash
Contraindications	Hypersensitivity
Drug interactions	Live vaccines
Remarks	Active immunization should be initiated simultaneously. The vaccine and HBIG should be administered in separate thighs

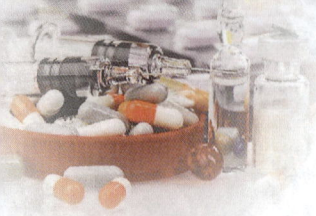

Human Milk Fortifier

Drug name	Human milk fortifier
Category	Nutritional supplement
Route	Oral
Strength	• 1 Sachet (1 g)—Contains whey proteins, milk solids, vitamins, minerals, medium chain triglycerides, emulsifiers, maltodextrins. • When 4 Sachets are mixed with 100 mL milk, an average amount of individual contents is as below: Energy: 150 Kcal, proteins: 4 g, calcium: 155 mg, phosphorous: 85 mg, iron 2.3 mg
Brands	Lactodex-HMF
Mechanism of action	Added to breast milk to make it energy dense along with adequate vitamin and mineral supplementation
Pharmacokinetics	Not known
Indications	To optimize nutrition of preterm infants who are unable to meet the required nutritional requirements with mother's feed alone
Dosage as per indications	1 sachet (1 g) to be mixed well with 25 mL of EBM before giving. Dosage to be individualized for each baby after calculating the required calorie, protein and fat requirement
Maximum dosage	Not known
Dose adjustments	Not known
Adverse effects	Delayed gastric emptying, feed intolerance, nephrocalcinosis, necrotizing enterocolitis, faster weight gain than required may lead to increased risk of cardiometabolic diseases
Contraindications	Hypersensitivity, feed intolerance
Drug interactions	Not known
Remarks	• Other vitamin and mineral supplementation should be done only if required, after calculating the total doses being received with addition of HMF to breast milk • To be started only after feeds reach 100 mL/kg/day • Regular monitoring of calcium, phosphorous and ALP should be done to avoid risk of nephrocalcinosis • Close growth monitoring to be done to avoid undernutrition or overnutrition

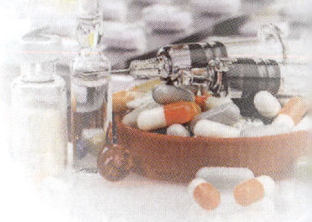

Hydralazine Hydrochloride

Drug name	Hydralazine hydrochloride
Category	Antihypertensive, Arterial vasodilator
Route	Oral, Intravenous
Strength	Tab (10 mg, 25 mg); Inj (20 mg/mL ampoule)
Brands	Corbetazine (Tab), Dralgeen (Inj)
Mechanism of action	Directly acting vasodilator mainly on the arterioles, resulting in low peripheral resistance and decreased arterial blood pressure. The use of hydralazine can result in sodium and fluid retention, producing edema and reduced urinary volume
Pharmacokinetics	Rapid and complete absorption after oral intake. Peak plasma levels noted in 30–90 minutes with plasma half-life 2–3 hours
Indications	Hypertensive crisis; Chronic hypertension
Dosage as per indications	• *Hypertensive crisis:* 0.1–0.2 mg/kg/dose IM or IV q 4–6 h, maximum 20 mg/dose • *Chronic hypertension:* Start at 0.75–1 mg/kg/day PO q 6–12 h (maximum 25 mg/dose). Can increase if needed to 5 mg/kg/day for infants, and 7.5 mg/kg/day for older children
Maximum dosage	• *IV:* 20 mg/dose • *Oral:* Starting maximum 25 mg/dose. Can be increased to maximum 200 mg/day
Dose adjustments	Needed in renal and hepatic impairment
Adverse effects	Lupus-like syndrome may be seen in patients with renal impairment. May cause reflex tachycardia, headache, hypotension, nausea, diarrhea, peripheral neuropathy
Contraindications	Hypersensitivity, severe tachycardia, high output heart failure, porphyria
Drug interactions	Antihypertensives, anesthetics, tricyclic antidepressants, drugs with central depressant effect, MAO inhibitors
Remarks	Use with caution in severe renal and cardiac disease

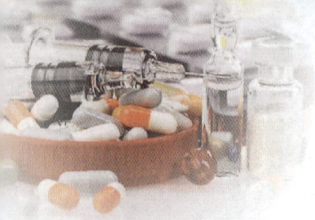

Hydrochlorothiazide

Drug name	Hydrochlorothiazide
Category	Thiazide
Route	Oral
Strength	Tab (25 mg, 50 mg)
Brands	Aquazide (Tab), Bpzide (Tab), Hydride (Tab)
Mechanism of action	It acts on the distal renal tubular and affects electrolyte reabsorption. It causes natriuresis. After oral use, diuresis begins within 2 hours, peaks in about 4 hours and lasts about 6–12 hours
Pharmacokinetics	Onset of action: 2 hours, peak: 4 hours, total duration: 6–12 hours, poorly metabolized, eliminated by kidneys. *Half-life:* 5–15 hours
Indications	Hypertension
Dosage as per indications	Antihypertensive, diuretic 2–4 mg/kg/day q 12 h, PO
Maximum dosage	• <2 years: 37.5 mg/day • 2–12 years: 100 mg/day
Dose adjustments	Use with caution in liver and renal disease
Adverse effects	Hyperuricemia, fluid, and electrolyte disturbances
Contraindications	Anuria, hypersensitivity
Drug interactions	Antihypertensives, antidiabetics, corticosteroids, NSAIDs
Remarks	May not be effective in patients with impaired creatinine clearance

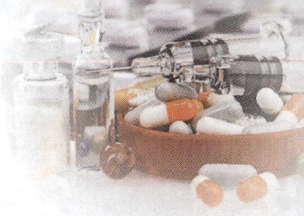

Hydrocortisone Sodium Succinate

Drug name	Hydrocortisone sodium succinate
Category	Steroid
Route	Intravenous, Oral
Strength	Inj (100 mg); Tab (5 mg, 10 mg)
Brands	Effcorlin (Inj), Histone (Tab), Primacort (Inj)
Mechanism of action	Acts by its metabolic and anti-inflammatory actions
Pharmacokinetics	Readily absorbed from gut. On intravenous administration, clinical effect is noted within 1 hour. Drug is eliminated mainly in urine, in around 12 hours. *Half-life:* 120–150 minutes, mainly excreted in urine
Indications	Asthma; Shock; Congenital adrenal hyperplasia (CAH)

Dosage as per indications	• *Asthma:*
	  – *Loading:* 4–8 mg/kg/dose IV, max: 250 mg
	  – *Maintenance:* 8 mg/kg/day divided 6-hourly IV
	• *Acute adrenal insufficiency:* 50 mg/m²/day
	• *CAH:* 10–15 mg/m²/day
	• *Anti-inflammatory:* 2.5–10 mg/kg/day divided 6-hourly

Maximum dosage	250 mg (IV) loading dose
Dose adjustments	Not known
Adverse effects	As other steroids
Contraindications	Hypersensitivity
Drug interactions	As other steroids
Remarks	Do not withdraw abruptly if given for >10–15 days

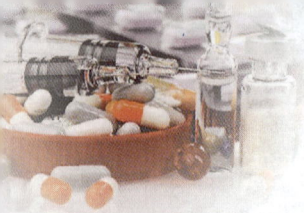

Hydroxyzine Hydrochloride

Drug name	Hydroxyzine hydrochloride
Category	Antihistamine
Route	Oral, Intramuscular
Strength	Tab (10 mg, 25 mg); Syp (10 mg/5 mL); Inj (25 mg/mL); Drops (6 mg/mL)
Brands	Atarax (Tab, Syp, Drops, Inj), H-Zine (Tab, Syp, Drops), Prugo (Tab, Syp)
Mechanism of action	Suppression of activity in certain key regions of the subcortical area of the central nervous system
Pharmacokinetics	Rapidly absorbed from GI tract, effect noted within 15–30 minutes of intake
Indications	Allergic manifestations; Anxiety
Dosage as per indications	Anxiolytic 0.6 mg/kg/dose q 6 h PO or 0.5–1 mg/kg/dose q 6 h intramuscular
Maximum dosage	2 mg/kg/day to max of 100 mg/day
Dose adjustments	Dose adjustment in hepatic and renal impairment
Adverse effects	Dry mouth, drowsiness, tremor, convulsions, blurred vision, hypotension
Contraindications	Any patient with underlying risk of QT prolongation, torsades de pointes
Drug interactions	Antidepressants, sedatives, drugs affecting QT interval
Remarks	Do not administer IV

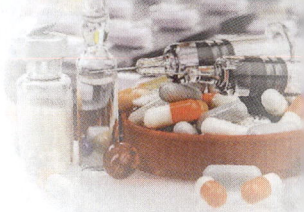

Hyoscine Butylbromide

Drug name	Hyoscine butylbromide
Category	Anticholinergic
Route	Oral, Intravenous, Intramuscular
Strength	Tab (10 mg); Inj (20 mg/mL)
Brands	Buscopan (Tab, Inj), Hyocimax (Tab, Inj), Buscogast (Tab, Inj)
Mechanism of action	It inhibits muscarinic actions of acetylcholine at postganglionic parasympathetic neuroeffector sites
Pharmacokinetics	Rapidly absorbed after IV or IM Inj. Crosses blood–brain barrier, metabolized by the liver, mainly excreted in the urine
Indications	Antispasmodic
Dosage as per indications	6–12 years: 10 mg/dose q 8 h PO, or 10–20 mg IV, IM bolus
Maximum dosage	20 mg/dose
Dose adjustments	Renal and hepatic impairment needs dose adjustment
Adverse effects	Glaucoma, dry mouth, dry skin, blurred vision, diarrhea, palpitations, flushing, difficulty in urinating
Contraindications	Porphyria, myasthenia gravis, glaucoma, and achalasia
Drug interactions	Tricyclic antidepressants, monoamine oxidase inhibitors (MAOIs), antihistamines, quinidine, amantadine, antipsychotics, nitrates, beta-adrenergic agents, metoclopramide, and domperidone

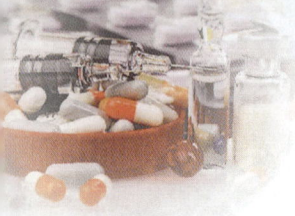

Ibuprofen

Drug name	Ibuprofen
Category	Nonsteroidal anti-inflammatory drug (NSAID)
Route	Oral, Intravenous
Strength	Syp (100 mg/5 mL); Tab (200 mg); Inj (10 mg/mL in 2 mL vials)
Brands	Ibugesic (Tab, Inj, Syp), Brufen (Tab, Inj, Syp), Cipgesic (Tab)
Mechanism of action	Has anti-inflammatory, analgesic and antipyretic action by inhibiting cyclo-oxygenase activity required for prostaglandin synthesis. It also inhibits ADP (adenosine diphosphate) or collagen stimulated platelet aggregation
Pharmacokinetics	Rapidly absorbed from the gut, peak serum levels: 1–2 hours after intake. Highly bound to plasma proteins. It is metabolized in the liver with an elimination half-life of around 2.5 hours. Predominantly excreted (90%) by the kidneys
Indications	Fever; Analgesia; Patent ductus arteriosus (PDA); JIA
Dosage as per indications	• *Fever/analgesia:* 10–15 mg/kg/dose q 4–6 h, maximum 40 mg/kg/day • *For JIA:* 30–70 mg/kg/day q 4–6 h PO • *Ductus closure:* 10 mg/kg IV followed by 5 mg/kg IV every 24 hours for 2 doses
Maximum dosage	40 mg/kg/day or 2400 mg/day
Dose adjustments	Hepatic and renal dysfunction
Adverse effects	Abdominal cramps, nausea, heartburn, fluid retention
Contraindications	Active GI bleeding and ulceration
Drug interactions	Increased risk of bleeding with other NSAIDs, corticosteroids, anticoagulants

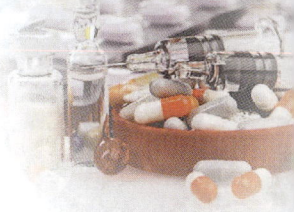

IgM Enriched Immunoglobulin

Drug name	IgM enriched immunoglobulin
Category	Immunoglobulin
Route	Intravenous
Strength	Inj (each mL has 50 mg plasma protein contains 6 mg IgM, 6 mg IgA, 38 mg IgG vial)
Brands	Pentaglobin
Mechanism of action	It is an IgM rich immunoglobulin. It has more potent antibacterial and immunomodulatory actions compared to normal immunoglobulin
Pharmacokinetics	Not known
Indications	Severe bacterial infection; Severe secondary immunodeficiency
Dosage as per indications	5 mL (0.25 g)/kg once a day for 3 days
Maximum dosage	Not known
Dose adjustments	Not needed in hepatic derangement. Not to be given in renal insufficiency
Adverse effects	Acute renal failure, thromboembolism, hemolytic disease, decreased leukocyte count, transient aseptic meningitis
Contraindications	Hypersensitivity, patients with selective IgA deficiency who developed antibodies to IgA
Drug interactions	Live vaccines, loop diuretics

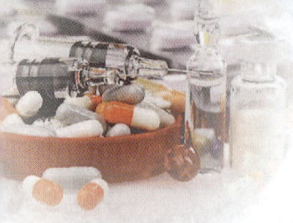

Imipenem-Cilastatin

Drug name	Imipenem-cilastatin
Category	Antibiotic (Carbapenem antibiotic and dehydropeptidase inhibitor combination)
Route	Intravenous
Strength	Inj (250 mg, 500 mg vials)
Brands	Carbinem (Inj), Cilanem (Inj), Iminem (Inj), Primaxin (Inj)
Mechanism of action	Bactericidal, inhibits bacterial cell wall synthesis in gram-positive and gram-negative bacteria through binding to penicillin-binding proteins (PBPs). Cilastatin sodium reversibly inhibits dehydropeptidase-I, thereby preventing metabolism and inactivation of imipenem in kidney
Pharmacokinetics	Peak concentration achieved in 20–30 minutes. Half-life for imipenem or cilastatin: 1 hour. Protein binding for imipenem is 20% and cilastatin is 40%
Indications	Drug of choice for extended-spectrum beta-lactamase (ESBL) producing microorganisms
Dosage as per indications	60–100 mg/kg/day q 6 h IV
Maximum dosage	4 g/day
Dose adjustments	Renal
Adverse effects	Pruritus, urticaria, GI symptoms, seizures, dizziness, hypotension, elevated LFTs, blood dyscrasias
Contraindications	Hypersensitivity, newborns
Drug interactions	Valproate, oral anticoagulants
Remarks	The drug is not preferred in infants and young children

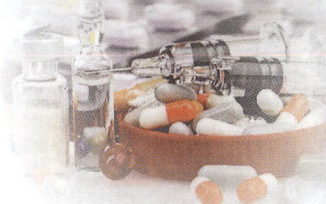

Imipramine Hydrochloride

Drug name	Imipramine hydrochloride
Category	Antidepressant
Route	Oral
Strength	Tab (25 mg, 75 mg)
Brands	Antidep (Tab), Depsonil (Tab), Depsin (Tab)
Mechanism of action	It blocks uptake of norepinephrine and serotonin at nerve endings
Pharmacokinetics	Rapidly and well absorbed when taken orally, peak levels in 2–6 hours, highly protein bound, mostly metabolized in liver, mainly excreted in the urine. *Half-life:* 12 hours
Indications	Depression; Childhood enuresis
Dosage as per indications	Given in children >6 years • *Depression:* 0.5 mg/kg/dose 8 hourly; increase gradually till max of 5 mg/kg/day • *Nocturnal enuresis:* Start with 10–25 mg/day can be increased over few weeks till 50–75 mg/day
Maximum dosage	*For depression:* • *Child:* 5 mg/kg/day; adolescent 100–200 mg/day *For enuresis:* • *6–12 years:* Lesser of 2.5 mg/kg/day or 50 mg/day • *>12 years:* 75 mg/24 h
Dose adjustments	Should be used with caution in patients with significantly impaired renal or hepatic function
Adverse effects	Arrhythmia, conduction defects, ECG changes
Contraindications	Concomitant use of monoamine oxidase inhibiting compounds
Drug interactions	TCAs, decongestants, MAO inhibitors

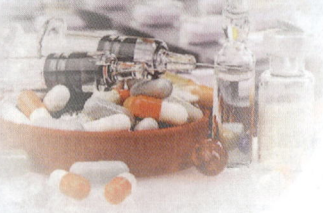

Indinavir

Drug name	Indinavir
Category	Antiretroviral, Protease inhibitor
Route	Oral
Strength	Tab (400 mg)
Brands	Indivan (Tab), Indivir (Tab)
Mechanism of action	It inhibits the activity of HIV-1 protease enzyme leading to formation of immature noninfectious viral particles
Pharmacokinetics	Rapid absorption, peak levels: 1 hour, >50% protein bound, half-life: 2 hours
Indications	AIDS/HIV infection
Dosage as per indications	234–500 mg/m^2 BSA along with ritonavir
Maximum dosage	800 mg/dose 8 hourly
Dose adjustments	Needed in hepatic derangement, not known in renal derangement
Adverse effects	Nausea, pain abdomen, headache, metallic taste, hyperbilirubinemia, lipid abnormalities, rash, stone formation
Contraindications	Not approved in <1 year. Generally avoided in children
Drug interactions	Midazolam, astemizole, ergot derivatives, sildenafil
Remarks	Fasting increases absorption

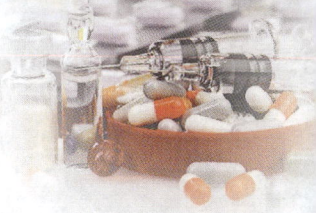

Indomethacin

Drug name	Indomethacin
Category	Nonsteroidal anti-inflammatory ©drug (NSAID)
Route	Oral, Intravenous
Strength	Cap (25 mg, 50 mg); Inj (1 mg)
Brands	Indocap (Cap), Indoflam (Cap), Artisid (Cap). Inj not available
Mechanism of action	Inhibits prostaglandin synthetase, preventing prostaglandin synthesis. This leads to anti-inflammatory, antipyretic, and analgesic effects
Pharmacokinetics	Rapid and complete absorption when orally administered, peak plasma levels: 30–120 minutes. Highly bound to plasma proteins
Indications	Analgesia; Fever; Closure of patent ductus arteriosus (PDA)
Dosage as per indications	• *Analgesia/fever:* 3 mg/kg/day q 8 h • *For duct closure in preterm neonate:* 0.2 mg/kg/dose IV 8 hours for three doses
Maximum dosage	200 mg/day oral
Dose adjustments	Dose adjustment in renal and cardiac impairment
Adverse effects	Decreased urine output, platelet dysfunction, decreased GI blood flow
Contraindications	Avoid in neonates with NEC, poor renal function, or active bleeding
Drug interactions	Other NSAIDs, cardiac glycosides, diuretics, antihypertensives

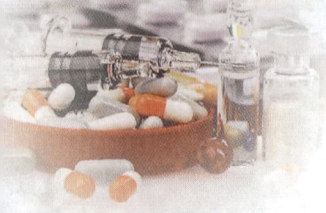

Insulin

Drug name	Insulin
Category	Antidiabetic
Route	Intravenous, Subcutaneous
Strength	Inj (40 IU/mL, 80 IU/mL, 100 IU/mL)
Brands	Actrapid, Huminsulin, Human Insulatard, Mixtard, Lantus
Mechanism of action	It lowers blood glucose by various mechanisms as stimulates peripheral glucose uptake, inhibits hepatic glucose production, inhibits lipolysis and proteolysis, enhances protein synthesis
Pharmacokinetics	• *Rapidly acting:* Onset: 5–15 minutes, peak effect: 1–2 hours, duration of action: 4–6 hours • *Regular:* Onset: 30 minutes, peak effect: 2–4 hours, duration of action: 6–8 hours • *Intermediate:* Onset: 1–2 hours, peak effect: 4–6 hours, duration of action: 12 hours • *Long acting:* Onset: 1.5–2 hours, peak effect: plateau effect, duration of action: 12–24 hours
Indications	Diabetes mellitus; Hyperglycemia
Dosage as per indications	• 0.7–1.5 U/kg/day • In <5 years start 0.2–0.4 U/kg/day, prepubertal: 0.5–0.8 U/kg/day, puberty: 0.8–1.5 U/kg/day • *DKA:* Start with 0.05–0.1U/kg/h
Maximum dosage	Not known
Dose adjustments	Use with caution in hepatic and liver dysfunction
Adverse effects	Hypoglycemia, hypokalemia, fluid retention, lipodystrophy
Contraindications	Hypersensitivity
Drug interactions	Drugs causing hypoglycemia

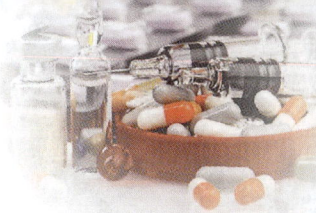

Intravenous Immunoglobulin (IVIG)

Drug name	Intravenous immunoglobulin (IVIG)
Category	Immunoglobulin (Human)
Route	Intravenous
Strength	Inj (0.25 g, 0.5 g, 1 g, 2 g, 5 g vials)
Brands	Bharglob (Inj), Gamma-Glob (Inj), Immunorel (Inj), Sandoglobulin (Inj)
Mechanism of action	Contains mainly immunoglobulin G (IgG) with a broad spectrum of antibodies against infectious agents
Pharmacokinetics	Rapid and complete bioavailability after intravenous administration
Indications	For prophylaxis and treatment of life-threatening gram-negative infections; Immunodeficiency states; Immune thrombo-cytopenic purpura (ITP); Guillain–Barré syndrome; and Kawasaki disease
Dosage as per indications	• *For Kawasaki disease/GBS:* 400 mg/kg/day IV infusion over 6 hours × 5 days, or 1 g/kg/day IV infusion over 2 hours × 2 days, or 2 g/kg IV infusion over 10–12 hours as single dose • *For acute ITP:* 0.8–1 g/kg IV as one or two doses • *For primary immunodeficiency:* 300–400 mg/kg IV once every 4 weeks
Maximum dosage	2 g/kg
Dose adjustments	None
Adverse effects	Headache, flushing, chills, myalgia, wheezing, tachycardia, lower back pain, nausea, and hypotension
Contraindications	IVIG should not be used in patients with IgA deficiency
Drug interactions	Live-attenuated virus vaccines cannot be given for 3–6 months
Remarks	• If hypotension/severe reactions happen during an infusion, the infusion should be stopped • Use with caution in patients with an increased risk of thrombosis

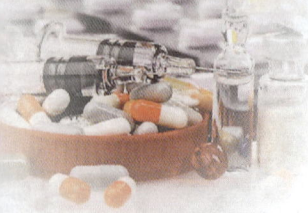

Ipratropium Bromide

Drug name	Ipratropium bromide
Category	Bronchodilator, Anticholinergic, Muscarinic antagonist
Route	Inhalation
Strength	Nebulizing sol (250 µg/mL); MDI (20 µg/puff)
Brands	Ipravent (Respule), Ipratop (Respule)
Mechanism of action	Has anticholinergic activity at the bronchial smooth muscle. Leads to bronchial smooth muscle relaxation by preventing intracellular increase in calcium
Pharmacokinetics	10–30% dose is deposited in lungs when inhaled, rest is swallowed traverses through the gut. The drug from the lungs is absorbed within minutes
Indications	Asthma
Dosage as per indications	*Nebulized dose* • *<1 year:* 125 µg/dose • *>1 year:* 250 µg/dose • *>12 years:* 500 µg/dose. Nebulized after dilution in 2–4 mL of saline and given over 10 minutes 6–8 hourly *Inhaler dose* • *<12 years:* 1–2 puffs three to four times a day • *≥12 years:* 2–3 puffs four times a day
Maximum dosage	500 µg/dose
Dose adjustments	Hypersensitivity
Adverse effects	Urinary retention, allergy, flushing, palpitations, glaucoma, blurred vision, dry mouth, headache
Contraindications	Contraindicated in glaucoma, intestinal obstruction, and achalasia
Drug interactions	Anticholinergics

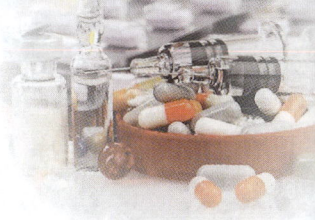

Isoniazid

Drug name	Isoniazid
Category	Antituberculous drug
Route	Oral
Strength	Tab (50 mg, 100 mg, 300 mg); Syp (100 mg/5 mL)
Brands	Isonex (Tab), Isonex forte (Tab), Solonex (Tab)
Mechanism of action	Bacteriostatic, acts on *Mycobacterium tuberculosis*
Pharmacokinetics	Rapid and complete absorption after oral administration. Plasma elimination half-life: 1.2 hours in rapid acetylators and 3.5 hours in slow acetylators. Mostly excreted in urine
Indications	Tuberculosis treatment; Prophylaxis
Dosage as per indications	8–15 mg/kg/day PO, once daily
Maximum dosage	300 mg/day
Dose adjustments	Liver dysfunction
Adverse effects	Peripheral neuropathy, optic neuritis, seizures, encephalopathy, psychosis, deranged LFTs
Contraindications	Liver failure, hypersensitivity
Drug interactions	It inhibits hepatic microsomal enzymes and decreases the dose of carbamazepine, phenytoin, and diazepam
Remarks	Change urine color to orange red

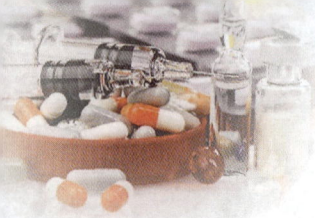

Isoprinosine (Inosine Pranobex)

Drug name	Isoprinosine (Inosine pranobex)
Category	Immunomodulator
Route	Oral
Strength	Tab (500 mg)
Brands	Inosiplex (Tab)
Mechanism of action	Increases T lymphocyte maturation and differentiation via Th1, increases IFN-γ secretion, decreases IL-4 levels
Pharmacokinetics	Rapid and complete absorption, elimination half-life: 3.5 hours, metabolized to xanthine and hypoxanthine, excreted in urine
Indications	Subacute sclerosing panencephalitis (SSPE)
Dosage as per indications	Subacute sclerosing panencephalitis 50–100 mg/kg/d q 12 h PO
Maximum dosage	4 g/day
Dose adjustments	Dose adjustment/monitoring needed in hepatic and renal derangement
Adverse effects	Transient elevation of uric acid levels in serum and urine, skin rash, GI disturbances, fatigue, nausea, arthralgia
Contraindications	Hypersensitivity, elevated uric acid/gout
Drug interactions	Xanthine oxidase inhibitors, immunomodulators
Remarks	To be taken with food

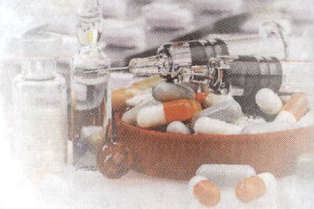

Isosorbide Dinitrate

Drug name	Isosorbide dinitrate
Category	Vasodilator
Route	Oral
Strength	Tab (5 mg, 10 mg, 20 mg)
Brands	Isordil, Sorbitrate
Mechanism of action	Acts by relaxing vascular smooth muscle leading to vasodilatation, both arterial and venous
Pharmacokinetics	Highly absorbed, but variable bioavailability. It undergoes extensive first pass metabolism, peak serum levels in an hour when taken orally
Indications	Angina pectoris
Dosage as per indications	0.1 mg/kg/day
Maximum dosage	2 mg/kg/day
Dose adjustments	In renal and hepatic dysfunction
Adverse effects	Hypotension, syncope, methemoglobinemia
Contraindications	Hypersensitivity
Drug interactions	Phosphodiesterase inhibitors, vasodilatory drugs
Remarks	Not routinely recommended in children

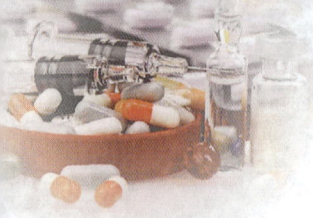

Itraconazole

Drug name	Itraconazole
Category	Antifungal, Triazole
Route	Oral, Inj
Strength	Cap (100 mg); Oral sol (10 mg/mL); Inj (10 mg/mL)
Brands	Canditral (Cap), Candistat (Cap), Sporanox (Cap)
Mechanism of action	It impairs the synthesis of ergosterol in fungal cells
Pharmacokinetics	Rapidly absorbed after oral administration, peak plasma levels: 2–5 hours after oral intake; extensively metabolized by the liver
Indications	Opportunistic fungal infections in HIV; Immunocompromised conditions
Dosage as per indications	• 200–400 mg/day q 12–24 h limited data for children • *Candida:* 5 mg/kg/day; higher doses of 5–10 mg/kg/day for treatment/prophylaxis of histoplasmosis, *Cryptococcus* and coccidioides infections
Maximum dosage	200–400 mg/day
Dose adjustments	Use with caution in renal and hepatic impairment
Adverse effects	Elevated liver enzymes, nausea, vomiting, convulsions, dry mouth, loss of appetite, mood disturbances, running nose, dizziness
Contraindications	Hypersensitivity
Drug interactions	Drugs affecting CYP3A4 enzyme
Remarks	Oral solution is used for treating oral candidiasis

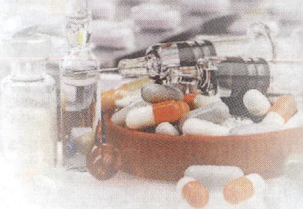

Ivermectin

Drug name	Ivermectin
Category	Antihelminthic
Route	Oral
Strength	Tab (3 mg, 6 mg, 12 mg)
Brands	Ivermect (Tab), Ivermectol (Tab), Vermectin (Tab)
Mechanism of action	Binds with glutamate-gated chloride ion channels in invertebrate nerve and muscle cells leading to increased cell membrane permeability. This causes imbalance of chloride ions leading to hyperpolarization followed by paralysis and death of parasite
Pharmacokinetics	Metabolized in liver, excreted in the feces, elimination time around 12 days. *Half-life:* 18 hours, peak serum levels: 4 hours
Indications	Scabies; Strongyloidiasis; Onchocerciasis
Dosage as per indications	• *Cutaneous larva migrans, scabies:* 0.2 mg/kg, single oral dose • *Strongyloidiasis:* 0.2 mg/kg PO for 2 days • *Onchocerciasis:* 0.15 mg/kg oral single dose
Maximum dosage	12 mg/dose
Dose adjustments	To be avoided in renal and hepatic derangement
Adverse effects	Hypotension, worsening of bronchial asthma, deranged liver enzymes
Contraindications	Hypersensitivity, contraindicated in children <6 years age or weighing <15 kg
Drug interactions	Warfarin

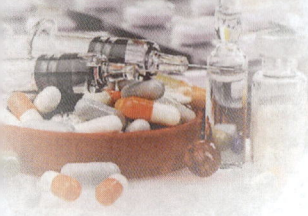

Kanamycin

Drug name	Kanamycin
Category	Antibiotic, Aminoglycoside
Route	Intravenous, Intramuscular, Oral
Strength	Inj (500 mg, 750 mg, 1 g vials)
Brands	Kanamac (Inj), Kanacin (Inj)
Mechanism of action	Binds to bacterial 30S ribosomal subunit, leading to RNA misreading
Pharmacokinetics	Not much available, rapidly absorption when given intramuscular, poor absorption orally, peak levels 1 hour after injection, half-life: 2.5 hours
Indications	Active against *Mycobacterium* infection; Gram-negative infection
Dosage as per indications	• *Used for MDR TB:* 15 mg/kg/day q 8–12 h IM, IV given over 30–60 minutes • *For bacterial overgrowth:* 150–250 mg/kg/day q 6 h PO
Maximum dosage	Not known, studies suggest 1 g/day
Dose adjustments	In renal derangement
Adverse effects	Nephrotoxic, ototoxic
Contraindications	Hypersensitivity
Drug interactions	Other nephrotoxic drugs
Remarks	Poor oral absorption. Given orally to treat bacterial overgrowth

Ketamine

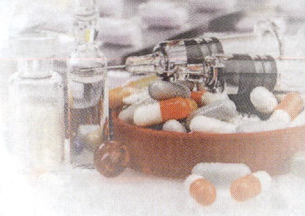

Drug name	Ketamine
Category	General anesthetic for sedation
Route	Intravenous, Intramuscular, Oral, Rectal
Strength	Inj (10 mg/mL, 50 mg/mL per vial)
Brands	Aneket (Inj), Ketalar (Inj), Ketam (Inj), Ketamax (Inj)
Mechanism of action	Acts by antagonism of N-methyl-D-aspartate (NMDA receptors) in the central nervous system producing dissociative anesthesia characterized by catalepsy, amnesia, and marked analgesia
Pharmacokinetics	Rapidly distributed all over including brain. Metabolized in liver and eliminated by kidney. Elimination half-life: 2–3 hours
Indications	Sedation
Dosage as per indications	• *For procedural sedation:* 0.5–1 mg/kg IV; 4 mg/kg IM • *IV induction:* 0.5–2 mg/kg at a rate not exceeding 0.5 mg/kg/min
Maximum dosage	4.5 mg/kg IV; 6 mg/kg IM
Dose adjustments	Dose adjustment in hepatic impairment
Adverse effects	Hallucinations, purposeless movements of limbs, raised intracranial tension, hypertension, amnesia, increased respiratory secretions
Contraindications	Hypertension, severe cardiovascular disease, stroke, brain trauma, cerebral edema, intracerebral hemorrhage, hyperthyroidism
Drug interactions	Not to be used with barbiturates, diazepam
Remarks	Rate of infusion to be <0.5 mg/kg/min, not less than 1 minute

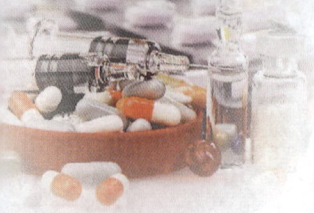

Ketoconazole

Drug name	Ketoconazole
Category	Imidazole
Route	Topical, Oral Antifungal
Strength	Tab (200 mg); also available as Cream, Shampoo, Sol for LA
Brands	Nizoral (Tab), Ketovate (Tab), Phytoral (Tab)
Mechanism of action	Blocks the synthesis of ergosterol required for cell wall synthesis by inhibiting lanosterol 14α-demethylase
Pharmacokinetics	Peak levels obtained in 1–2 hours, elimination is biphasic; first half life of 2 hours in first 10 hours and thereafter 8 hours; further metabolized and excreted mainly through bile
Indications	Fungal infection
Dosage as per indications	3.5–6.5 mg/kg/day OD
Maximum dosage	200 mg/day
Dose adjustments	Hepatic derangement
Adverse effects	Nausea, vomiting, pruritus, raised liver enzymes, headache, fever
Contraindications	Do not use it concomitantly with cisapride, terfenadine, astemizole
Drug interactions	Has many drug interactions including those affecting P450, those causing QT prolongation

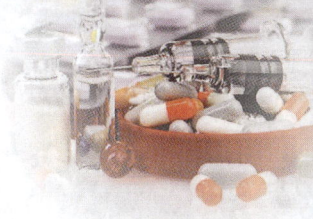

Ketotifen

Drug name	Ketotifen
Category	Antiallergic
Route	Oral
Strength	Tab (1 mg); Syp (1 mg/5 mL)
Brands	Aryfen (Tab, Syp), Asthafen (Tab), Ketasma (Tab), Ketovent (Tab)
Mechanism of action	*Inhibits:* • Effects of inflammatory mediators • Airway hyperreactivity • Accumulation of eosinophils and platelets by acting on PAF
Pharmacokinetics	High and fast absorption. High first pass metabolism leading to low bioavailability (50%). Peak plasma levels: 2–4 hours. Metabolized in liver
Indications	Add on medication for asthma
Dosage as per indications	• *6 months to 3 years:* 0.05 mg/kg • *>3 years:* 1 mg twice a day
Maximum dosage	1 mg/dose
Dose adjustments	Not known
Adverse effects	Convulsions, sedation, dry mouth, excitability, nervousness
Contraindications	Hypersensitivity
Drug interactions	Sedatives, hypnotics, oral antidiabetic agents
Remarks	Continue other medications of asthma. Tapering of steroid should be very gradual to avoid acute adrenal insufficiency

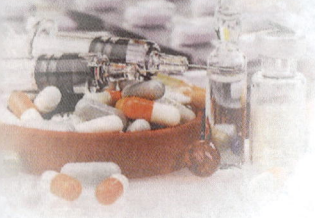

Labetalol

Drug name	Labetalol
Category	Adrenergic agonist (Alpha and beta)
Route	Oral, Intravenous
Strength	Tab (50, 100 mg); Inj (5 mg/mL ampoule)
Brands	Lobet (Tab, Inj), Normadate (Tab)
Mechanism of action	Blocks peripheral arteriolar alpha-adrenoceptors, thereby reducing the peripheral resistance, and inhibition of reflex sympathetic drive
Pharmacokinetics	Nearly 50% drug is protein bound. Well absorbed from gut after oral administration but has high first pass metabolism. Metabolized by conjugating to glucuronide metabolites, plasma half-life: 6–8 h
Indications	Hypertension; Hypertensive emergency
Dosage as per indications	• *Oral:* 2 mg/kg/dose 12 h; maximum dose 12 mg/kg/day or 1,200 mg/24 h • *Hypertensive emergency:* IV 0.2–1 mg/kg/dose q 10 min; max: 40 mg/dose Infusion: 0.4–1 mg/kg/h to maximum of 3 mg/kg/h; can initiate with 0.2–1 mg/kg bolus, maximum 40 mg bolus
Maximum dosage	• *Oral maximum dose:* 12 mg/kg/day or 1,200 mg/24 h • *IV max:* 40 mg/dose • *Infusion:* Maximum of 3 mg/kg/h; maximum 40 mg bolus
Dose adjustments	Dose adjustment needed in hepatic impairment
Adverse effects	Light headedness, cold extremities, rash, tiredness, mood changes, bradycardia
Contraindications	Contraindicated in asthma, heart block, cardiogenic shock, pulmonary edema
Drug interactions	Antiarrhythmics, calcium antagonist

Lactulose

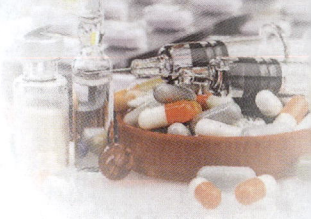

Drug name	Lactulose
Category	Synthetic sugar
Route	Oral
Strength	Syp (10 g/15 mL)
Brands	Duphalac (Syp), Livoluk (Syp), Looz (Syp)
Mechanism of action	It is formed from D-galactose and fructose. In the colon, it gets converted to short chain fatty acids by bacterial enzymes. Production of lactic acid, acetic acid, methane and hydrogen leads to a lowering of pH and increase in osmotic pressure stimulating peristalsis
Pharmacokinetics	Mainly remains unabsorbed, metabolized in the colon by the bacterial flora
Indications	Constipation
Dosage as per indications	1–2 mL/kg/day q 6–8 h
Maximum dosage	Not known
Dose adjustments	Not known
Adverse effects	Flatulence, belching, abdominal discomfort, cramps, nausea, vomiting, diarrhea
Contraindications	Hypersensitivity, inflammatory bowel disease, intestinal obstruction
Drug interactions	Thiazides, cardiac glycosides
Remarks	Antacids can decrease its efficacy, if coadministered

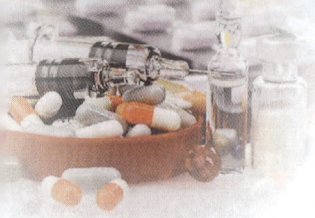

Lamivudine (3TC)

Drug name	Lamivudine (3TC)
Category	Antiretroviral, Nucleotide reverse transcriptase inhibitor (NRTI)
Route	Oral
Strength	Available in fixed dose combination with Lamivudine as Combivir (300 mg AZT + 150 mg 3TC), or with Abacavir (300 mg 3TC + 600 mg ABC), or both (150 mg 3TC + 300 mg AZT + 300 mg ABC); Tab (150 mg, 300 mg); Sol (5 mg/mL, 10 mg/mL)
Brands	Epivir (Tab), Lamivir (Tab), Lavir (Tab), Virolam (Tab)
Mechanism of action	Majority is eliminated unchanged in urine
Pharmacokinetics	Has high bioavailability, only one-third of the drug is protein bound
Indications	AIDS/HIV infection
Dosage as per indications	4 mg/kg/dose BID
Maximum dosage	150 mg/dose
Dose adjustments	Not known completely but may require adjustment in renal and hepatic derangement
Adverse effects	Headache, fatigue, nausea, diarrhea, skin rash, pancreatitis, abdominal pain, peripheral neuropathy, decreased neutrophil count, and increased liver enzymes
Contraindications	Pancreatitis, hepatic disease, and hypersensitivity to lamivudine
Drug interactions	Sorbitol

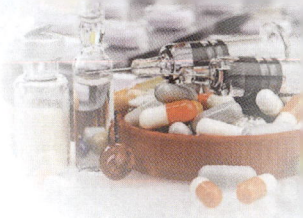

Lamotrigine

Drug name	Lamotrigine
Category	Anticonvulsant
Route	Oral
Strength	Tab (5 mg, 25 mg, 50 mg, 100 mg)
Brands	Lamepil (Tab), Lametec (Tab), Lamictal (Tab)
Mechanism of action	Voltage-dependent blockage of voltage-gated sodium channels thereby inhibiting sustained repetitive firing of neurons and release of glutamate
Pharmacokinetics	Rapidly absorbed from gut, 55% bound to plasma proteins, plasma half-life around 7 hours
Indications	Partial seizures; Generalized seizures; Atypical absence; Atonic generalized; Tonic-clonic seizures
Dosage as per indications	Start at 0.6 mg/kg/day q 12–24 h for initial 2 weeks, followed by 1.2 mg/kg/day the next for 2 weeks followed by 5–15 mg/kg/day q 12 h
Maximum dosage	15 mg/kg/day or 400 mg/day
Dose adjustments	Use with caution in renal derangement
Adverse effects	Ataxia, blurred vision, diplopia, dizziness, headache, rhinitis, rash, fever
Contraindications	Hypersensitivity
Drug interactions	Inducers or inhibitors of CYP3A4 cytochrome P450 enzyme
Remarks	• Started in low dose to lessen incidence of rash • Decrease dose to one-fourth in patients on valproate

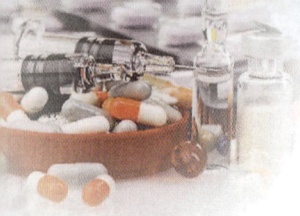

Lansoprazole Junior

Drug name	Lansoprazole Junior
Category	Proton pump inhibitor
Route	Oral
Strength	Tab (15 mg, 30 mg)
Brands	Lanzol (Tab), Lancid (Tab), Prevacid (Tab), Zapacid (Tab)
Mechanism of action	Proton pump inhibitor; dose-dependent reversible inhibition of H^+/K^+ ATPase of the parietal cells in stomach
Pharmacokinetics	High bioavailability, peak levels in 1.5–2 hours, extensively metabolized in liver, excreted by renal and biliary route
Indications	Gastritis
Dosage as per indications	1 mg/kg/day
Maximum dosage	60 mg/day; daily doses of up to 180 mg/day (not >120 mg/dose) have been tried in adults
Dose adjustments	Dose adjustment in liver derangement
Adverse effects	Headache, diarrhea, constipation, abdominal pain, nausea, drowsiness
Contraindications	Hypersensitivity
Drug interactions	Protease inhibitors, digoxin, warfarin
Remarks	Bioavailability decreases if taken after food

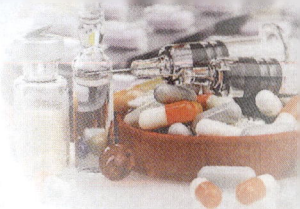

Ledipasvir/Sofosbuvir Oral

Drug name	Ledipasvir/Sofosbuvir oral
Category	Antiviral
Route	Oral
Strength	Tab (Ledipasvir 90 mg and Sofosbuvir 400 mg)
Brands	Harvoni (Tab), Ledifos (Tab)
Mechanism of action	Ledipasvir inhibits HCV NS5A protein, whereas sofosbuvir inhibits HCV NS5B RNA-dependent RNA polymerase
Pharmacokinetics	Peak levels of ledipasvir noted 4–5 hours after oral administration, whereas sofosbuvir peaks in 1 hour. Highly bound to human plasma proteins. Metabolized in the liver. Ledipasvir excreted mainly in feces, sofosbuvir excreted in urine
Indications	Hepatitis C virus (HCV) infection
Dosage as per indications	Given as fixed dose combination (FDC 90/400 mg) for treatment of genotypes 1, 4, 5, and 6 chronic hepatitis C (HCV) infection for 12–24 weeks
Maximum dosage	Not known
Dose adjustments	In severe renal derangement, not needed in hepatic/mild to moderate renal derangement
Adverse effects	Vomiting, cough, pyrexia
Contraindications	Hypersensitivity
Drug interactions	Amiodarone, antacids, digoxin, anticonvulsants
Remarks	Not recommended for children below 12 years or weight below 30 kg

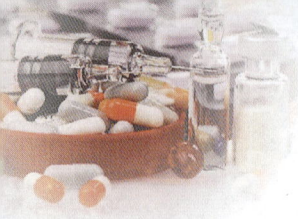

Leuprolide Acetate

Drug name	Leuprolide acetate (Gonadotropin-releasing hormone)
Category	Hormone
Route	Intramuscular
Strength	Inj (1 mg, 4 mg, 11.25 mg)
Brands	Lupride (Inj), Leuprofact (Inj)
Mechanism of action	It reversibly inhibits gonadotropin secretion when given as continuation therapy though initially there is stimulation
Pharmacokinetics	Not much known. It has a biphasic absorption, with peak levels 4 hours after administration
Indications	Central precocious puberty
Dosage as per indications	• *<25 kg:* 7.5 mg IM once a month • *25–37.5 kg:* 11.25 mg IM once a month • *>37.5 kg:* 15 mg IM once a month
Maximum dosage	Not known
Dose adjustments	Not known
Adverse effects	Convulsions, pseudotumor cerebri, fever, Inj site pain/erythema, bronchospasm
Contraindications	Hypersensitivity
Drug interactions	Antiarrhythmics
Remarks	Serum luteinizing hormone (LH) levels should initially be measured every 1–2 monthly to check for adequate suppression

Levamisole Hydrochloride

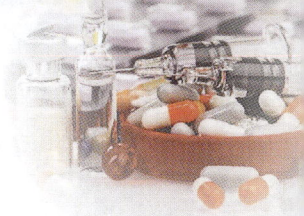

Drug name	Levamisole hydrochloride
Category	Antihelminthic, Immunostimulant, Antiviral
Route	Oral
Strength	Tab (50 mg, 150 mg); Syp (50 mg/5 mL)
Brands	Dewormis (Syp), Dicaris (Syp), Vermisol (Syp)
Mechanism of action	• Acts on L nicotinic acetylcholine receptors in nematodes. To control the reproductive muscle • Acts as immunomodulator to increase NK cell and T-cell activity
Pharmacokinetics	Rapidly absorbed, 25% bound to plasma protein, mainly metabolized in liver; half-life: 4–6 hours
Indications	Ascariasis; Hookworm infection; Frequently relapsing nephrotic syndrome; Steroid-dependent nephrotic syndrome
Dosage as per indications	• *Ascariasis:* 2 mg/kg/day PO single dose; • *Frequently relapsing nephrotic syndrome and steroid-dependent nephrotic syndrome:* 2–2.5 mg/kg on alternate days with low dose steroids on alternate days for 12–18 months duration
Maximum dosage	150 mg/day
Dose adjustments	In renal derangement
Adverse effects	Leukopenia, agranulocytosis, thrombocytopenia, abdominal pain, nausea, headache, convulsions
Contraindications	Contraindicated in preexisting blood disorders, pregnancy and lactation and severe renal impairment
Drug interactions	Albendazole, ivermectin
Remarks	Take empty stomach

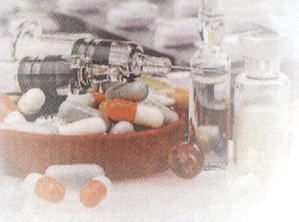

Levetiracetam

Drug name	Levetiracetam
Category	Antiepileptic
Route	Oral, Intravenous
Strength	Syp (100 mg/5 mL, 200 mg/5 mL); Tab (250 mg, 500 mg, 750 mg, 1 g); Inj (100 mg/mL)
Brands	Levera (Inj, Syp, Tab), Levesam (Inj, Syp, Tab), Levipil (Inj, Syp, Tab)
Mechanism of action	Selectively binds to synaptic vesicle protein 2A, also affects GABAergic neurotransmission. This helps in inhibiting hypersynchronized epileptiform burst firing without affecting normal neuronal transmission
Pharmacokinetics	Rapidly and almost completely absorbed; 65–70% drug eliminated in the urine, plasma half-life: 6–8 hours
Indications	Partial seizures; GTCS

Dosage as per indications	• *Partial seizures:*
	  – *1–6 months:* 15 mg/kg/day in two divided doses; can be increased by 15 mg/kg/day every 2 weeks up to 40 mg/kg/day
	  – *6 months–4 years:* 20 mg/kg/day in 2 divided doses; can be increased by 20 mg/kg/day every 2 weeks up to 50 mg/kg/day
	  – *4–16 years:* 20 mg/kg/day in 2 divided doses; can be increased by 20 mg/kg/day every 2 weeks up to 60 mg/kg/day
	• *GTCS:*
	  – *6–16 years:* 20 mg/kg/day in 2 divided doses; can be increased by 20 mg/kg/day every 2 weeks up to 60 mg/kg/day

Maximum dosage	3,000 mg/day (in children >4 years/>40 kg)
Dose adjustments	Dose adjustment needed in renal derangement, not required in hepatic derangement
Adverse effects	Fatigue, aggression, nasal congestion, decreased appetite, and irritability
Contraindications	Hypersensitivity
Drug interactions	Benzodiazepine
Remarks	Sudden stoppage can lead to withdrawal seizures

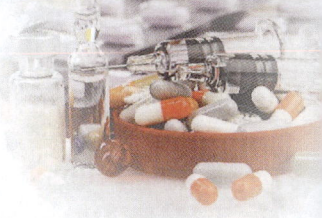

Levocetirizine

Drug name	Levocetirizine
Category	Antiallergic
Route	Oral
Strength	Tab (5 mg, 10 mg); Syp (2.5 mg/5 mL, 5 mg/5 mL)
Brands	Levocet (Tab), LCZ (Tab, Syp), Lecope (Tab, Syp)
Mechanism of action	Acts by blocking H1 receptors and preventing histamine action
Pharmacokinetics	Rapid and high absorption after oral intake. Peak levels around 1 hour after intake. Highly protein bound. Metabolized in liver via CYP 3A4. Excreted mainly via urine
Indications	Allergic rhinitis; Allergic cough
Dosage as per indications	- *>12 years:* 5 mg once a day - *6–11 years:* 2.5 mg once a day
Maximum dosage	10 mg/day
Dose adjustments	Dose adjustment in renal impairment
Adverse effects	Fatigue, dry mouth
Contraindications	Hypersensitivity
Drug interactions	Azithromycin, cimetidine, erythromycin, ketoconazole

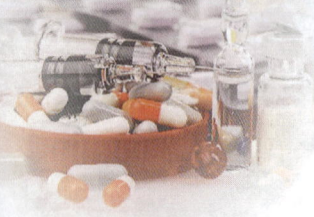

Levofloxacin

Drug name	Levofloxacin
Category	Antibiotic
Route	Oral
Strength	Tab (250 mg, 500 mg, 750 mg)
Brands	Levloc (Tab), Levoflox (Tab)
Mechanism of action	Inhibition of bacterial topoisomerase IV and DNA gyrase
Pharmacokinetics	Rapid and complete absorption after oral administration. Poorly metabolized, excreted unchanged in urine. Elimination half-life: 6–8 hours
Indications	Acts against gram-negative; Gram-positive bacteria
Dosage as per indications	8 mg/kg/dose bid
Maximum dosage	250 mg/dose
Dose adjustments	In renal dysfunction
Adverse effects	Peripheral neuropathy, myopathy, tendinitis, hepatotoxic, arthropathy, QT interval prolongation
Contraindications	Hypersensitivity
Drug interactions	Warfarin, antidiabetics, antacids, digoxin, cyclosporine

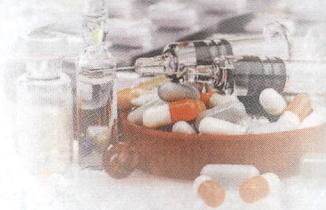

Levosalbutamol

Drug name	Levosalbutamol
Category	Beta-2 agonist, Bronchodilator
Route	Oral, Inhalational
Strength	Syp (1 mg/5 mL); Nebulizing Respules (0.31, 0.63, 1.2 mg/2.5 mL); MDI (50 μg)
Brands	Levolin (Syp, Respule, Inhaler MDI and Rotacap), Aerozest (Respule, Inhaler)
Mechanism of action	Acts as an agonist on β2 adrenergic receptors on airway smooth muscle causing adenylate cyclase activation and increased cAMP thus inducing muscle relaxation
Pharmacokinetics	Inhalation delivers the medication directly into the airways and lungs, thereby minimizing side effects because of reduced systemic absorption of the inhaled medications. It is excreted in urine
Indications	Asthma; Reactive airway disease
Dosage as per indications	• *Oral:* 0.05–0.1 mg/kg/dose 2–3 times/day • *Nebulization:* 0.075 mg/kg/dose • *MDI:* 1–2 puffs 6–8 hourly
Maximum dosage	Oral 8 mg/dose, inhalational: 1.2 mg/dose
Dose adjustments	Use with caution in renal derangement
Adverse effects	Tremors, tachycardia, muscular cramps, diarrhea
Contraindications	Hypersensitivity
Drug interactions	Anesthetic agents

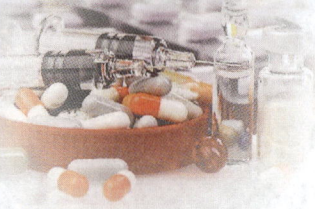

Levothyroxine

Drug name	Levothyroxine
Category	Thyroxine
Route	Oral
Strength	Tab (12.5 µg, 25 µg, 50 µg, 100 µg)
Brands	Eltroxin (Tab), Thyronorm (Tab)
Mechanism of action	It acts like endogenous thyroxine and exerts similar control on DNA transcription and protein synthesis
Pharmacokinetics	Highly protein bound, around 40–80% drug absorbed from gut. Mainly metabolized via deiodination, monodeiodination converts peripheral T4 to T3. Liver is the major site of degradation for both T4 and T3. Main route of elimination is via kidneys
Indications	Hypothyroidism

Dosage as per indications	• Synthetic levo isomer of thyroxine
	  – *1–3 months:* 10–15 µg/kg/dose OD
	  – *3–6 months:* 8–10 µg/kg/dose OD
	  – *6–12 months:* 6–8 µg/kg/dose OD
	  – *1–5 years:* 5–6 µg/kg/dose OD
	  – *6–12 years:* 4–5 µg/kg/dose OD
	• *>12 years:*
	  – *Incomplete growth and prepuberty:* 2–3 µg/kg/dose OD
	  – *Complete growth and puberty:* 1.7 µg/kg/dose OD

Maximum dosage	200–300 µg/day
Dose adjustments	Not required
Adverse effects	Chest pain, congestive heart failure, flushing, tachycardia, irregular heartbeat, arthralgia
Contraindications	Uncorrected adrenal insufficiency
Drug interactions	Steroids, cardiac glycosides, oral contraceptives, antiepileptics
Remarks	Administer empty stomach, do not take along with iron calcium and antacid supplement within 4 hours

Lignocaine Hydrochloride

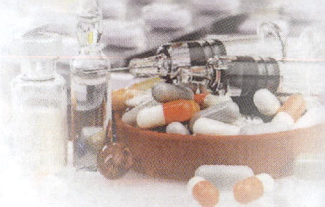

Drug name	Lignocaine hydrochloride
Category	Antiarrhythmic
Route	Intravenous
Strength	Inj 2%; Sol (20 mg/mL)
Brands	Gesicard (Inj), Xylocard (Inj)
Mechanism of action	Stabilizes neuronal membrane by inhibiting ionic refluxes required for the initiation and conduction of impulses. Decreases electrical excitability, conduction rate and force of contraction in the myocardium
Pharmacokinetics	Highly bound to plasma proteins, crosses blood-brain, metabolized in the liver, eliminated via kidneys
Indications	Antiarrhythmic
Dosage as per indications	1 mg/kg/dose IV slowly (can repeat in 5–10 min × 2; maximum 3 mg/kg) loading followed by 20–50 µg/kg/min as maintenance
Maximum dosage	3 mg/kg for local infiltration
Dose adjustments	Multiple doses need adjustment in hepatic derangement
Adverse effects	Hypotension, asystole, seizures and respiratory arrest
Contraindications	Stokes-Adams attacks, SA, AV, or intraventricular heart block without pacemaker
Drug interactions	Antiarrhythmics, anticonvulsants

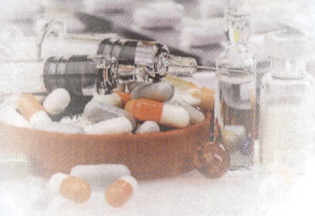

Lincomycin

Drug name	Lincomycin
Category	Antibiotic
Route	Oral, Intravenous
Strength	Inj (300 mg/mL); Cap (250 mg, 500 mg); Syp (125 mg/mL)
Brands	Linc (Inj, Cap), Lincin (Inj, Cap), Lincocin (Inj, Cap), Lynx (Inj, Cap, Syp)
Mechanism of action	Lincomycin inhibits bacterial protein synthesis by binding to the 23S RNA of the 50S subunit of the bacterial ribosome
Pharmacokinetics	Not much known, peak levels: 1 hour, half-life 5.5–6.5 hours
Indications	Gram-positive bacteria; Anaerobes; *Clostridium perfringens*

Dosage as per indications	• Children >1 month:
	  – 10–20 mg/kg/day divided 12 hourly IV
	  – 10–20 mg/kg/dose oral 8 hourly

Maximum dosage	Not known
Dose adjustments	In renal and hepatic derangement
Adverse effects	Hypersensitivity
Contraindications	Diarrhea, vomiting, nausea, toxic epidermal necrolysis (TEN), altered renal and hepatic functions
Drug interactions	Droperidol, doxycycline, atracurium

Linezolid

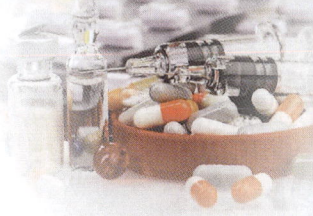

Drug name	Linezolid
Category	Antibiotic, Oxazolidinone
Route	Oral, Intravenous
Strength	Tab (300 mg, 600 mg); Inj (600 mg/300 mL)
Brands	Linospan (Inj, Tab), Linox (Inj, Tab), Lizoforce (Inj, Tab)
Mechanism of action	It binds on the bacterial 23S ribosomal RNA of the 50S subunit thereby preventing bacterial translation
Pharmacokinetics	Rapidly and extensively absorbed after oral dosing. Maximum plasma concentrations: 1–2 hours after dosing, nearly 100% bioavailability
Indications	Resistant gram-positive infections including MRSA
Dosage as per indications	For treatment of resistant gram-positive infections, especially MRSA and VRSA infections: 10 mg/kg/dose q 12 h PO/IV
Maximum dosage	600 mg/dose 12 hourly
Dose adjustments	Not needed in renal and hepatic derangement
Adverse effects	Thrombocytopenia, diarrhea, nausea, vomiting, taste disturbances, oral thrush
Contraindications	Hypersensitivity
Drug interactions	Linezolid has monoamine oxidase inhibitor activity and hence should be used cautiously when co-administered with adrenergic or serotonergic drugs

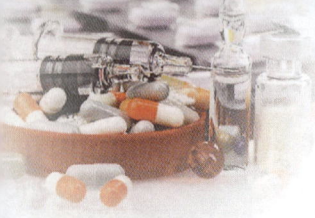

Lisinopril

Drug name	Lisinopril
Category	Antihypertensive
Route	Oral
Strength	Tab (2.5 mg, 5 mg, 10 mg, 20 mg)
Brands	Linvas (Tab), Listril (Tab), Lisoral (Tab)
Mechanism of action	Suppresses renin-angiotensin system by inhibiting angiotensin-converting enzyme (ACE) hence stopping conversion of angiotensin I to angiotensin II
Pharmacokinetics	Peak serum levels 7 hours after oral intake, half-life: 12 hours, poorly metabolized, excreted primarily through kidneys
Indications	Hypertension
Dosage as per indications	0.07 mg/kg once a day (up to 5 mg) initially, increase gradually
Maximum dosage	0.61 mg/kg or 40 mg/day
Dose adjustments	In renal dysfunction
Adverse effects	Hyperkalemia, hypotension, hypoglycemia
Contraindications	Hypertrophic cardiomyopathy/aortic stenosis; impaired renal function, bilateral renal artery stenosis
Drug interactions	Diuretics, antidiabetics, NSAIDs
Remarks	Used in children >6 years

Lithium

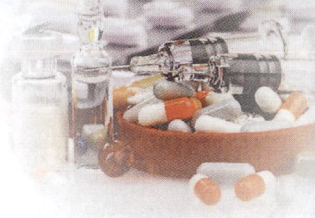

Drug name	Lithium
Category	Antidepressant
Route	Oral
Strength	Tab (150 mg, 300 mg)
Brands	Lithocap (Tab), Lithocarb (Tab)
Mechanism of action	Affects sodium transport in nerve and muscle cells affecting intraneuronal metabolism of catecholamines. It decreases sodium reabsorption in renal tubules
Pharmacokinetics	Rapidly and completely absorbed, poorly metabolized, elimination half-life: 24 hours, excreted in urine which is proportional to its plasma concentration
Indications	Bipolar disorder; Depression
Dosage as per indications	15–60 mg/kg/day in 3–4 divided doses
Maximum dosage	Not known
Dose adjustments	Renal disease
Adverse effects	Diarrhea, vomiting, muscle weakness, ataxia, blurred vision, drowsiness
Contraindications	Hypersensitivity, cardiovascular disease, severe dehydration
Drug interactions	Haloperidol, NSAID, diuretics
Remarks	• Risk of lithium toxicity, worsening of hypothyroidism • Maintain blood levels between 0.6 and 1.5 mEq/L

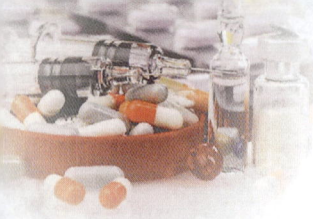

Lopinavir/Ritonavir (LPV/r)

Drug name	Lopinavir/Ritonavir (LPV/r)
Category	Antiretroviral
Route	Oral
Strength	Sol (80 mg/20 mg LPV/r per mL); Tab (100 mg/25 mg, 200 mg/50 mg LPV/r)
Brands	Lopimune (Tab, Syp), Ritomax L (Cap)
Mechanism of action	Lopinavir is antiretroviral protease inhibitor whereas ritonavir is a potent inhibitor of the enzymes responsible for lopinavir metabolism
Pharmacokinetics	Lopinavir metabolized by CYP3A, highly protein bound. Ritonavir is a potent CYP3A inhibitor. Lopinavir is excreted in feces, half-life: 5–9 hours
Indications	AIDS/HIV infection
Dosage as per indications	300 mg/75 mg per m^2 of BSA per dose twice daily
Maximum dosage	Maximum dose 400 mg/100 mg twice daily
Dose adjustments	In hepatic derangement, not well studied in renal derangement
Adverse effects	Diarrhea, headache, asthenia, nausea and vomiting, rash, and hyperlipidemia, especially hypertriglyceridemia, fat maldistribution
Contraindications	Hypersensitivity
Drug interactions	CYP3A4 inducers
Remarks	Once a day dosing not preferred due to high variability and risk of diarrhea

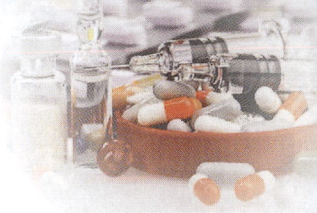

Loratadine

Drug name	Loratadine
Category	Antihistaminic (Second generation)
Route	Oral
Strength	Tab (5 mg, 10 mg); Syp (5 mg/5 mL)
Brands	Loridin (Tab), Alaspan (Tab, Syp), Tirlor (Tab)
Mechanism of action	It selectively inhibits peripheral histamine H1-receptor activity
Pharmacokinetics	Highly protein bound, metabolized by cytochrome P450 3A4 (CYP3A4), eliminated in urine and feces, elimination half-life: 10 hours
Indications	Allergic rhinitis; Urticaria
Dosage as per indications	• *<30 kg:* 5 mg/24 h • *>30 kg:* 10 mg/24 h
Maximum dosage	10 mg/day
Dose adjustments	Hepatic derangement
Adverse effects	Diarrhea, nervousness, fatigue, stomatitis, rash, earache, viral infection, flulike symptoms, dry mouth, headache, insomnia, somnolence
Contraindications	Phenylketonuria
Drug interactions	Erythromycin, ketoconazole, cimetidine
Remarks	Should be avoided in patients with phenylketonuria, if tablet contains phenylalanine

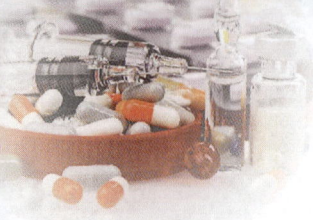

Lorazepam

Drug name	Lorazepam
Category	Anticonvulsant (Benzodiazepine)
Route	Oral, Intravenous, Intramuscular, Per Rectal
Strength	Tab (1 mg, 2 mg); Inj (2 mg/mL, 10 mg/mL ampoules)
Brands	Almazine (Inj, Tab), Lorez (Inj, Tab), Zepnap (Inj, Tab), Lopez (Inj, Tab)
Mechanism of action	Acts on γ-aminobutyric acid (GABA)-benzodiazepine receptor complex
Pharmacokinetics	Completely and rapidly absorbed, peak levels: 3 hours, conjugated to the 3-O-phenolic glucuronide in the liver, undergoes enterohepatic recirculation
Indications	Uncontrolled status epilepticus; Anxiety; Insomnia
Dosage as per indications	*Status epilepticus:* 0.05–0.2 mg/kg/dose over 2–5 minutes IV or per rectal, may repeat after 10–15 minutes
Maximum dosage	4 mg/dose
Dose adjustments	Needed in renal impairment
Adverse effects	Drowsiness, dizziness, blurred vision, muscle weakness, nausea, rash
Contraindications	Respiratory depression, hypersensitivity
Drug interactions	Along with other CNS depressants
Remarks	Duration of action is longer than diazepam

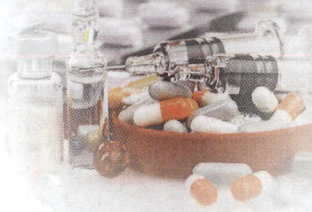

Losartan

Drug name	Losartan
Category	Antihypertensive
Route	Oral
Strength	Tab (25 mg, 50 mg)
Brands	Alsartan (Tab), Loscar (Tab), Losar (Tab)
Mechanism of action	Selectively blocks the binding of angiotensin II to the AT1 receptor
Pharmacokinetics	Well absorbed on oral administration with high first pass metabolism. Has one-third bioavailability. Terminal half-life: 2 hours
Indications	Hypertension
Dosage as per indications	0.7 mg/kg once daily
Maximum dosage	1.4 mg/kg or 100 mg/day
Dose adjustments	In hepatic and renal disease
Adverse effects	Congestion, dizziness, leg cramps
Contraindications	Hypersensitivity
Drug interactions	Phenobarbitone, rifampicin, fluconazole, erythromycin

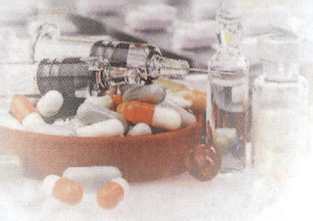

Magnesium Sulfate

Drug name	Magnesium sulfate
Category	Bronchodilator
Route	Intravenous, Intramuscular, Oral
Strength	Inj (50% Sol; 1 mL = 500 mg ampoule)
Brands	Magnesium sulfate (Inj)
Mechanism of action	It blocks neuromuscular transmission by decreasing acetylcholine secreted at the end-plate
Pharmacokinetics	Not much known, eliminated by kidneys, elimination rate proportional to the plasma concentration
Indications	Status asthmaticus; Protein energy malnutrition (PEM)
Dosage as per indications	• *Bronchodilator:* 25–50 mg/kg/dose IV infusion over 20 minutes • *For PEM:* 1–2 mL stat intramuscular dose followed by 0.2–0.3 mL/kg orally for next 13 days
Maximum dosage	2 g/dose
Dose adjustments	In renal derangement
Adverse effects	Respiratory depression, if given in overdose
Contraindications	Heart block, myocardial damage
Drug interactions	CNS depressants, cardiac glycosides, neuromuscular blockers
Remarks	• Normal plasma magnesium levels range from 1.5 to 2.5 mEq/L • Plasma magnesium >4 mEq/L: Deep tendon reflexes disappear; >10 mEq/L: Respiratory paralysis occurs • *Antidote:* Calcium gluconate

Mannitol

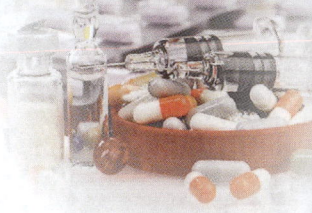

Drug name	Mannitol
Category	Diuretic
Route	Intravenous
Strength	20% Bottles 100 mL
Brands	Mannitol (Inj)
Mechanism of action	Parenteral obligatory osmotic diuretic
Pharmacokinetics	Mostly remains extracellular, poorly metabolized, excreted by kidneys. Has a diuretic effect by increasing glomerular filtrate osmolarity
Indications	Raised intracranial tension
Dosage as per indications	5 mL/kg IV over 30 minutes (loading dose) followed by 2 mL/kg/dose q 6 h IV for 2 days
Maximum dosage	Not known
Dose adjustments	Dose adjustment in renal derangement
Adverse effects	Electrolyte imbalance, circulatory overload
Contraindications	Intracranial bleed, dehydration, pulmonary edema, severe renal disease
Drug interactions	Nephrotoxic drugs, diuretics

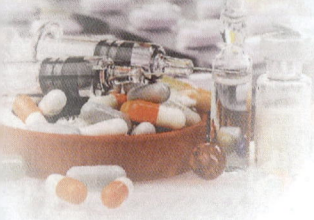

Mebendazole

Drug name	Mebendazole
Category	Antihelminthic, Benzimidazole
Route	Oral
Strength	Tab (100 mg); Susp (100 mg/5 mL)
Brands	Mebex (Tab, Syp), Wormin (Tab, Syp)
Mechanism of action	Interferes in cellular tubulin formation in the helminth intestine, affecting digestive and reproductive functions and ultimately leading to death of the helminth
Pharmacokinetics	Highly protein bound, acts locally in gut, metabolized mainly by the liver, eliminated in feces. *Half-life:* 2.5–5.5 hours
Indications	Helminthic infections
Dosage as per indications	• *Ascariasis:* 100 mg twice a day × 3 days • *Enterobius infection:* 100 mg single dose, repeat after 2 weeks • *Tapeworms and mixed infections:* 200 mg BD × 3 days; repeat course after 2–4 weeks • *Hydatid cyst:* 30 mg/kg/day q 8 h, oral, for 4 weeks
Maximum dosage	500 mg/day
Dose adjustments	Dose adjustment in hepatic derangement
Adverse effects	Diarrhea, abdominal cramp, rash, deranged liver enzymes
Contraindications	Hypersensitivity
Drug interactions	Metronidazole (risk of SJS)
Remarks	Not recommended in children below 2 years

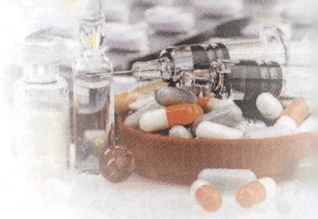

Mefenamic Acid

Drug name	Mefenamic acid
Category	Nonsteroidal anti-inflammatory drug (NSAID)
Route	Oral
Strength	Tab (100 mg); Cap (250 mg, 500 mg); Susp (100 mg/5 mL, 50 mg/5 mL)
Brands	Mefacid (Tab, Syp), Meftal/Meftal-P (Tab, Syp)
Mechanism of action	Inhibition of cyclo-oxygenase (COX-1 and COX-2) producing anti-inflammatory effect
Pharmacokinetics	Rapidly absorbed after oral intake. Highly protein bound, elimination half-life: 2 hours
Indications	Fever; JIA
Dosage as per indications	• *For arthritis:* 25 mg/kg/day q 6 h • *For fever:* 3 mg/kg/dose
Maximum dosage	500 mg/dose; 1,000 mg per day
Dose adjustments	Dose adjustment in renal and hepatic impairment
Adverse effects	Diarrhea, skin rash, and gastritis
Contraindications	Seizures
Drug interactions	Other NSAIDs, anticoagulants
Remarks	Administer with food. Avoid in patients having seizures

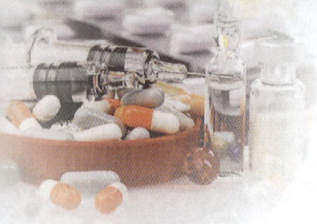

Mefloquine Hydrochloride

Drug name	Mefloquine hydrochloride
Category	Antimalarial
Route	Oral
Strength	Tab (250 mg)
Brands	Facital (Tab), Mefque (Tab), Larimef (Tab)
Mechanism of action	Mefloquine is an antimalarial agent which acts as a blood schizonticide
Pharmacokinetics	High bioavailability, extensively metabolized by liver, half-life: 12–14 days, eliminated in bile and feces
Indications	Malaria prophylaxis; Treatment
Dosage as per indications	• Used as combination therapy with artesunate as: 25 mg/kg divided as 15 mg/kg on D1 and 10 mg/kg on D2 OD • Used as single drug for prophylaxis as 3.5 mg/kg of base weekly
Maximum dosage	250 mg/dose
Dose adjustments	Hepatic derangement
Adverse effects	Headache, syncope, dizziness, seizures, psychiatric illness
Contraindications	Active depression, psychiatric disease, seizures
Drug interactions	QTc prolonging drugs

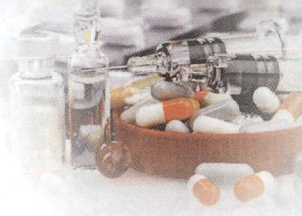

Melatonin

Drug name	Melatonin
Category	Sedative
Route	Oral
Strength	Tab (3 mg)
Brands	Meloset (Tab), Melanew (Tab)
Mechanism of action	Melatonin inhibits adenylate cyclase and activates phospholipase C. It also acts on melatonin receptors in suprachiasmatic nucleus to induce sleep. Production of melatonin is stimulated by darkness and inhibited by light. High levels of melatonin induce sleep
Pharmacokinetics	Variable absorption and bioavailability. Metabolized in liver. *Half-life:* 1 hour
Indications	Insomnia, as sedative for EEG

Dosage as per indications	• *For children:*
	  – *3–5 years:* 0.5–1 mg/day
	  – *5–10 years:* 1–3 mg/day
	• *Adolescents:* 3–5 mg/day

Maximum dosage	5 mg/day
Dose adjustments	Not known
Adverse effects	Headache, dizziness, nausea
Contraindications	Hypersensitivity
Drug interactions	Amlodipine, gabapentin, fluvoxamine
Remarks	Start with the lowest doses, can be increased gradually

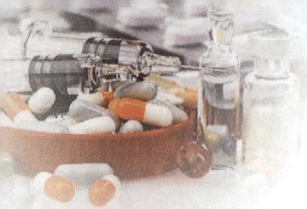

Meropenem

Drug name	Meropenem
Category	Antibiotic, Carbapenem
Route	Intravenous
Strength	Inj (500 mg, 1,000 mg vials)
Brands	Carbapen M, Merocrit, Meromac (Inj)
Mechanism of action	Bactericidal; inhibits cell wall synthesis by binding to penicillin-binding-protein (PBP). Mostly resistant to hydrolysis by beta-lactamases, both penicillinases and cephalosporinases
Pharmacokinetics	Has low plasma protein binding. Elimination half-life: 1 hour; mainly excreted by kidney
Indications	Severe gram-positive; Gram-negative infections except MRSA
Dosage as per indications	• *Sepsis:* 60 mg/kg/day q 8 h • *Meningitis:* 120 mg/kg/day q 8 h • *Neonatal sepsis:* 20 mg/kg/dose q 12 h
Maximum dosage	2 g/dose
Dose adjustments	Renal derangement
Adverse effects	Nausea, vomiting, rash, deranged liver enzymes
Contraindications	Do not use in neonates
Drug interactions	Valproate, probenecid
Remarks	Increases the risk of seizures when given in meningitis and CNS disorders

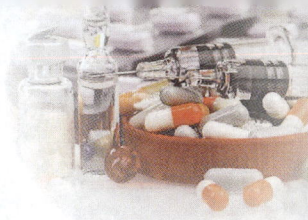

Metformin

Drug name	Metformin
Category	Antihyperglycemic, Biguanide
Route	Oral
Strength	Tab (500 mg, 850 mg, 1,000 mg)
Brands	Glumet (Tab), Zomet (Tab), Fortmet (Tab)
Mechanism of action	It decreases hepatic glucose production and intestinal absorption of glucose. It also increases peripheral glucose uptake and utilization
Pharmacokinetics	Around 50% absorbed, poorly protein bound, not metabolized, mostly eliminated by kidneys in an unchanged form, plasma elimination half-life: 6 hours
Indications	Diabetes mellitus type 2
Dosage as per indications	• *10–16 years:* Start with 500 mg BID; can be increased by 500 mg/24 h weekly in two divided doses • *17 years and above:* Start 500 mg PO BID; increase dose weekly by 500 mg/24 h divided in two doses
Maximum dosage	• *10–16 years:* 2,000 mg/24 h • *>17 years:* 2,500 mg/24 h
Dose adjustments	Renal and hepatic derangement
Adverse effects	Decreased vitamin B_{12} levels, lactic acidosis, abdominal discomfort, diarrhea, vomiting
Contraindications	Severe renal damage, hepatic impairment, CHF, metabolic acidosis, radiology studies using iodinated contrast media
Drug interactions	Oral hypoglycemics, insulin, carbonic anhydrase
Remarks	Administer with food

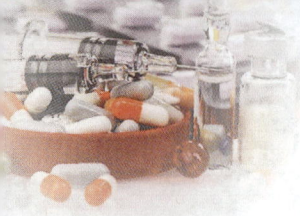

Methadone

Drug name	Methadone
Category	Opioid analgesic
Route	Oral, Subcutaneous, Intravenous, Intramuscular
Strength	Tab (5 mg)
Brands	Dolophine, Methadose (Indian brand not found, though available in India under specific government establishments)
Mechanism of action	Synthetic opioid (mu-agonist), acts similar to opioid
Pharmacokinetics	Variable bioavailability but can go as high as 100%, peak plasma levels obtained in 1–7 hours
Indications	Opioid addiction treatment
Dosage as per indications	*Child:* 0.7 mg/kg/24 h q 4–6 h PO, SC, IM, IV
Maximum dosage	10 mg/dose
Dose adjustments	Required in both renal and hepatic insufficiency, not much studied
Adverse effects	Respiratory depression, sedation, hypotension, bradycardia
Contraindications	Hypersensitivity, severe bronchial asthma, severe respiratory depression, suspected paralytic ileus
Drug interactions	CYP3A4 inducers and inhibitors, antiretroviral drugs, arrhythmogenic drugs
Remarks	Avoid in children with asthma

Methimazole

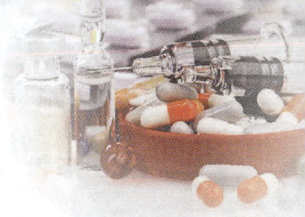

Drug name	Methimazole
Category	Antithyroid
Route	Oral
Strength	Tab (5 mg, 10 mg)
Brands	Methimez, Methimercazole
Mechanism of action	Inhibits the synthesis of thyroid hormone, by affecting thyroid peroxidase enzyme
Pharmacokinetics	Highly absorbed after oral administration, metabolized in liver, excreted in urine, half-life: 3–5 hours
Indications	Hyperthyroidism
Dosage as per indications	Initially 0.4 mg/kg/day in 3 divided doses; maintenance dose around 50% of the initial dose
Maximum dosage	30 mg/day
Dose adjustments	No dose adjustments. Stop the drug if hepatic dysfunction noted
Adverse effects	Agranulocytosis, liver toxicity, prolong prothrombin time
Contraindications	Hypersensitivity
Drug interactions	Anticoagulants, theophylline, β-adrenergic blocking drugs

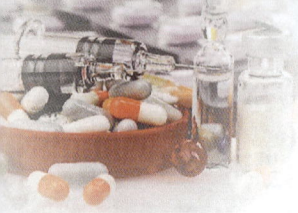

Methotrexate

Drug name	Methotrexate
Category	Immunosuppressant
Route	Oral, Intravenous, Intrathecal
Strength	Inj (5 mg, 15 mg, 25 mg); Tab (2.5 mg, 5 mg, 7.5 mg)
Brands	Altrex (Inj, Tab), Biotrexate, Oncotrex
Mechanism of action	It is a dihydrofolate reductase inhibitor. It inhibits DNA synthesis and repair by inhibiting synthesis of purine nucleotides required for DNA formation
Pharmacokinetics	Around 50% bioavailability after oral administration, 50% protein bound, elimination half-life: 3–10 hours. The drug is metabolized in liver and intestine and excreted by kidney via glomerular filtration and tubular secretion
Indications	Acute leukemias; Psoriasis; Rheumatoid arthritis; Lymphoma
Dosage as per indications	• *JIA:* 5–10 mg/m^2/week PO; given along with folic acid/leucovorin • *ALL:* As per the regime used, given as oral/IV/intrathecal in various phases
Maximum dosage	• *JIA:* 25 mg/week • *ALL:* Varies based on age and phase of chemotherapy
Dose adjustments	In renal disease
Adverse effects	Secondary infections, malignancy, bone marrow suppression, liver damage
Contraindications	Hypersensitivity, severe infections
Drug interactions	Immunosuppressants
Remarks	Do not give live vaccines

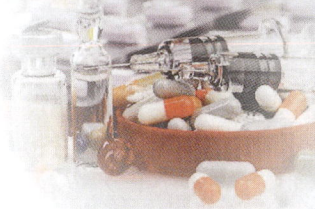

Methylcobalamin

Drug name	Methylcobalamin
Category	Vitamin B_{12}
Route	Oral, Sublingual, Intravenous, Intramuscular
Strength	Inj (500 µg/mL); Tab (500 µg, 1,000 µg, 1500 µg)
Brands	Alnerve (Inj, Tab), Neurokind (Inj, Tab), Neucobal (Inj, Tab)
Mechanism of action	Essential for formation of tetrahydrofolate needed for conversion of methylmalonate to succinate and synthesis of methionine from homocysteine
Pharmacokinetics	Rapid absorption after intramuscular/subcutaneous Inj. Binds to plasma proteins, stored in the liver. Excreted in the bile; undergoes enterohepatic recycling. Vitamin B_{12} bound to intrinsic factor during transit through the stomach; separates in the terminal ileum from where it enters the mucosal cell for absorption
Indications	Vitamin B_{12} deficiency; Megaloblastic anemia

Dosage as per indications	• *Vitamin B_{12} deficiency, treatment:*
	  – Oral:
	    - Infants: 500 µg, children: 1000 µg daily for 7 days, alternate day for 7 days, every other day for next 7 days, twice for a week, once for a week, once every 15 days followed by once a month to complete 3 months of therapy
	  – Intramuscular/SC/IV:
	    - Child: 25 µg/day for 2–3 days, followed by 100 µg (50 µg in infants) for 7–21 days (higher duration if neurological signs present), followed by 100 µg thrice/week and lastly 1000 µg once/week (can be given oral) for 1 month
	• *Pernicious anemia:*
	  – Child (IM): 30–50 µg/24 h for at least 14 days to a total dose of 1,000–5,000 µg
	  – Maintenance: 100 µg/month

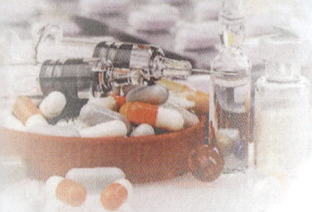

Maximum dosage	Intravenous 1,000 µg/day
Dose adjustments	Not known
Adverse effects	Hypokalemia, hypersensitivity, pruritus, vascular thrombosis
Contraindications	Hypersensitivity, optic atrophy
Drug interactions	Colchicine, methotrexate, or pyrimethamine, para-aminosalicylic acid (PAS). Avoid antacids when on B_{12} supplementation
Remarks	Protect from light. IV route not preferred due to more rapid elimination

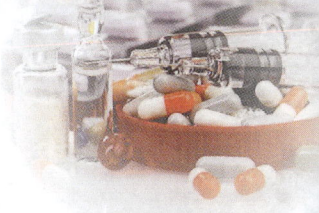

Methylene Blue

Drug name	Methylene blue
Category	Antidote
Route	Intravenous
Strength	Inj (10 mg/mL)
Brands	Corblue (Inj), Urolene Blue (Inj)
Mechanism of action	Methylene blue reduces the ferric iron of MetHb to the ferrous state of normal hemoglobin
Pharmacokinetics	*Half-life:* 24 hours, metabolism: UGT-mediated conjugation by UGT1A4 and UGT1A9. 40–50% excreted in urine
Indications	Methemoglobinemia
Dosage as per indications	1–2 mg/kg/dose or 25–50 mg/m^2/dose IV over 5 minutes, dose may be repeated after 1 hour
Maximum dosage	Not known
Dose adjustments	Dose adjustment in renal and hepatic impairment
Adverse effects	Nausea, vomiting, dizziness, headache, serotonin syndrome with SSRI, SNRI
Contraindications	Use with caution in G6PD deficiency or renal insufficiency
Drug interactions	Serotonergic drug, drugs metabolized via cytochrome P450
Remarks	At high doses, may cause methemoglobinemia

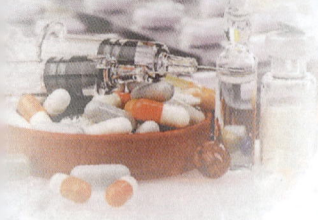

Methylphenidate

Drug name	Methylphenidate
Category	Stimulant
Route	Oral
Strength	Tab (5 mg, 10 mg, 20 mg)
Brands	Ritalin (Tab), Addwize (Tab), Methadate (Tab), Concerta (Tab) (extended release)
Mechanism of action	It blocks norepinephrine and dopamine reuptake into the presynaptic neuron leading to increased concentration in extraneuronal space
Pharmacokinetics	Low plasma protein binding, high first pass metabolism, average half-life: 2.5 hours, majorly eliminated in urine
Indications	Attention-deficit hyperactivity disorder (ADHD)
Dosage as per indications	For ADHD immediate release preparation • *Initial:* 0.3 mg/kg/dose (or 2.5–5 mg/dose), increase 0.1 mg/kg/dose PO (or 5–10 mg/24 h) weekly until maintenance dose achieved • *Maintenance:* 0.3–1 mg/kg/24 h
Maximum dosage	2 mg/kg/24 h or 60 mg/24 h for ≤50 kg and 100 mg/24 h >50 kg
Dose adjustments	Not known
Adverse effects	Nausea, vomiting, restlessness, tachycardia, palpitations, liver enzymes derangement, leukopenia, thrombocytopenia
Contraindications	<6 years, glaucoma, anxiety disorders, motor tics, Tourette's syndrome, hypersensitivity, MAO inhibitors
Drug interactions	Antacids, dopamine agonist, coumarin anticoagulants, anticonvulsants

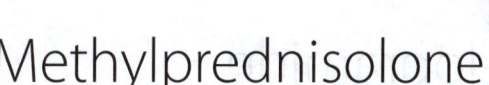

Methylprednisolone

Drug name	Methylprednisolone
Category	Anti-inflammatory
Route	Intravenous, Intramuscular, Oral
Strength	Tab (2 mg, 4 mg, 8 mg, 16 mg, 32 mg); Inj (125 mg, 500 mg, 1 g)
Brands	Solu-Medrol (Inj), Medrol (Inj, Tab)
Mechanism of action	Potent anti-inflammatory steroid; more anti-inflammatory but less salt and water retaining property than prednisolone
Pharmacokinetics	Effect starts within 1 hour of IV administration. Eliminated within 12 hours. High absorption intramuscular also
Indications	As immunosuppressant in inflammatory diseases; Asthma
Dosage as per indications	• *Immunosuppressive:* 0.5–1.7 mg/kg/24 h q 6 h • *Asthma:* Child ≤12 years: 1–2 mg/kg/24 h q 12 h (max dose: 60 mg/24 h), >12 years: 40–60 mg/24 h
Maximum dosage	60 mg/day
Dose adjustments	Use with caution, no adjustment needed
Adverse effects	Hypertension, pseudotumor cerebri, acne, Cushing syndrome, adrenal axis suppression, GI bleeding, hyperglycemia, osteoporosis
Contraindications	Not recommended in active infections
Drug interactions	Live vaccines, immunomodulators

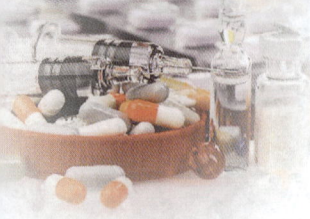

Metoclopramide Hydrochloride

Drug name	Metoclopramide hydrochloride
Category	Antiemetic
Route	Oral, Intravenous
Strength	Tab (10 mg); Syp (5 mg/5 mL); Inj (5 mg/mL ampoule)
Brands	Metanorm (Tab, Inj), Normide (Tab), Perinorm (Inj, Tab)
Mechanism of action	Stimulates GI motility but not secretions, gastric contractions intestinal peristalsis, increases lower esophageal sphincter tone
Pharmacokinetics	Around 30% bound to plasma proteins, undergoes metabolism in liver, elimination half-life: 5–6 hours, mostly eliminated in urine
Indications	Emesis; Gastroesophageal reflux (GER); Chemotherapy-induced nausea and vomiting (CINV)
Dosage as per indications	• *For GER or GI dysmotility:* – *Neonates:* 0.03–0.1 mg/kg/dose q 8 h – *Children:* 0.1–0.2 mg/kg/dose q 8 h – *Antiemetic effect:* 1–2 mg/kg/dose q 2–6 h IV/IM/PO • For CINV 2–3 mg/kg/dose before and after chemotherapy
Maximum dosage	0.8 mg/kg/24 h or 10 mg/dose
Dose adjustments	Renal and hepatic derangement
Adverse effects	Headache, anxiety, depression, extrapyramidal symptoms
Contraindications	Seizure disorder, GI obstruction, pheochromocytoma
Drug interactions	Cyclosporine, phenobarb, aspirin, phenytoin, ketoconazole
Remarks	Premedicate with diphenhydramine to reduce extrapyramidal side effects

Metoprolol

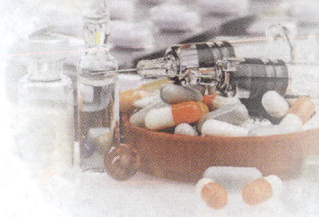

Drug name	Metoprolol, Antihypertensive
Category	Beta-1 receptor blocker
Route	Oral
Strength	Tab (50 mg, 100 mg); Inj (1 mg/mL)
Brands	Betaloc (Inj, Tab), Actocard (Tab), Metolar (Inj, Tab)
Mechanism of action	Beta-adrenergic receptor blocking agent to reduce heart rate, reflex tachycardia, cardiac output, and BP
Pharmacokinetics	Rapid and complete after oral administration. Has high first pass metabolism, bioavailability 100% after IV and 40–50% after oral intake. Peak levels: 20 minutes after IV, 1–2 hours after oral. Mainly excreted via kidneys
Indications	Hypertension
Dosage as per indications	Oral 1–5 mg/kg/day q 12 h; intravenous: 0.1 mg/kg/dose
Maximum dosage	200 mg/day oral
Dose adjustments	Impaired hepatic function
Adverse effects	Heart block, heart failure, bradyarrhythmia, dizziness, depression
Contraindications	Congestive heart failure, cardiogenic shock, first-degree block
Drug interactions	Catecholamine depleting drugs

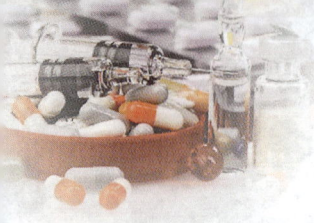

Metronidazole

Drug name	Metronidazole
Category	Antihelminthic, Nitroimidazole
Route	Oral, Intravenous
Strength	Syp (200 mg/5 mL); Tab (200 mg, 400 mg); Inj (5 mg/mL vial)
Brands	Flagyl (Tab, Syp), Metrogyl (Tab, Syp, Inj)
Mechanism of action	Has antibacterial action against anaerobes. It inhibits DNA synthesis by attaching to bacterial DNA and causing DNA degradation
Pharmacokinetics	Well absorbed orally, peak levels 1–2 hours after administration. Nearly three-fourths of the dose eliminated via urine
Indications	Amebiasis; Giardiasis; Anaerobic infections
Dosage as per indications	• *Amebiasis:* 30–50 mg/kg/day q 8 h for 10 days • *Trichomoniasis:* 15 mg/kg/day q 8 h for 5 days • *Anaerobic infections:* 20 mg/kg/day q 8 hourly for 7–10 days
Maximum dosage	4 g/day
Dose adjustments	Dose reduction needed in severe hepatic derangement
Adverse effects	Nausea, vomiting, metallic taste, diarrhea, dry mouth
Contraindications	Hypersensitivity, disulfiram intake in last 2 weeks, Cockayne syndrome
Drug interactions	Drugs prolonging QT interval, disulfiram, alcohol, warfarin, anticoagulants, lithium
Remarks	Avoid in severe renal/hepatic disease

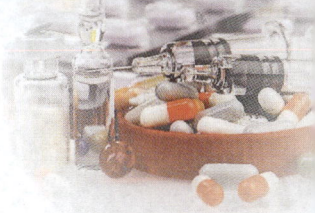

Mexiletine

Drug name	Mexiletine
Category	Antiarrhythmic (Class 1B)
Route	Oral, Intravenous
Strength	Inj (250 mg); Cap (50 mg, 150 mg)
Brands	Mexitil (Cap, Inj)
Mechanism of action	Inhibits the inward sodium movement in cardiac myocytes and nerve cells reducing the refractory period in Purkinje fibers
Pharmacokinetics	Well absorbed, metabolized in liver, 50% protein bound, half-life: 10–12 hours
Indications	Ventricular tachycardia; Symptomatic premature ventricular beats; Prevention of ventricular fibrillation
Dosage as per indications	1.5–5 mg/kg/dose 8 hourly PO
Maximum dosage	Not known
Dose adjustments	In renal and hepatic disease
Adverse effects	Nausea, vomiting, arrhythmias, hypotension, tremors, ataxia
Contraindications	Hypersensitivity, cardiogenic shock, heart block
Drug interactions	Aminophylline, phenytoin, fluvoxamine, terbinafine

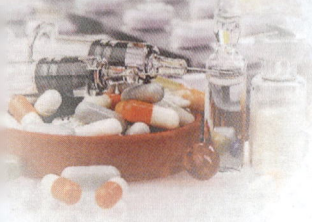

Micafungin

Drug name	Micafungin
Category	Antifungal, Echinocandin
Route	Intravenous
Strength	Inj (50 mg, 100 mg/vial)
Brands	B-cagin (Inj), Mycamine (Inj), Micedge (Inj)
Mechanism of action	Inhibits the synthesis of 1, 3-beta-D-glucan, required for fungal cell wall synthesis
Pharmacokinetics	Highly protein bound, metabolized to M-1 (catechol form) by arylsulfatase, further to M-2 (methoxy form) by catechol-O-methyltransferase, fecal excretion is the major route of elimination
Indications	Systemic fungal infection
Dosage as per indications	For invasive candidiasis • *Neonates:* 4 mg/kg IV once daily • Duration of therapy for candidemia, without metastatic complications, is 2 weeks after documented clearance of *Candida* from the bloodstream and resolution of symptoms
Maximum dosage	<30 kg: 100 mg/day, >30 kg: 150 mg/day
Dose adjustments	Not required in renal/mild liver derangement. Not known in severe liver derangement
Adverse effects	SJS, rash, nausea, vomiting, blood dyscrasia
Contraindications	Hypersensitivity
Drug interactions	Sirolimus, nifedipine
Remarks	Protect from light

Midazolam

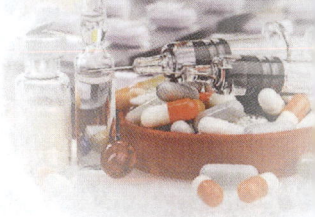

Drug name	Midazolam
Category	Benzodiazepine, Anticonvulsant, Sedative
Route	Intravenous, Intranasal
Strength	Inj 1 mg/1 mL, 0.5 mg per spray
Brands	Midaz (Inj), Midacip nasal spray
Mechanism of action	Short-acting CNS depressant. Also acts as anesthetic induction agent, needing 1.5 minutes for onset with opioid premedication and 2–2.5 minutes without premedication
Pharmacokinetics	Metabolized in liver, eliminated via urine
Indications	Sedation; Status epilepticus
Dosage as per indications	*Status epilepticus:* – *Loading:* 0.15 mg/kg IV – *Maintenance:* Continuous infusion of 1–7 µg/kg/min • *Sedation:* – *Intermittent:* 0.05–0.15 mg/kg/dose – *Continuous infusion:* 1–2 µg/kg/min
Maximum dosage	<5 years: 6 mg/dose, >5 years: 10 mg/dose. This is maximum total dose when given for procedural sedation
Dose adjustments	Renal and hepatic impairment
Adverse effects	Respiratory depression, bradycardia, hypotension
Contraindications	Use with caution in CHF, pulmonary disease, hepatic derangement
Drug interactions	Sedatives, muscle relaxants
Remarks	To be administered slowly over 10 minutes at a concentration of 1–5 mg/mL

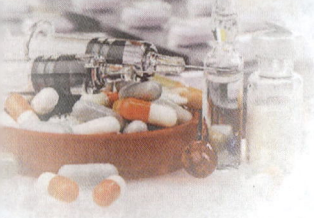

Milrinone

Drug name	Milrinone
Category	Pulmonary vasodilator
Route	Intravenous
Strength	Inj (1 mg/mL)
Brands	Primacor (Inj), Milrneon (Inj)
Mechanism of action	Phosphodiesterase 3 inhibitor; is a positive inotrope and vasodilator, selectively inhibits cAMP phosphodiesterase isozyme in cardiac and vascular muscle
Pharmacokinetics	Effect begins in 1 minute, peaks in 2–5 minutes, around 70% protein bound, terminal elimination half-life: 2–2.5 hours, primarily excreted via urine
Indications	Congestive heart failure (CHF)
Dosage as per indications	- *Loading dose:* 50 µg/kg - *Continuous infusion:* 0.25–1 µg/kg/min
Maximum dosage	Not known
Dose adjustments	Needed in renal derangement
Adverse effects	Dysrhythmia, hypotension, hypokalemia, hepatitis
Contraindications	Severe aortic stenosis, severe pulmonic stenosis, acute MI
Drug interactions	Not known

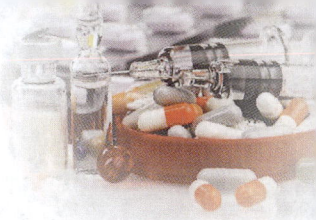

Miltefosine

Drug name	Miltefosine
Category	Antileishmanial
Route	Oral
Strength	Cap (10 mg, 50 mg)
Brands	Miltex (Cap), Mitepran (Cap)
Mechanism of action	Inhibits cytochrome-c oxidase leading to mitochondrial dysfunction, also inhibits phosphatidylcholine biosynthesis and protein kinase B
Pharmacokinetics	Variable absorption, highly protein bound, metabolized and eliminated by degradation via phospholipase D, terminal half-life around 30 days
Indications	Leishmaniasis
Dosage as per indications	• *30–44 kg:* Cap 50 mg twice a day • *>45 kg:* Cap 50 mg thrice a day for 28 consecutive days
Maximum dosage	150 mg/day
Dose adjustments	Not known
Adverse effects	Pain, pruritus, somnolence, elevated transaminases, and elevated creatinine
Contraindications	Hypersensitivity, Sjögren–Larsson syndrome
Drug interactions	Not known
Remarks	Used for children >12 years/>30 kg

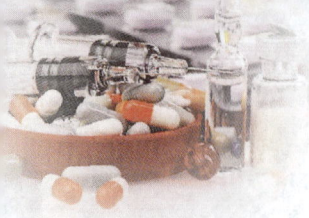

Minocycline

Drug name	Minocycline
Category	Antibiotic
Route	Oral
Strength	Cap (50 mg, 100 mg)
Brands	Minocin, Minomycin
Mechanism of action	Bacteriostatic drug; acts by inhibiting protein synthesis by binding to bacterial 30S ribosomal subunit. Active against many gram-positive and gram-negative organisms along with atypical organisms
Pharmacokinetics	*Half-life:* 11–22 hours, >70% protein bound, metabolized to 9-hydroxy minocycline, eliminated via biliary route
Indications	Rickettsial disease; Brucellosis; Syphilis; Chlamydia
Dosage as per indications	4 mg/kg initially followed by 2 mg/kg every 12 hours
Maximum dosage	200 mg/day
Dose adjustments	Renal and hepatic disease
Adverse effects	Dress, hepatic dysfunction, azotemia, tooth discoloration
Contraindications	Hypersensitivity
Drug interactions	Anticoagulants, antacids, penicillin
Remarks	Avoid in children <8 years

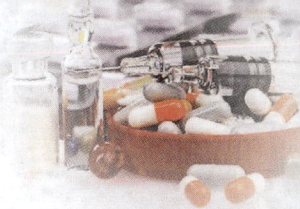

Minoxidil

Drug name	Minoxidil
Category	Direct vasodilator, Antihypertensive
Route	Oral
Strength	Tab (2.5 mg, 5 mg, 10 mg); Gel/Sol
Brands	Inoxl (Tab), Mintop (Sol), Tugain (Sol)
Mechanism of action	Direct acting peripheral vasodilator, decreases peripheral vascular resistance to reduce blood pressure
Pharmacokinetics	High absorption after oral intake. Peak plasma levels: 1 hour. Average plasma half-life: 4.2 hours. Metabolized after conjugation by glucuronidation
Indications	Hypertension
Dosage as per indications	Starting dose 0.2 mg/kg/day PO as single dose; can be increased till 5 mg/day. Increase by 0.1–0.2 mg/kg/day at 3-day intervals. Usual effective dose: 0.25–1 mg/kg/day PO q 12–24 h
Maximum dosage	• *<12 years:* 5 mg/kg/day or 50 mg/day • *>12 years:* 100 mg/day
Dose adjustments	Renal adjustment
Adverse effects	Dizziness, CHF, pulmonary edema, pericardial effusion, Stevens–Johnson syndrome, leukopenia, and hypertrichosis (reversible)
Contraindications	Acute MI, aortic aneurysm, pheochromocytoma
Drug interactions	Guanethidine

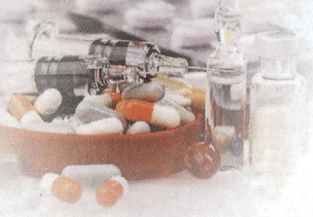

Mometasone

Drug name	Mometasone
Category	Steroid
Route	Nasal
Strength	Nasal spray (50 µg, 100 µg)
Brands	Momate (Nasal spray), Metaspray (Nasal spray)
Mechanism of action	Inhibits inflammatory mediators like other steroids
Pharmacokinetics	Very poor bioavailability, highly protein bound, metabolized in liver, elimination half-life: 6 hours, mainly excreted via bile
Indications	Allergic rhinitis
Dosage as per indications	• *Adults and adolescents (12 years and older):* 2 sprays in each nostril once daily • *Children (2–11 years):* 1 spray (50 µg) in each nostril once daily
Maximum dosage	2–11 years: 100 µg/day; >11 years: 200 µg/day
Dose adjustments	Not known
Adverse effects	Epistaxis, nasal ulceration, nasal septal perforation, infections
Contraindications	Hypersensitivity
Drug interactions	Concomitant administration of CYP3A4 inhibitors

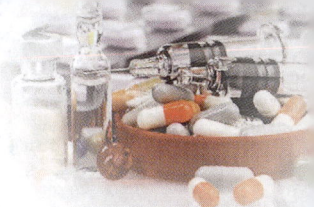

Montelukast Sodium

Drug name	Montelukast sodium
Category	Leukotriene inhibitor
Route	Oral
Strength	Tab (4 mg, 5 mg, 10 mg)
Brands	Almont (Tab), Montair (Tab), Montelast (Tab), Romilast (Tab)
Mechanism of action	Binds with high affinity and selectivity to the CysLT1 receptor and inhibits physiologic actions of LTD4 at the CysLT1 receptor without any agonist activity
Pharmacokinetics	Rapidly absorbed following oral administration. Highly bound to plasma proteins, extensively metabolized, mean plasma half-life: 2.7–5.5 hours
Indications	Allergic rhinitis; Add-on therapy asthma
Dosage as per indications	• *<5 years:* 4 mg once in the evening • *6–14 years:* 5 mg once in the evening • *>15 years:* 10 mg once in the evening
Maximum dosage	10 mg/day
Dose adjustments	Renal impairment
Adverse effects	Headache, dizziness, fatigue, elevated liver enzymes
Contraindications	Hypersensitivity
Drug interactions	Not known
Remarks	Chewable form not to be given in phenylketonuria

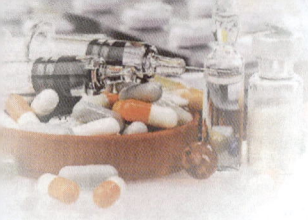

Morphine Sulfate

Drug name	Morphine sulfate
Category	Sedative, Hypnotic, Analgesic, Opioid
Route	Subcutaneous, Oral, Intravenous
Strength	Tab (2 mg, 4 mg, 5 mg, 10 mg, 15 mg); Inj (25 mg/mL ampoule); extended release Tab (60 mg)
Brands	Vermor-10 (Tab), Mitigo (Tab, Inj), Rumorf (Tab, Inj)
Mechanism of action	Selectively binds to mu-opioid receptor producing analgesia. Also reduces the responsiveness of brain stem respiratory centers causing respiratory depression
Pharmacokinetics	Around one-third is protein bound, metabolized by glucuronide conjugation to morphlne-3-glucuronide (M3G) and morphine-6-glucuronide (M6G). *Half-life:* 2 hours after IV administration
Indications	Analgesia; Cyanotic spell

Dosage as per indications	• *<28 days:* 4–6 hourly as needed
	  – *IV/IM/SC:* 0.05–0.2 mg/kg/dose
	  – *Oral:* 0.08–0.2 mg/kg/dose
	• *1–6 months:* 4–6 hourly as needed
	  – *PO:* 0.08–0.1 mg/kg/dose
	  – *IV:* 0.025–0.03 mg/kg/dose
	• *>6 months:* 4–6 hourly as needed
	  – *PO:* 0.2–0.5 mg/kg/dose
	  – *IM/IV/SC:* 0.1–0.2 mg/kg/dose
	
	For continuous infusion in neonates 0.01–0.02 mg/kg/h, infants and children 0.025–0.2 mg/kg/h IV

Maximum dosage	• *Oral (>6 months):* 15 mg/dose
	• *IV/IM/SC:*
	  – *<1 year:* 2 mg/dose
	  – *1–6 years:* 4 mg/dose
	  – *7–12 years:* 8 mg/dose
	• *Adolescent:* 10 mg/dose

Dose adjustments	Renal and hepatic
Adverse effects	Respiratory depression, hypotension, drowsiness, bradycardia

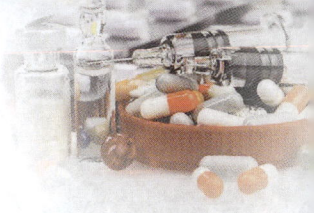

Contraindications	Contraindicated in children below 2 years, head injury, raised intracranial pressure, epilepsy, respiratory depression and renal failure
Drug interactions	Serotonergic drugs, MAO inhibitors, muscle relaxants

Morphine Sulfate

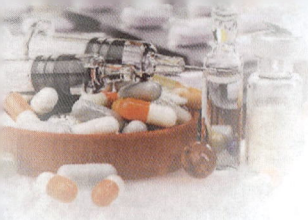

Moxifloxacin

Drug name	Moxifloxacin
Category	Antibiotic
Route	Oral, Intravenous
Strength	Tab (400 mg)
Brands	Moxiflox (Tab), Moxicip (Inj, Tab)
Mechanism of action	Inhibits topoisomerase II and IV
Pharmacokinetics	Well absorbed after oral administration, high bioavailability, 50% protein bound. Some is eliminated unchanged and rest metabolized via glucuronide and sulfate conjugation before elimination. Eliminated mainly in the feces, rest in urine
Indications	MDR TB
Dosage as per indications	10 mg/kg/day
Maximum dosage	400 mg/day
Dose adjustments	Not needed in renal dysfunction
Adverse effects	Nausea, vomiting, diarrhea, pain abdomen
Contraindications	Hypersensitivity
Drug interactions	Antacids, theophylline, warfarin, digoxin

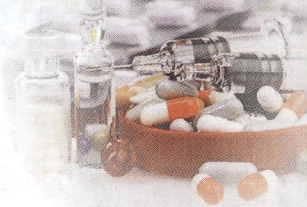

Mycophenolate Mofetil

Drug name	Mycophenolate mofetil
Category	Inosine monophosphate dehydrogenase inhibitor, Immunosuppressant
Route	Oral, Intravenous
Strength	Susp (200 mg/mL); Tab (250 mg, 500 mg)
Brands	CellCept (Tab, Syp), Mycofit 500 (Tab), MMF 500 (Tab), Mofilet (Tab)
Mechanism of action	Inhibits inosine monophosphate dehydrogenase (IMPDH) reversibly thereby affecting guanosine nucleotide synthesis
Pharmacokinetics	Rapidly and completely absorbed after oral intake, hydrolyzed to form MPA, which is the active metabolite
Indications	Organ transplant; Nephrotic syndrome
Dosage as per indications	• *For preventing organ rejection following kidney transplant:* 600 mg/m^2/dose orally 2 times a day up to a maximum of 2 g per day • *For liver transplant recipients:* 10–20 mg/kg/dose twice daily PO • *For steroid-resistant (SR) and steroid-dependent (SD) nephrotic syndrome:* 200–600 mg/m^2/dose body surface/dose (maximum 1 g), twice daily PO for 6–12 months
Maximum dosage	• *Organ transplant:* 2 g/day • *Nephrotic syndrome:* 1 g/day
Dose adjustments	Hepatic and renal derangement
Adverse effects	Dizziness, thrombocytopenia, diarrhea, asthma, herpes simplex infection, oral candidiasis, abdominal pain, vomiting, sepsis, myelosuppression, swelling of legs and ankles
Contraindications	Live vaccine
Drug interactions	Acyclovir, antacids, oral contraceptives, cyclosporine
Remarks	Take oral medicine on an empty stomach, either 1 hour before or 2 hours after a meal

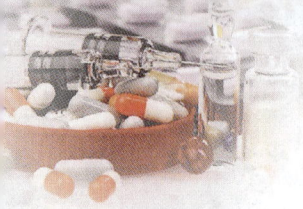

N-acetylcysteine

Drug name	N-acetylcysteine
Category	Antidote, Mucolytic
Route	Intravenous, Oral, For nebulization
Strength	Tab (200 mg, 400 mg, 600 mg); Inj (200 mg/mL), Syp (600 mg/15 mL); Nebulizing Sol (1000 mg/5 mL)
Brands	Fluimucil (Syp), Gluton (Cap), Mucare (Inj), Mucomyst (Inj), Mucotab (Tab), Mucyst 20% (Neb Sol)
Mechanism of action	Restores glutathione levels by providing cysteine. Best effect when given within 10–12 hours of acetaminophen toxicity
Pharmacokinetics	Highly protein bound, elimination half-life: 11 hours in newborns, decreases to 5 hours in adults. Deacetylated and converted to cysteine. Eliminated in urine and feces
Indications	Paracetamol poisoning; Mucolysis
Dosage as per indications	• *Antidote for acetaminophen (paracetamol) toxicity:* Administered PO in a loading dose of 140 mg/kg and followed by 70 mg/kg 4 hourly (diluted to 5% solution) for additional 17 doses • *Also used in nebulized routes for mucolytic effects:* Nebulized into a face mask, mouth piece, or tracheostomy: Recommended dosage: 3–5 mL of 20% solution, or 6–10 mL of 10% solution, 3–4 times a day
Maximum dosage	Not known
Dose adjustments	Hepatic derangement
Adverse effects	Nausea, vomiting, and diarrhea or constipation. Inhaled route may rarely cause swelling in the mouth, runny nose, drowsiness, clamminess, and chest tightness
Contraindications	Hypersensitivity
Drug interactions	Not known
Remarks	The critical ingestion to treatment interval is 0–8 hours for maximal protection against severe hepatic injury following acetaminophen overdose. Determine serum acetaminophen level at least 4 hours after ingestion of suspected overdose to determine the need for treatment with acetylcysteine

Nalidixic Acid

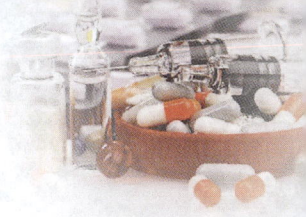

Drug name	Nalidixic acid
Category	Antibiotic, Quinolone
Route	Oral
Strength	Tab (125 mg, 500 mg); Susp (300 mg/5 mL)
Brands	Gramoneg (Tab, Syp), Negadix (Tab, Syp), Ordixic (Susp)
Mechanism of action	Blocks DNA replication by inhibiting a subunit of DNA gyrase
Pharmacokinetics	Rapidly absorbed following oral administration, partially metabolized in the liver, rapidly eliminated via kidneys; half-life: 90 minutes
Indications	Active against gram-negative infections
Dosage as per indications	50–55 mg/kg/day q 6–8 h PO
Maximum dosage	4 g/day
Dose adjustments	Renal and liver derangement
Adverse effects	Pseudotumor cerebri
Contraindications	Avoid in infants below 3 months. Avoid in children with history of seizures, G6PD deficiency
Drug interactions	Quinolone, cyclosporine, theophylline

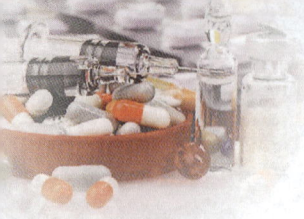

Naloxone Hydrochloride

Drug name	Naloxone hydrochloride
Category	Narcotic antagonist
Route	Intravenous
Strength	Inj (0.4 mg/mL, 0.02 mg/mL)
Brands	Narcan (Inj), Narcotan (Inj)
Mechanism of action	Opioid antagonist, competes for the same receptor sites as opioid. Reverses respiratory depression, sedation, hypotension, and other opioid effects
Pharmacokinetics	Onset of action: 2 minutes, most rapid response with IV administration. Half-life: 1.5 hours, metabolized in liver, mainly eliminated in urine
Indications	Opioid intoxication
Dosage as per indications	• *Neonates, infants and children <20 kg:* 0.1–0.2 mg/kg/dose IM/IV/SC/ETT. May repeat every 2–3 minutes • *Children ≥20 kg or >5 years:* 2 mg/dose, may repeat every 2–3 minutes
Maximum dosage	Not known
Dose adjustments	Use with caution in renal and hepatic derangement
Adverse effects	Abrupt reversal of narcotic dependence can lead to nausea, vomiting, tachycardia, hypertension, and tremulousness
Contraindications	To be used cautiously in patients with chronic cardiac disease
Drug interactions	CNS depressants
Remarks	• In case of chronic opioid dependence, it can lead to narcotic withdrawal syndrome • Lack of response after a cumulative dose of 10 mg warrants detailed evaluation to look for alternate diagnosis

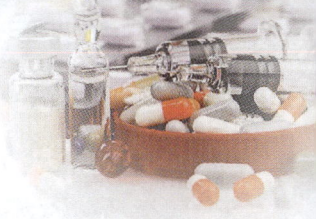

Naproxen

Drug name	Naproxen
Category	Nonsteroidal anti-inflammatory drug (NSAID)
Route	Oral
Strength	Tab (250 mg, 500 mg, 750 mg); Syp (125 mg/5 mL)
Brands	Arthopan (Tab), Naprosyn (Tab, Syp), Spirox (Tab)
Mechanism of action	Has anti-inflammatory action by inhibiting prostaglandin synthesis
Pharmacokinetics	Well absorbed after oral administration, peak plasma levels 5 hours, half-life 15 hours, metabolized in liver, excreted in urine
Indications	Analgesic; JIA
Dosage as per indications	• *For analgesia:* 5–7 mg/kg/dose q 8–12 h PO • *For juvenile idiopathic arthritis (JIA):* 10–20 mg/kg/day q 12 h PO
Maximum dosage	1,000 mg/day
Dose adjustments	Renal disease, not recommended in severe renal derangement
Adverse effects	Dizziness, rash, gastric irritation
Contraindications	Peptic ulcer disease
Drug interactions	NSAIDs, anticoagulants

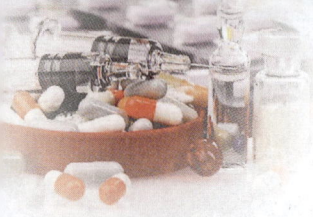

Nelfinavir (NFV)

Drug name	Nelfinavir (NFV)
Category	Antiviral, Protease inhibitor
Route	Oral
Strength	Tab (250 mg)
Brands	Emnel (Tab), Nelvir (Tab)
Mechanism of action	Inhibitor of the HIV-1 protease, preventing cleavage of the gag and gag-pol polyprotein resulting in the production of immature, noninfectious virus
Pharmacokinetics	Well-absorbed orally, extensively protein-bound, terminal half-life: 3.5–5 hours, poorly metabolized, excreted mostly unchanged via feces
Indications	AIDS/HIV infection
Dosage as per indications	• *Neonates:* 40 mg/kg/dose PO BID • *Children (>3 months):* 25–30 mg/kg/dose PO TID
Maximum dosage	750 mg/day
Dose adjustments	Not known
Adverse effects	Diarrhea, asthenia, abdominal pain, rash, hyperglycemia, exacerbation of chronic liver disease
Contraindications	Hypersensitivity
Drug interactions	Terfenadine, astemizole, midazolam, amiodarone, quinine, antiepileptics
Remarks	It should be taken with food

Neomycin Sulfate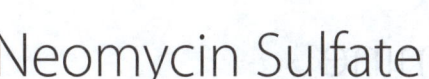

Drug name	Neomycin sulfate
Category	Aminoglycoside and ammonium desiccant
Route	Oral, Topical Antibiotic
Strength	Tab (350 mg, 500 mg); Cream (0.5%); Ointment (0.5%); Sol (125 mg/5 mL)
Brands	Nebasulf Skin Ointment, Neomycin (Tab)
Mechanism of action	Bactericidal mainly gram-negative bacilli; acts by inhibiting the synthesis of protein in susceptible bacterial cells
Pharmacokinetics	Poorly absorbed after oral administration. Absorbed fraction is mainly eliminated by kidney and unabsorbed by feces
Indications	Active against gram-negative bacteria
Dosage as per indications	• *Diarrhea:* 50 mg/kg/day q 6 h PO • *Hepatic encephalopathy:* 50–100 mg/kg/day q 6–8 h PO × 5 days • *Topical:* Apply one to four times to the affected area
Maximum dosage	1 g/day
Dose adjustments	Reduce dose in renal failure
Adverse effects	Nephrotoxic, ototoxic. When applied topically may cause itching, redness, edema, colitis, candidiasis or poor wound healing
Contraindications	Contraindicated in intestinal obstruction
Drug interactions	Nephrotoxic and ototoxic drugs

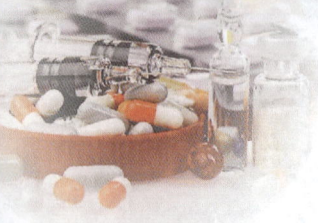

Neostigmine

Drug name	Neostigmine
Category	Anticholinesterase (Cholinergic) agent
Route	Intramuscular, Intravenous, Subcutaneous
Strength	Tab (15 mg); Inj (0.25 mg/mL, 0.5 mg/mL, 1 mg/mL)
Brands	Prostigmin (neostigmine bromide) (Tab) Bloxiverz (Inj)
Mechanism of action	• It is a competitive cholinesterase inhibitor. • It reduces acetylcholine breakdown thereby increasing acetylcholine in the synaptic cleft • It attaches on the same site as of nondepolarizing neuromuscular blocking agents, and hence reverses the neuromuscular blockade
Pharmacokinetics	Metabolized in liver by microsomal enzymes. Around 20% bound to protein. Elimination half-life: 30 minutes to 2 hours
Indications	Myasthenia gravis
Dosage as per indications	• *Myasthenia gravis:* – *IV/SC/IM:* 0.01–0.04 mg/kg/dose q 2–3 h – *Oral:* 2 mg/kg/day q 3–4 h • *Reversal of nondepolarizing neuromuscular blockade (co-administered with atropine or glycopyrrolate):* 0.025–0.08 mg/kg/dose IV
Maximum dosage	Maximum total dosage up to 5 mg/dose when given IV/SC/IM when used for reversal of neuromuscular blockade
Dose adjustments	Renal and hepatic impairment
Adverse effects	May cause cholinergic crisis, bronchospasm, salivation, nausea, vomiting, diarrhea, miosis, bradycardia, hypotension, fatigue, seizures, lacrimation, sweating, and respiratory depression
Contraindications	Contraindicated in GI and urinary obstruction
Drug interactions	Muscle relaxants, cholinergic and anticholinergic drugs
Remarks	*Antidote:* Atropine 0.01–0.04 mg/kg/dose IV

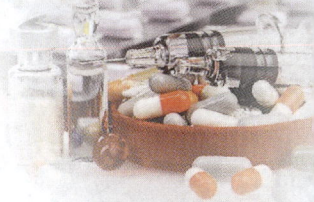

Netilmicin Sulfate

Drug name	Netilmicin sulfate
Category	Antibiotic, Aminoglycoside
Route	Intravenous, Intramuscular
Strength	Inj (10 mg/mL, 25 mg/mL, 50 mg/mL, 100 mg/mL ampoules)
Brands	Netromycin (Inj), Netromax (Inj)
Mechanism of action	Acts like other aminoglycosides, inhibits protein synthesis by binding to ribosome 30 subunit in bacteria
Pharmacokinetics	Rapidly absorbed after parenteral administration, poorly protein bound, peak levels in 1 hour, half-life 2.5 hours
Indications	Acts against gram-negative; Gram-positive bacteria
Dosage as per indications	5–7.5 mg/kg/day q 8–12 h (infants 7.5–10 mg/kg/day) for 7–14 days
Maximum dosage	Not known
Dose adjustments	In renal derangement
Adverse effects	Headache, malaise, visual disturbances, palpitation, thrombocytosis, hepatic dysfunction, anemia
Contraindications	Hypersensitivity
Drug interactions	Vancomycin, other nephrotoxic/ototoxic drugs, muscle relaxants

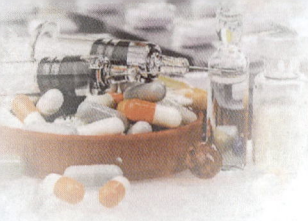

Nevirapine (NVP)

Drug name	Nevirapine (NVP)
Category	Antiviral, Protease inhibitor
Route	Oral
Strength	Tab (200 mg), Syp (10 mg/5 mL)
Brands	Nevimune (Tab), Nevir (Tab, Syp), Nevivir (Tab)
Mechanism of action	It is a non-nucleoside reverse transcriptase inhibitor (NNRTI) of HIV-1 virus. Nevirapine binds to reverse transcriptase (RT) enzyme and blocks the RNA-dependent and DNA-dependent DNA polymerase
Pharmacokinetics	Readily absorbed after oral administration, >50% protein bound
Indications	AIDS/HIV infection

Dosage as per indications	• *Initial:* 120 mg/m^2 once a day for 2 weeks
	• *Maintenance:* 120 mg/m^2/dose BID, if no rash or other side effects
	• *For prevention of mother to child transmission (PMTCT):*
	  – *Birth weight <2 kg:* 2 mg/kg PO started within 24 hours of birth and given for 6 weeks of life
	  – *Birth weight 2–2.5 kg:* 10 mg, PO, OD
	  – *Birth weight ≥2.5 kg:* 15 mg, PO, OD

Maximum dosage	400 mg/day
Dose adjustments	In severe renal and hepatic derangement
Adverse effects	Nausea, liver toxicity, pain abdomen, skin rash, low neutrophil count
Contraindications	Hypersensitivity
Drug interactions	Drugs affecting CYP450 enzyme, indinavir, ritonavir, saquinavir, rifampicin, rifabutin
Remarks	NVP should be taken with food to decrease gastrointestinal irritation

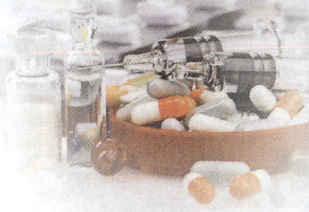

Niclosamide

Drug name	Niclosamide
Category	Antihelminthic
Route	Oral
Strength	Tab (500 mg)
Brands	Niclosan (Tab), Niclesone (Tab)
Mechanism of action	It inhibits oxidative phosphorylation in the parasite's mitochondria, leads to death of the scolex and adjoining segments. As a result, the segment loses its grip and is eliminated from the intestine during bowel movement
Pharmacokinetics	Poorly absorbed from the gut after oral administration
Indications	*Infestations with Taenia saginata; Taenia solium; Diphyllobothrium latum; Hymenolepis nana*
Dosage as per indications	The whole initial dose of 2 g to be given in 2 parts. 1 g empty stomach followed by another dose after 1 hour. A brisk purgative is given after 2 hours of last dose. For dwarf tapeworm (*H. nana*), single dose as above followed by half dose for the next 6 days. Use half of this dose in children <6 years. In children <2 years, initial dose in 500 mg.
Maximum dosage	Initial dose: • <2 years: 500 mg • 2–6 years: 1 g • >7 years: 2 g
Dose adjustments	None in hepatic and renal derangement
Adverse effects	Nausea, vomiting, abdominal pain, constipation, itching, dizziness, skin rash, drowsiness, perianal itching, or an unpleasant taste
Contraindications	Hypersensitivity
Drug interactions	Not known
Remarks	Niclosamide tablets should be thoroughly chewed or crushed and then swallowed with a small amount of water

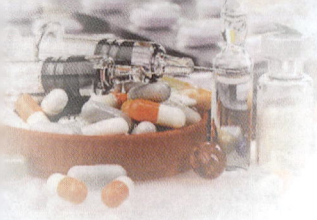

Nifedipine

Drug name	Nifedipine
Category	Calcium channel blocker
Route	Oral
Strength	Cap (5 mg, 10 mg, 20 mg); Tab (10 mg, 20 mg)
Brands	Calcigard (Cap, Tab), Depin (Cap, Tab), Nicardia (Cap, Tab)
Mechanism of action	Inhibits the transmembrane influx of calcium ions into cardiac muscle and smooth muscle
Pharmacokinetics	Rapid and high absorption after oral administration. Effect begins in 10 minutes and peak blood levels noted in 30 minutes. Bioavailability increases with increasing dose
Indications	Hypertension
Dosage as per indications	• *For hypertensive emergency/hypertension:* 0.25–0.5 mg/kg/dose q 4–6 h. 300–500 μg/kg/dose sublingual for severe hypertension • *For hypertrophic cardiomyopathy:* 0.5–0.9 mg/kg/d q 6–8 h PO/SL
Maximum dosage	10 mg/dose
Dose adjustments	Dose adjustment in hepatic derangement, not needed in renal impairment
Adverse effects	Hypotension, flushing, tachycardia, headache, dizziness, and nausea
Contraindications	Hypersensitivity
Drug interactions	Avoid concurrent beta blockers
Remarks	For sublingual administration, capsule to be punctured and liquid expressed in mouth. Do not chew/crush sustained release tablets

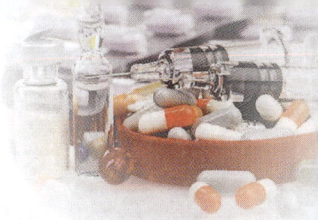

Nitazoxanide

Drug name	Nitazoxanide
Category	Antiparasitic, Antiviral
Route	Oral
Strength	Tab (100 mg, 500 mg); Syp (100 mg/5 mL)
Brands	Nozoa (Tab, Syp), Nitadox (Tab, Syp)
Mechanism of action	Disrupts energy metabolism in anaerobic microbes by inhibition of the pyruvate: ferredoxin/flavodoxin oxidoreductase (PFOR) cycle
Pharmacokinetics	Mostly bound to proteins, metabolism by glucuronidation after being hydrolyzed to tizoxanide, excreted in urine, bile and feces
Indications	For ascariasis; Cryptosporidium; Giardiasis infection in children
Dosage as per indications	• *2–3 years:* 100 mg BD × 3 days • *4–11 years:* 200 mg BD × 3 days • *>12 years:* 500 mg BD × 3 days
Maximum dosage	1 g/day
Dose adjustments	In severe renal/hepatic impairment
Adverse effects	Abdominal pain, diarrhea, nausea, anorexia, flatulence, fever, pruritus
Contraindications	Hypersensitivity
Drug interactions	Digitalis, anticoagulants
Remarks	• Food increases its absorption • Also shown efficacy in chronic hepatitis B and C infection

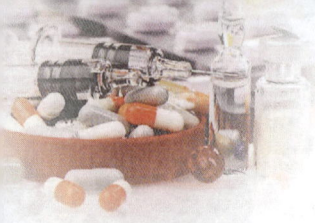

Nitrazepam

Drug name	Nitrazepam
Category	Benzodiazepine
Route	Oral
Strength	Tab (5 mg, 10 mg)
Brands	Nitavan, Nitraplan (Tab)
Mechanism of action	It is a centrally acting drug which enhances GABA binding activity at central benzodiazepine receptors. It also binds to voltage-dependent sodium channels and exerts anticonvulsant action
Pharmacokinetics	Not much known. Bioavailability highly variable, from 50 to 95% after oral administration, elimination half-life 25–26 hours
Indications	Sedative; Anticonvulsant
Dosage as per indications	0.5–1 mg/kg/day in 1–2 divided doses
Maximum dosage	1 mg/kg/day
Dose adjustments	Not needed in renal and mild-moderate hepatic dysfunction
Adverse effects	Drowsiness, irritability, respiratory depression
Contraindications	Hypersensitivity, severe hepatic insufficiency
Drug interactions	CNS depressants, antipsychotics

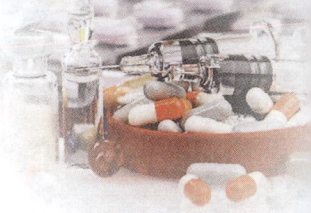

Nitrofurantoin

Drug name	Nitrofurantoin
Category	Antibiotic, Nitrofuran
Route	Oral
Strength	Tab (50 mg, 100 mg); Syp (25 mg/5 mL)
Brands	Urifast (Tab, Syp), Furadantin (Tab, Syp), Martifur (Tab, Syp)
Mechanism of action	Bactericidal in urine, inactivate or alter bacterial ribosomal proteins resulting in hampering protein synthesis, DNA and RNA synthesis
Pharmacokinetics	High bioavailability, with nearly 40% excreted in urine, around three-fourths of drug is metabolized in liver, bactericidal in bladder in levels achieved in urine
Indications	Urinary tract infections (Treatment and Prophylaxis)
Dosage as per indications	• *Treatment:* 5–7 mg/kg/day q 6–8 h, with meals, PO • *Prophylaxis:* 1–2 mg/kg/day HS
Maximum dosage	400 mg/day
Dose adjustments	Required in renal and hepatic derangement
Adverse effects	Nausea, hypersensitivity, vomiting, cholestatic jaundice, polyneuropathy, and hemolytic anemia
Contraindications	Avoid in G6PD deficiency, infants and pregnant females
Drug interactions	Quinolones
Remarks	May result in false-positive urine glucose tested using dipstick method. Preferably give with food or milk

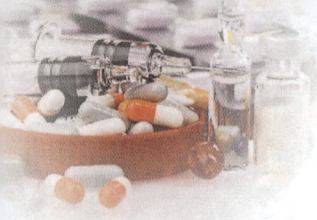

Nitroprusside

Drug name	Nitroprusside
Category	Vasodilator, Antihypertensive drug
Route	Intravenous
Strength	Inj (50 mg ampoule)
Brands	Nipride, Sonide (Inj)
Mechanism of action	Sodium nitroprusside combines with oxyhemoglobin and produces nitric oxide (NO). NO produces cGMP with the help of guanylate cyclase. cGMP relaxes smooth muscle by reducing intracellular calcium. It also causes dilatation of peripheral vessels, veins more than arteries
Pharmacokinetics	The effect starts within 1–2 minutes. Half-life: 2 minutes. Eliminated from body via urine in the form of thiocyanate
Indications	Hypertension
Dosage as per indications	Start continuous infusion at a dose 0.3–0.5 µg/kg/min, titrate according to clinical effect. Usual dose 3–4 µg/kg/min
Maximum dosage	10 µg/kg/min
Dose adjustments	Needed in renal and hepatic derangement
Adverse effects	Metabolic acidosis, methemoglobinemia
Contraindications	Raised intracranial pressure, hypertension due to coarctation of aorta or secondary to arteriovenous shunts
Drug interactions	Lidocaine, morphine, fentanyl

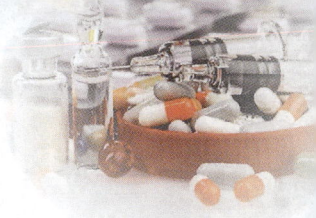

Nizatidine

Drug name	Nizatidine
Category	Antacid
Route	Oral
Strength	Cap (150 mg, 300 mg); Syp (75 mg/5 mL)
Brands	Axid (Cap), Nizatect (Cap), Nizatidine (Cap/Syp)
Mechanism of action	Competitive and reversible inhibitor at H_2 histamine receptors in gastric parietal cells
Pharmacokinetics	Bioavailability after oral administration around 70%. Elimination half-life 1–2 hours, protein binding 35%, mainly eliminated in urine with >50% as unchanged drug
Indications	Esophagitis; GERD
Dosage as per indications	>12 years: 150 mg twice a day
Maximum dosage	300 mg/day
Dose adjustments	In renal derangement
Adverse effects	Headache, dizziness, rash
Contraindications	Hypersensitivity
Drug interactions	Indinavir, ketoconazole, cefpodoxime
Remarks	Not used in children <12 years

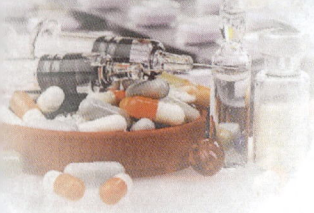

Norepinephrine

Drug name	Norepinephrine
Category	Adrenergic agonist
Route	Intravenous
Strength	Inj (1 mg/mL ampoule)
Brands	Norad (Inj), Veralin (Inj), Adrenor (Inj)
Mechanism of action	Alpha- and beta-adrenergic action leading to peripheral vasoconstriction, cardiac stimulation and coronary artery dilatation with reduced flow to abdominal organs and skeletal muscle
Pharmacokinetics	Rapid response with steady state within 5 minutes. The pressor action stops within 1–2 minutes of discontinuation of the drug. Metabolized in liver
Indications	Shock
Dosage as per indications	As continuous intravenous infusion. Start at 0.05–0.1 µg/kg/min
Maximum dosage	2 µg/kg/min
Dose adjustments	As per the response
Adverse effects	Cardiac arrhythmia, headache
Contraindications	Hypersensitivity
Drug interactions	Other ionotropic drugs
Remarks	To be given by central line only. Extravasation causes severe tissue necrosis

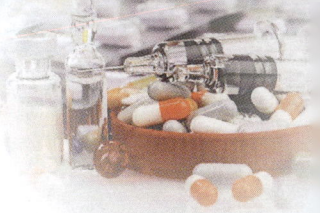

Norfloxacin

Drug name	Norfloxacin
Category	Antibiotic, Quinolone
Route	Oral
Strength	Tab (100 mg, 200 mg, 400 mg); Susp (100 mg/5 mL)
Brands	Bacigyl (Tab), Norflox (Tab, Syp), Norspan (Tab)
Mechanism of action	Bactericidal, inhibits bacterial DNA synthesis by inhibition of the ATP-dependent DNA supercoiling reaction, inhibition of the relaxation of supercoiled DNA, and promotion of double-stranded DNA breakage. The above actions occur due to inhibition of Topoisomerase II and IV
Pharmacokinetics	Rapid absorption, peak levels: 1 hour, half-life: 3–4 hours, eliminated through biliary and renal excretion
Indications	Active mainly against gram-negative bacteria; Some gram-positive bacteria
Dosage as per indications	10–15 mg/kg/day q 12 h
Maximum dosage	400 mg/dose
Dose adjustments	In renal derangement
Adverse effects	Arthropathy
Contraindications	Hypersensitivity
Drug interactions	Warfarin
Remarks	Administer empty stomach

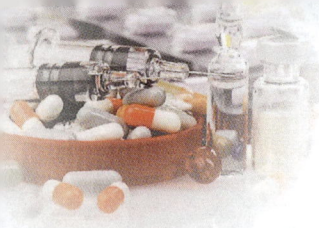

Nystatin

Drug name	Nystatin
Category	Antifungal
Route	Oral, Topical, Oral mouth rinse for oral candidiasis
Strength	Tab (500,000 U); Susp (100,000 U/mL); Cream/Ointment (100,000 U/g); Vaginal Tab (100,000 U)
Brands	Mycostatin (Tab, Syp, Cream), Nystatin (Tab, Oint)
Mechanism of action	Fungistatic and fungicidal, acts by binding to sterols in the cell membrane of susceptible *Candida* species, alters membrane permeability, leads to leakage of intracellular components
Pharmacokinetics	Negligible absorption from gut. Most passes unchanged via feces
Indications	Oral candidiasis; Vaginal candidiasis; Fungal diarrhea
Dosage as per indications	• *Children:* 400,000–600,000 U QID • *Neonates:* 50,000–100,000 U QID • *Vaginal:* 1 tablet HS × 14 days • *Topical:* Apply BD-QID • *Diarrhea due to Candida albicans:* 1 million U/day
Maximum dosage	Not known
Dose adjustments	Renal impairment
Adverse effects	Diarrhea, nausea, vomiting, rash, tachycardia, bronchospasm
Contraindications	Hypersensitivity
Drug interactions	Not known
Remarks	Oral suspension should be swished in mouth and retained for as long as possible before swallowing

Octreotide

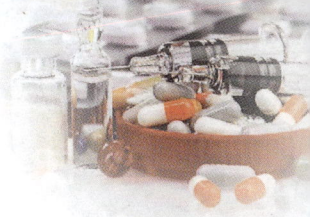

Drug name	Octreotide
Category	Somatostatin analog
Route	Intravenous, Subcutaneous
Strength	Inj (50 μg, 100 μg)
Brands	Humtide (Inj), Octride (inj), Sandostatin (Inj)
Mechanism of action	Inhibits growth hormone (GH), glucagon, and insulin. It also affects GIT by decreasing splanchnic blood flow, and inhibiting serotonin, gastrin, vasoactive intestinal peptide, secretin, motilin, and pancreatic polypeptide release
Pharmacokinetics	Rapid and high absorption from injection site when given subcutaneously. Elimination half-life: 1.7–1.9 hours
Indications	Portal hypertension-related variceal bleeding; Chylothorax; Hyperinsulinemic hypoglycemia
Dosage as per indications	• *Hyperinsulinemic hypoglycemia:* 1 μg/kg/dose every 6 hours SC or IV; titrate upward till desired effect • *Chylothorax:* Begin at 1 μg/kg/h IV continuous infusion or SC injection; can be titrated upward • *Portal hypertension-related variceal bleeding:* 1 μg/kg bolus, then 1 μg/kg/h infusion; taper by 50% when no active bleeding for 24 hours
Maximum dosage	10 μg/kg/dose
Dose adjustments	Use cautiously in hepatic and renal derangement
Adverse effects	Cholelithiasis, pancreatitis, B_{12} malabsorption, hyperhidrosis, arthralgia, increased blood glucose, vomiting, sinus bradycardia, low TSH, AV block
Contraindications	Hypersensitivity
Drug interactions	Cyclosporine, insulin, calcium and beta blockers
Remarks	Avoid in cardiac failure

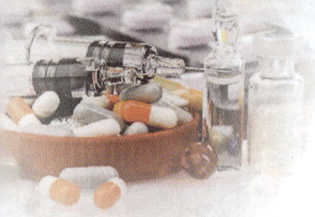

Ofloxacin

Drug name	Ofloxacin
Category	Antibiotic, Fluoroquinolone
Route	Oral, Intravenous
Strength	Tab (200 mg, 400 mg); Susp (100 mg/5 mL); Inj (200 mg/100 mL, 400 mg/100 mL)
Brands	Bestoflox (Inj, Syp, Tab), Inflobid (Syp, Tab), Oflomac (Syp, Tab, Inj)
Mechanism of action	Inhibits bacterial topoisomerase IV and DNA gyrase thereby preventing DNA replication
Pharmacokinetics	Almost complete bioavailability after oral administration. Peak levels: 1–2 hours after oral administration. Almost three-fourths of the dose excreted unchanged after 48 hours in urine through the kidneys
Indications	Acts mostly against gram-negative; Some gram positive bacteria
Dosage as per indications	• *Oral:* 15 mg/kg/day q 12 h • *Intravenous:* 5–10 mg/kg/day q 12 h
Maximum dosage	400 mg/dose
Dose adjustments	Renal derangement
Adverse effects	Nausea, vomiting, headache, dizziness, skin itching, change in sense of taste, diarrhea, vaginal pruritus
Contraindications	Avoid use in patients with myasthenia gravis
Drug interactions	Antiretroviral, warfarin, methotrexate

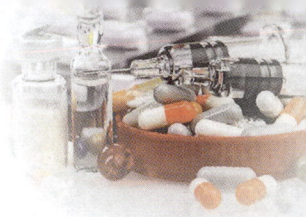

Olanzapine

Drug name	Olanzapine
Category	Antipsychotic
Route	Oral
Strength	Tab (2.5 mg, 5 mg, 7.5 mg, 10 mg, 15 mg)
Brands	Dopin (Tab), Jolyon-MD (Tab), Lanopin (Tab)
Mechanism of action	Has dual action. Acts as dopamine and serotonin type 2 (5HT2) antagonist
Pharmacokinetics	Well absorbed, high first pass metabolism, highly bound to plasma proteins, mainly metabolized in liver, mainly eliminated in liver after metabolized, half-life around 30 hours
Indications	Bipolar disorder; Schizophrenia
Dosage as per indications	Start with 2.5–5 mg/day and increase gradually till clinical improvement or reaches target of 10 mg/day
Maximum dosage	20 mg/day
Dose adjustments	Needed in liver derangement
Adverse effects	Hyperglycemia, dyslipidemia, neuroleptic malignant syndrome
Contraindications	Hypersensitivity
Drug interactions	Diazepam, fluvoxamine, carbamazepine, dopamine agonist

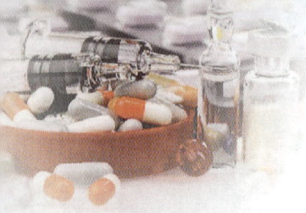

Olmesartan

Drug name	Olmesartan
Category	Antihypertensive
Route	Oral
Strength	Tab (10 mg, 20 mg, 40 mg)
Brands	Olbet (Tab), Olmetor (Tab), Olsar (Tab), Pinom (Tab)
Mechanism of action	It is an angiotensin II receptor blocker. It prevents angiotensin II to bind to AT1 receptor thus preventing vasoconstriction in vascular smooth muscle
Pharmacokinetics	Converted to active form during absorption from the gut, highly bound to plasma proteins, eliminated in both urine and feces in a biphasic manner, terminal elimination half-life around 13 hours
Indications	Hypertension
Dosage as per indications	• *20–35 kg:* 10 mg once a day • *>35 kg:* 20 mg once a day • Dose titration may be considered after 2 weeks of therapy
Maximum dosage	• *20–35 kg:* 20 mg once a day • *>35 kg:* 40 mg once a day
Dose adjustments	Use with caution in hepatic and renal derangement
Adverse effects	Diarrhea, cough, hypertriglyceridemia, cough, headache
Contraindications	Hypersensitivity, infants, bilateral renal artery stenosis
Drug interactions	NSAIDs, diuretics
Remarks	Avoid in <6 years old children

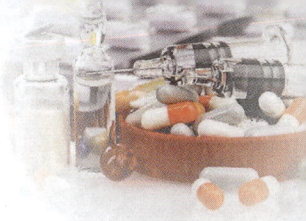

Omalizumab

Drug name	Omalizumab
Category	Anti-IgE antibody
Route	Subcutaneous
Strength	Inj (150 mg)
Brands	Bolstran (Inj), Xolair (Inj), Omalirel (Inj)
Mechanism of action	Recombinant DNA-derived humanized IgG1κ monoclonal antibody. It selectively binds to human immunoglobulin E. This prevents IgE to bind to its receptor present on mast cells and basophils
Pharmacokinetics	Well absorbed, bioavailability around 60%. After SC administration, omalizumab was absorbed with an average absolute bioavailability of 62%. The complexes are degraded and cleared by liver, reticuloendothelial system and endothelial cells. Serum elimination half-life: 24–26 days
Indications	Moderate to severe persistent asthma; Chronic idiopathic urticaria
Dosage as per indications	*Used in >6 years* • Serum IgE – ≥30–100 IU/mL: <30 kg: 75 mg, >30 kg: 150 mg 4 weekly – 100–200 IU/mL: <30 kg: 150 mg, >30 kg: 300 mg every 4 weekly – ≥200–300 IU/mL: <30 kg: 150 mg, 30–60 kg: 300 mg 4 weekly, >60 kg: 225 mg 2 weekly – ≥300–400 IU/mL: 225 mg 2 weekly – 400–500 IU/mL: 300 mg 2 weekly – ≥500–600 IU/mL: 30–60 kg: 300 mg 2 weekly, >60 kg: 375 mg 2 weekly – >600 IU/mL: 375 mg 2 weekly
Maximum dosage	150 mg on one site
Dose adjustments	Not known

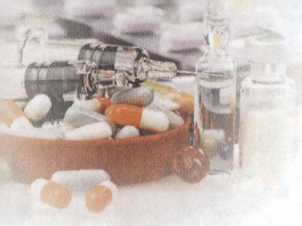

Adverse effects	Nasopharyngitis, headache, fever, pain abdomen, otitis media, epistaxis. Some added side-effects seen in ≥12 years of age were arthralgia, generalised pain, tiredness, dizziness, fracture, pruritus and dermatitis
Contraindications	Hypersensitivity
Drug interactions	Not known
Remarks	Increases risk of malignancy. Not effective in acute attack

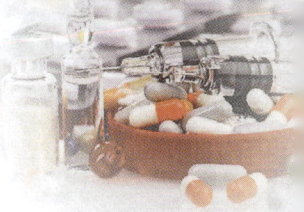

Omeprazole

Drug name	Omeprazole
Category	Proton pump inhibitor
Route	Oral
Strength	Cap (10 mg, 20 mg)
Brands	Ocid, Omepral, Omez
Mechanism of action	Inhibits H^+/K^+ ATPase to inhibit secretion from gastric parietal cell
Pharmacokinetics	Effect starts within 1 hour of oral intake, peak effect in 2 hours. Acid secretion decreases by 50% in 24 hours. It is rapidly absorbed after oral intake, highly protein bound, metabolized in liver via cytochrome P450 system and eliminated mostly in urine
Indications	Gastritis; Duodenal; Gastric ulcer
Dosage as per indications	• 5–9 kg: 5 mg • 10–19 kg: 10 mg • >20 kg: 20 mg
Maximum dosage	20 mg/day
Dose adjustments	In liver derangement
Adverse effects	Headache, abdominal pain, nausea, diarrhea, vomiting, and flatulence
Contraindications	Hypersensitivity
Drug interactions	Antiretroviral drugs (saquinavir, nelfinavir), anticoagulant drugs, drugs metabolized by cytochrome P450
Remarks	Not used in infants

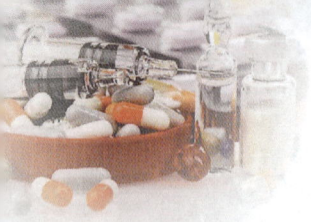

Ondansetron Hydrochloride

Drug name	Ondansetron hydrochloride
Category	Antiemetic, 5HT3 antagonist
Route	Oral, Intravenous, Intramuscular
Strength	Tab (4 mg, 8 mg); Syp (4 mg/5 mL); Inj (2 mg/mL ampoule)
Brands	Emset (Inj, Syp, Tab), Ondem (Inj, Syp, Tab), Vomikind (Inj, Syp, Tab)
Mechanism of action	Selective 5-HT3 receptor antagonist. Does not allow serotonin to stimulate vagal afferents through 5-HT3 receptors to initiate vomiting
Pharmacokinetics	Around 50% bioavailability after oral dose. Extensively metabolized by hydroxylation followed by glucuronidation. Half-life around 3–4 hours
Indications	Vomiting
Dosage as per indications	• IV 0.15 mg/kg/dose q 6–8 h • PO 0.1–0.2 mg/kg/dose q 6–8 h • *For chemotherapy-induced nausea and vomiting (CINV):* 0.15–0.45 mg/kg/dose at 30 minutes before and 4 and 8 hours after emetogenic drugs
Maximum dosage	8 mg/dose oral
Dose adjustments	Hepatic impairment, severe renal impairment
Adverse effects	Bronchospasm, tachycardia, hypokalemia, seizures, constipation or diarrhea, transient increase in liver enzymes
Contraindications	Avoid in QT syndrome
Drug interactions	CYP 3A4 inducers, antacids

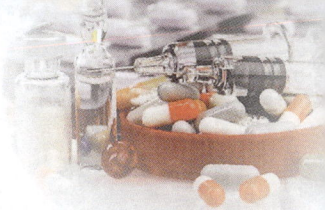

Oral Rehydration Salt (ORS)

Drug name	Oral rehydration salt (ORS)
Category	Rehydrating fluid
Route	Oral
Strength	Powder (to reconstitute in 1 L); Tetra pack (200 mL)
Brands	Electral (Powder), ORS (Powder), Prolyte ORS (Solution), Electrorush (Powder, Solution)
Mechanism of action	Acts by replacing fluids and electrolytes. Contains sodium chloride 2.6 g, trisodium citrate 2.9 g, potassium chloride 1.5 g, glucose 13.5 g per liter of fluid. In mEq/L, sodium 75 mEq/L, chloride 65 mEq/L, potassium 20 mEq/L, glucose 75 mOsm/L (WHO formulation)
Pharmacokinetics	Well absorbed from gut after oral administration. Glucose facilitates sodium absorption
Indications	Diarrhea with or without dehydration
Dosage as per indications	• *No dehydration:* Replace as 5–10 mL/kg per loose stool • *Some dehydration:* 75 mL/kg over 4 hours along with replacement of the ongoing losses
Maximum dosage	Not known
Dose adjustments	Not needed
Adverse effects	Dyselectrolytemia, if not prepared as per the instructions
Contraindications	Persistent vomiting, decreased consciousness, paralytic ileus, intestinal obstruction
Drug interactions	Warfarin, cimetidine, phenobarbitone, rifampin

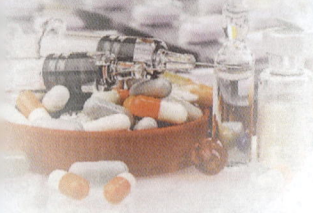

Ornidazole

Drug name	Ornidazole
Category	Antihelminthic
Route	Oral
Strength	Tab (500 mg); Susp (125 mg/5 mL)
Brands	Ornida (Inj, Tab, Susp), OZ (Tab)
Mechanism of action	It is a nitroimidazole, inhibit nucleic acid synthesis through the nitro group
Pharmacokinetics	Rapidly absorbed, peak levels in 3 hours, poorly protein bound, metabolized in liver, half-life 13 hours
Indications	Giardiasis; Intestinal amebiasis
Dosage as per indications	• *Giardiasis:* 40 mg/kg for 2 days • *Intestinal amebiasis:* 40 mg/kg for 3 days
Maximum dosage	Not known
Dose adjustments	In severe liver derangement
Adverse effects	Dizziness, vertigo, tremors, seizures
Contraindications	Hypersensitivity, CNS disorder
Drug interactions	Anticoagulants, antiepileptics
Remarks	Avoid in blood dyscrasia

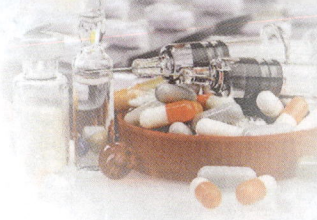

Oseltamivir

Drug name	Oseltamivir
Category	Neuraminidase inhibitor
Route	Oral
Strength	Cap (30 mg, 45 mg, 75 mg); Syp (12 mg/mL)
Brands	Fluvir (Cap, Syp), Antiflu (Cap, Syp), Tamiflu (Cap, Syp)
Mechanism of action	Inhibits neuraminidase enzyme of influenza virus thus preventing release of viral particles
Pharmacokinetics	Well-absorbed after oral dose, converted to oseltamivir carboxylate by hepatic esterases which is the active circulating form. Most of the drug eliminated as oseltamivir carboxylate. Half-life: 1–3 hours
Indications	Influenza H1N1
Dosage as per indications	*Antiflu agent:* • *<15 kg:* 30 mg BD • *15–23 kg:* 45 mg BD • *23–40 kg:* 60 mg BD • *>40 kg:* 75 mg BD. For 5 days duration
Maximum dosage	75 mg/dose
Dose adjustments	Renal derangement
Adverse effects	Vomiting, diarrhea, headache, insomnia, seizures, neuropsychiatric disturbances
Contraindications	Hypersensitivity
Drug interactions	Influenza vaccine
Remarks	It must be preferably started within 48 hours of first symptoms of infection

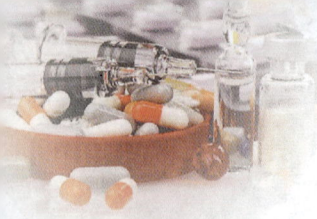

Oxcarbazepine

Drug name	Oxcarbazepine
Category	Anticonvulsant
Route	Oral
Strength	Tab (150 mg, 300 mg, 600 mg); Syp (300 mg/5 mL)
Brands	Oleptal (Tab), Oxcarb (Tab), Oxeptal (Tab, Syp)
Mechanism of action	Blocks voltage-sensitive sodium channels, stabilizes hyperexcited neural membranes, inhibits repetitive neuronal firing, and decreases propagation of synaptic impulses
Pharmacokinetics	Well absorbed after oral dose; extensively metabolized in liver, half-life: 9 hours, predominantly eliminated by the kidneys
Indications	Partial and generalized tonic-clonic seizures; Mood stabilizing drug
Dosage as per indications	Start at 8–10 mg/kg/day q 12 h; increase to 30–45 mg/kg/day over next 2 weeks, usual increments of 10 mg/kg/week
Maximum dosage	1,800 mg/day
Dose adjustments	In renal impairment
Adverse effects	Nausea, vomiting, dizziness, headache, double vision, anaphylaxis
Contraindications	Hypersensitivity
Drug interactions	Oral contraceptives, calcium channel blockers, antiepileptics

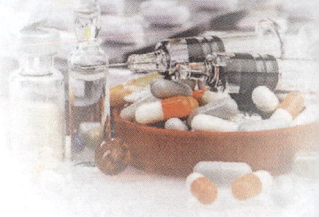

Palonosetron

Drug name	Palonosetron
Category	Serotonin-3 (5-HT3) receptor antagonist
Route	Intravenous
Strength	Inj (0.25 mg/5 mL)
Brands	Palnox (Inj), Palzen (Inj)
Mechanism of action	It is a 5-HT3 serotonin receptor antagonist. It acts peripherally on the nerve terminals of the vagus and centrally in the chemoreceptor trigger zone of the area postrema where the receptors are located
Pharmacokinetics	Around 60% plasma protein bound, terminal half-life 40 hours, mainly eliminated through renal route
Indications	Antiemetic
Dosage as per indications	20 µg/kg/dose
Maximum dosage	1.5 mg/dose
Dose adjustments	Not needed
Adverse effects	QT prolongation, bradycardia, headache, and constipation
Contraindications	Hypersensitivity
Drug interactions	Serotonergic drugs, can lead to serotonin syndrome

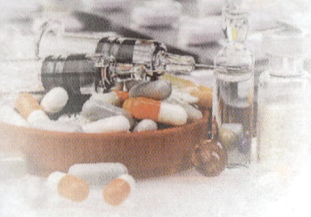

Pancuronium

Drug name	Pancuronium
Category	Muscle relaxant
Route	Intravenous
Strength	Inj (2 mg/mL)
Brands	Pavulon, Neocuron, Panuron (Inj)
Mechanism of action	Nondepolarizing neuromuscular blocking agent, acts by competing for cholinergic receptors at the motor end-plate
Pharmacokinetics	Onset of action: 1–2 min; Elimination half-life: 1.5–3 hours. Nearly 40% eliminated from urine, 10% from bile
Indications	Paralytic agent; Anesthetic (for intubation and ventilation)
Dosage as per indications	*Intermittent dosing:* • *Neonate:* Initial: 0.02 mg/kg/dose IV; maintenance: 0.05–0.1 mg/kg/dose IV q 0.5–4 h PRN • *1 month to adult:* Initial: 0.04–0.1 mg/kg/dose IV; maintenance: 0.015–0.1 mg/kg/dose IV q 30–60 min *Continuous IV infusion:* • *Neonate:* 0.02–0.04 mg/kg/h • *Child:* 0.03–1 mg/kg/h • *Adolescent and adult:* 0.02–0.04 mg/kg/h
Maximum dosage	Not known
Dose adjustments	Liver and renal derangement
Adverse effects	Tachycardia, salivation, anaphylaxis
Contraindications	Hypersensitivity
Drug interactions	Neuromuscular blocking drugs, anesthetic agents, antibiotics like aminoglycosides
Remarks	Antidote: neostigmine; avoid in severe renal impairment

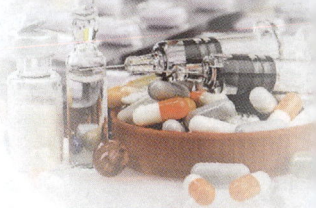

Pantoprazole

Drug name	Pantoprazole
Category	Proton pump inhibitor
Route	Oral, Intravenous
Strength	Inj (40 mg/vial); Tab (40 mg, 80 mg)
Brands	Pantop (Tab, Inj), PAN (Tab, Inj), Pantocid (Tab, Inj)
Mechanism of action	Binds to (H^+, K^+)-ATPase enzyme system in the gastric parietal cell leading to inhibition of gastric acid secretion
Pharmacokinetics	Terminal elimination half-life: 1 hour. Highly protein bound, metabolized in liver via cytochrome P450 (CYP) system
Indications	Erosive gastritis; Gastroesophageal reflux disorder (GERD)
Dosage as per indications	1 mg/kg/day up to 8 weeks duration • *Weight 15–40 kg:* 20 mg OD • *Weight ≥40 kg:* 40 mg OD
Maximum dosage	40 mg/dose
Dose adjustments	No dose adjustment needed in renal and hepatic derangement
Adverse effects	Long-term use causes vitamin B_{12} deficiency, stomach ache, rash, arthralgia, kidney problems
Contraindications	Hypersensitivity
Drug interactions	Methotrexate, antifungal, ampicillin
Remarks	Pantoprazole tablets are taken by mouth, with or without food. The oral granules should be taken 30 minutes before a meal

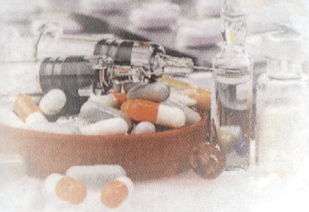

Para-amino Salicylic Acid

Drug name	Para-amino salicylic acid
Category	Antibacterial
Route	Oral
Strength	Tab (1 g)
Brands	Monopas (Tab)
Mechanism of action	It has bacteriostatic action, mainly used for *Mycobacterium tuberculosis*. It acts by competing with para-aminobenzoic acid (PABA) for dihydropteroate synthetase (DHP) required for folate synthesis
Pharmacokinetics	It is 50% plasma protein bound, acetylated in the liver to the inactive metabolite. Plasma half-life: 1 hour, eliminated from kidneys by glomerular filtration and tubular secretion
Indications	MDR TB
Dosage as per indications	150 mg/kg per day, divided in two doses
Maximum dosage	4 g/dose
Dose adjustments	In hepatic and renal derangement
Adverse effects	Nausea, vomiting, giddiness, rash, liver injury, malabsorption syndrome
Contraindications	Hypersensitivity
Drug interactions	Vitamin B_{12}, digoxin, ethionamide, antiretrovirals
Remarks	Increases risk of hypothyroidism in HIV positive patients

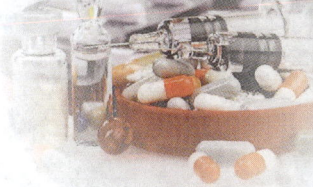

Paracetamol (PCM)

Drug name	Paracetamol (PCM)
Category	Acetaminophen
Route	Oral, Intravenous, Rectal
Strength	Tab (500 mg, 650 mg); Syp/Susp (250 mg/5 mL, 125 mg/5 mL); Drops (50 mg/mL, 100 mg/mL); Inj (150 mg/mL ampoule)
Brands	Calpol (Tab, Syp), Crocin (Tab, Syp), Dolo (Tab, Syp, Inj)
Mechanism of action	*Central:* Inhibits prostaglandin synthesis; peripheral: blocks pain impulse generation
Pharmacokinetics	*Oral absorption:* Rapid and complete, predominantly metabolized in liver, half-life 1–4 hours, elimination by renal route
Indications	Fever; Pain; Inflammation
Dosage as per indications	Oral: 10–15 mg/kg/dose, intravenous: 5 mg/kg/dose, rectal: 15 mg/kg/dose 4–6 hourly
Maximum dosage	90 mg/kg/day, not exceeding 4 g/day
Dose adjustments	Maximum daily dose not to exceed 3 g/day in hepatocellular insufficiency, chronic malnutrition; keep minimum interval of 6 hours between 2 doses in those with Cr clearance <30 mL/min
Adverse effects	Liver failure with overdosage, chronic hepatic necrosis, acute pancreatitis, blood dyscrasia, hypersensitivity
Contraindications	Drug allergy
Drug interactions	• Increased absorption with metoclopramide, domperidone • Increased elimination with drugs inducing hepatic microsomal enzymes • Increased risk of bleeding with warfarin/coumarin derivatives
Remarks	• *Risk factors for liver damage with PCM:* Overdose, those on drugs inducing liver enzymes, regular ethanol consumption, glutathione depletion • *Antidote:* N-acetyl cysteine

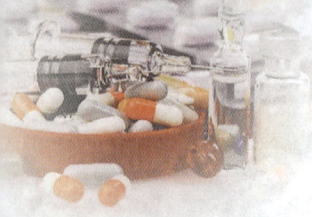

Paraldehyde

Drug name	Paraldehyde
Category	Sedative
Route	Oral, Inj, Per Rectal (PR)
Strength	Inj (5 mL, 1 g/mL ampoules)
Brands	Paraldehyde (Inj, Oral, PR)
Mechanism of action	Decreases release of acetylcholine during neuronal depolarization
Pharmacokinetics	Rapidly absorbed after oral ingestion. More than three-fourths metabolized to CO_2 and exhaled. Half-life 7–8 hours
Indications	Hypnotic-sedative with antiepileptic effects; Used in uncontrolled status epilepticus
Dosage as per indications	0.1–0.2 mL/kg/dose deep IM, 0.3 mg/kg/dose PR mixed 3:1 with coconut oil. Additional dosing may be given after 30 minutes and then every 4–6 hours
Maximum dosage	Not known
Dose adjustments	In liver derangement
Adverse effects	Unpleasant taste, imparts smell to breath; skin rashes, headache, nausea
Contraindications	Contraindicated in hepatic and pulmonary disease
Drug interactions	Additive sedative effects and/or respiratory depression with other CNS depressants (e.g., barbiturates, ethanol, narcotic analgesics, and other sedatives

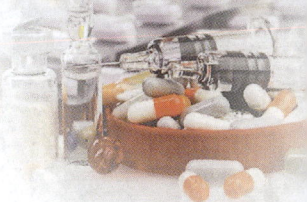

Paromomycin Sulfate

Drug name	Paromomycin sulfate
Category	Aminoglycoside antibiotic
Route	Oral
Strength	Cap (250 mg)
Brands	Humatin (Cap)
Mechanism of action	Amebicide which acts in the intestinal lumen by inhibiting protein synthesis in susceptible bacteria at the 30S segment of the ribosome
Pharmacokinetics	Poorly known. It is poorly absorbed after oral administration. Predominantly eliminated in feces as unchanged drug
Indications	Intestinal amebiasis, cryptosporidiosis associated diarrhea; Tapeworm infestation (*Taenia solium; T. saginata; D. latum; H. nana*), hepatic coma
Dosage as per indications	• 25–35 mg/kg body weight daily, administered in 3 doses for 7–10 days • *For tapeworm infections:* 11 mg/kg/dose orally Q15 min for 4 doses • *For Dwarf tapeworm:* 45 mg/kg/dose OD for 5–7 days
Maximum dosage	Not known, up to 4 g/day used in adults
Dose adjustments	Not needed in mild to moderate hepatic disease, use with caution in renal and severe hepatic disease
Adverse effects	Nausea, abdominal cramps, and diarrhea have
Contraindications	Hypersensitivity
Drug interactions	Not known
Remarks	Not effective in extra-intestinal amebiasis

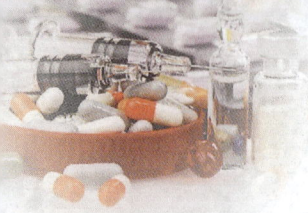

Pefloxacin

Drug name	Pefloxacin
Category	Quinolone antibiotic
Route	Oral, Intravenous
Strength	Tab (400 mg); Inj (100 mg/50 mL)
Brands	Pefbid, Pefcin, Peflobid (Inj, Tab)
Mechanism of action	Inhibits DNA gyrase and topoisomerase IV required for transcription and replication of bacterial DNA
Pharmacokinetics	Well absorbed, poorly bound to protein, most metabolized in liver, half-life 8–9 hours
Indications	Active against gram-negative; Gram-positive bacteria
Dosage as per indications	15–20 mg/kg/day in two divided doses oral; IV doses not well studied
Maximum dosage	400 mg/dose
Dose adjustments	Not much known, not required in hepatic derangement
Adverse effects	Nausea, vomiting, headache, rash
Contraindications	Hypersensitivity
Drug interactions	Vincristine, foscarnet, NSAID, cimetidine, probenecid, cyclosporine
Remarks	Not used in children <12 years

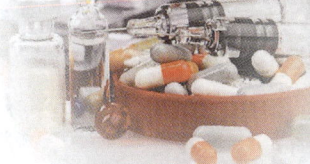

Penicillin G Aqueous

Drug name	Penicillin G aqueous
Category	Antibiotic
Route	Oral, Intravenous
Strength	Tab (2 lakh units, 4 lakh units, 8 lakh units); Inj (5 lakh units, 10 lakh units vial)
Brands	Bistrepen (Inj), Kaypen (Tab), Pentids (Tab)
Mechanism of action	Bactericidal, inhibits biosynthesis of cell wall mucopeptide, is not resistant to penicillinase-producing bacteria
Pharmacokinetics	Bound to plasma protein, rapidly absorbed. Eliminated via kidneys. Half-life around 45 minutes
Indications	Bacterial infections; Rheumatic fever
Dosage as per indications	• 1–2 lakh units/kg/day IV/IM infusion q 4–6 h • *For meningitis and endocarditis:* 2–3 lakh units/kg/day IV/IM q 4 h (maximum dose 24 million U/day) • *For rheumatic fever prophylaxis:* 2 lakh units (125 mg) BD oral
Maximum dosage	24 M U/day IV/IM
Dose adjustments	Dose adjustment in renal failure
Adverse effects	Urticaria, hemolytic anemia, interstitial nephritis, Jarisch Herxheimer reaction
Contraindications	Hypersensitivity
Drug interactions	Aminoglycosides, allopurinol

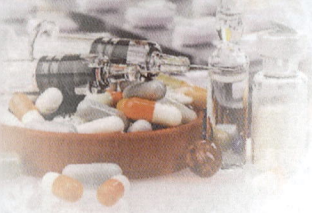

Penicillin G Benzathine

Drug name	Penicillin G benzathine
Category	Antibiotic, Penicillin
Route	Intramuscular
Strength	Inj (1.2, 2.4 million units vial)
Brands	Benzylpenicillin (Inj)
Mechanism of action	Bactericidal acts through the inhibition of biosynthesis of cell-wall peptidoglycan
Pharmacokinetics	Released slowly from the IM site due to low solubility. Half-life around 15 days, eliminated by kidneys
Indications	Secondary prophylaxis of rheumatic fever
Dosage as per indications	• <6 years: 0.6 MU IM every 21 days • >6 years: 1.2 MU IM every 21 days
Maximum dosage	1.2 MU/dose
Dose adjustments	Dose adjustment in renal and hepatic derangement
Adverse effects	Urticaria, hemolytic anemia, interstitial nephritis, Jarisch–Herxheimer reaction
Contraindications	Never give IV as it may result in cardiac arrest and death
Drug interactions	Aminoglycosides, allopurinol
Remarks	To be given only after a test dose; can cause severe anaphylaxis

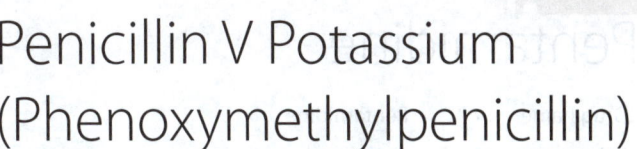

Penicillin V Potassium (Phenoxymethylpenicillin)

Drug name	Penicillin V potassium (Phenoxymethylpenicillin)
Category	Antibiotic, Penicillin
Route	Oral
Strength	Tab (125 mg, 250 mg)
Brands	Kaypen (Tab)
Mechanism of action	Bactericidal acts through the inhibition of biosynthesis of cell-wall peptidoglycan
Pharmacokinetics	Resistant to gastric acid, highly protein bound. Tissue levels are highest in the kidneys, half-life around 30 minutes, eliminated via kidneys
Indications	Bacterial infections; Rheumatic fever

Dosage as per indications	• *Infants:* 62.5–125 mg/dose q 6 h
	  – *<5 years:* 125 mg/dose q 6 h
	  – *>5 years:* 250 mg/dose q 6 h
	• *For rheumatic fever prophylaxis:* 250 mg BD; 250 mg is equivalent to 4 lakh units

Maximum dosage	2 g/day
Dose adjustments	Dose adjustment in renal failure
Adverse effects	Urticaria, hemolytic anemia, interstitial nephritis, Jarisch–Herxheimer reaction
Contraindications	Hypersensitivity
Drug interactions	Allopurinol
Remarks	Administer 30 minutes before or 2 hours after meals

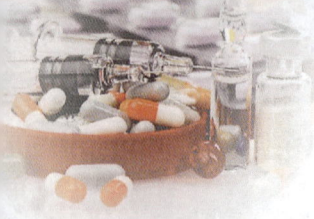

Pentamidine

Drug name	Pentamidine
Category	Antifungal
Route	Intramuscular, Intravenous, Inhalational
Strength	Inj (300 mg/3 mL)
Brands	Pentam, NebuPent (Indian brand not available)
Mechanism of action	It inhibits DNA, RNA, phospholipid and protein synthesis required for microbial nuclear metabolism
Pharmacokinetics	Limited data available. After IV/IM administration: Half-life 6–9 hours based on route. Mainly eliminated from kidneys
Indications	Systemic leishmaniasis; Prevention; Treatment of *Pneumocystis carinii* pneumonia
Dosage as per indications	• 4 mg/kg/day intramuscular for resistant leishmaniasis • 4 mg/kg/day IV for treatment of Pneumocystis in children >4 months of age • Aerosolized pentamidine 300 mg once every 4 weeks used for prevention of *Pneumocystis pneumonia* in children >5 years and who do not tolerate co-trimoxazole
Maximum dosage	300 mg/day
Dose adjustments	Use with caution in renal and liver disease
Adverse effects	Hypoglycemia, risk of developing diabetes mellitus, torsades de pointes, hypotension, kidney injury
Contraindications	Hypersensitivity
Drug interactions	Nephrotoxic drugs
Remarks	Reconstitute in sterile water only

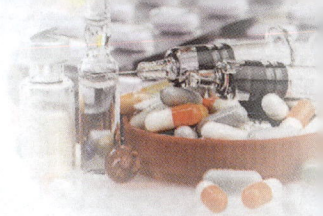

Pentazocine Hydrochloride

Drug name	Pentazocine hydrochloride
Category	Opioid
Route	Oral, Intravenous, Intramuscular
Strength	Tab (25 mg); Inj (30 mg/mL ampoule)
Brands	Fortwin (Inj, Tab), Pentawin (Inj, Tab), Forstar (Inj, Tab)
Mechanism of action	Mixed agonist-antagonist at opioid receptors. Pentazocine is partial agonist at the mu opioid receptor and an agonist at the kappa opioid receptor
Pharmacokinetics	Metabolized in the liver and excreted primarily in the urine
Indications	Analgesic
Dosage as per indications	Opioid analgesic 0.5–1.0 mg/kg/d q 4 h oral, IM or IV
Maximum dosage	30 mg/dose IV
Dose adjustments	Dose adjustment in renal and hepatic derangement
Adverse effects	Drowsiness, respiratory and cardiac depression
Contraindications	Contraindicated in raised intracranial tension, head injury
Drug interactions	Concomitant use with benzodiazepines and other CNS depressants can lead to excessive sedation and respiratory depression
Remarks	Use of pentazocine in pregnancy can lead to neonatal opioid withdrawal syndrome

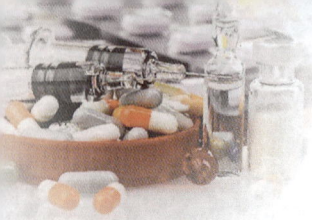

Permethrin

Drug name	Permethrin
Category	Scabicidal drug
Route	Topical
Strength	Permite (Cream 5%; Liquid Cream Rinse 1%)
Brands	Elimite
Mechanism of action	Dysregulates membrane depolarization by disrupting the sodium channel current on cell membrane
Pharmacokinetics	Not known
Indications	Scabies; Pediculosis capitis; *Pthirus pubis*
Dosage as per indications	• *Scabies:* Apply 5% cream neck downward to the toes, leave on for 12–24 hours and wash off with water and scrubbing bath. May repeat course after 7 days. Generally, a single application will suffice • *Pediculosis:* Saturate hair/scalp with 1% cream (leave on for 10 minutes). Rinse after shampooing, rinsing and towel drying. May repeat every 7–10 days
Maximum dosage	Not known
Dose adjustments	Not known
Adverse effects	Pruritus, hypersensitivity, stinging, erythema and rash
Contraindications	Hypersensitivity
Drug interactions	Not known
Remarks	Contact with eyes may cause local irritation

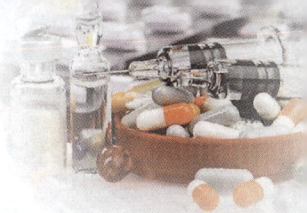

Pethidine Hydrochloride

Drug name	Pethidine hydrochloride
Category	Opioid agonist
Route	Subcutaneous, Oral, Intramuscular
Strength	Inj (50 mg/mL)
Brands	Pethidine (Inj), Verpat (Inj)
Mechanism of action	Synthetic opiate agonist which acts similar to morphine but being less potent but faster onset of action and shorter duration of action. It acts by inhibiting adenylate cyclase and decreasing intracellular cAMP. It also inhibits release of some other neurotransmitters such as substance P, GABA, dopamine, acetylcholine and noradrenaline
Pharmacokinetics	Around 50% bioavailability after oral intake, extensive first-pass metabolism, 60–80% bound to plasma proteins. Metabolized in the liver, excreted mainly in urine, terminal elimination half-life 3–5 hours
Indications	Pain; Sedation
Dosage as per indications	1–1.5 mg/kg/dose 4–6 hourly PO/SC/IM
Maximum dosage	Not known in children. Up to 400 mg/24 hours have been used in adults
Dose adjustments	Required in renal and hepatic derangement
Adverse effects	Nausea vomiting, hypotension, seizures, bradycardia, dependence
Contraindications	Hypersensitivity, MAO inhibitors in last 2 weeks, respiratory depression
Drug interactions	CNS depressants drugs affecting CYP3A4 enzyme

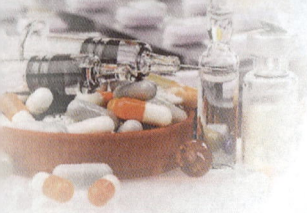

Pheniramine Maleate

Drug name	Pheniramine maleate
Category	Antihistamine with anticholinergic effects
Route	Oral, Intramuscular, Intravenous
Strength	Tab (25 mg, 50 mg); Syp (15 mg/mL); Inj (22.75 mg/mL)
Brands	Avil (Inj, Syp, Tab)
Mechanism of action	Inverse agonist at H1 receptor. Decreased H1 receptor activity helps in reducing itching, redness and edema by decreasing vasodilation and capillary leakage
Pharmacokinetics	Eliminated by metabolism and via renal excretion. Pheniramine undergoes N-dealkylation in liver, peak levels: 1–2.5 hours, elimination half-life 8–17 hours
Indications	Allergic reaction
Dosage as per indications	0.5 mg/kg/day q 8 h PO, IM or IV
Maximum dosage	Not known
Dose adjustments	In liver derangement
Adverse effects	• Dry mouth, constipation, CNS depression, bradycardia • Overdose may lead to seizures
Contraindications	Hypersensitivity
Drug interactions	MAO inhibitors

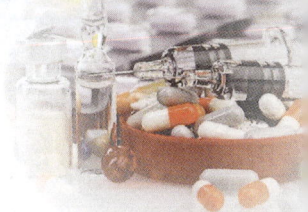

Phenobarbitone Sodium

Drug name	Phenobarbitone sodium
Category	Barbiturate, Anticonvulsant
Route	Intravenous, Oral
Strength	Syp (20 mg/5 mL); Tab (30 mg, 60 mg); Inj (200 mg/mL ampoule)
Brands	Luminal (Inj, Tab), Gardenal (Inj, Tab, Syp), Phenobarb (Inj, Tab)
Mechanism of action	Acts by enhancing and/or mimicking the synaptic action of gamma-aminobutyric acid (GABA), an inhibitory neurotransmitter. Also inhibits conduction in the reticular resulting in sedative action
Pharmacokinetics	Rapid and complete absorption after oral intake. Better absorption as sodium salts, liquid preparation. When given IV, starts acting within 5 minutes. High concentrations noted in the brain, liver and kidney, slowly metabolized and/or conjugated in the liver and then eliminated via kidney. Half-life varies with age: neonates 45–100 hours, infants 20–133 hours, children 37–73 hours
Indications	Tonic clonic; Akinetic; and Partial seizures in children. Also for neonatal seizures. May be used in febrile seizure

Dosage as per indications	• *Loading dose:* 15–20 mg/kg IV over 15–20 min @ 1 mg/kg/min as slow IV bolus. May administer additional bolus 5 mg/kg/dose every 15–30 minutes up to a maximum of 30 mg/kg
	• *Maintenance dose:* PO, IV
	  – *Neonates:* 3–5 mg/kg/day q 12 h
	  – *Infants:* 5–6 mg/kg/day q 12–24 h
	  – *Children 1–5 years:* 6–8 mg/kg/day q 12–24 h
	  – *Children 6–12 years:* 4–6 mg/kg/day q 12–24 h
	  – *Children >12 years:* 1–3 mg/kg/day q 12–24 h

Maximum dosage	30 mg/kg as bolus
Dose adjustments	Use with caution in hepatic or renal disease

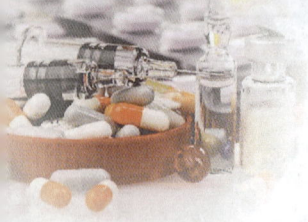

Adverse effects	Drowsiness, hypotension, respiratory depression, megaloblastic anemia, apnea, hepatitis
Contraindications	Porphyria, severe respiratory disease with dyspnea or obstruction
Drug interactions	Other antiepileptics, sedatives
Remarks	*Therapeutic levels:* 15–40 µg/mL

Phenytoin Sodium

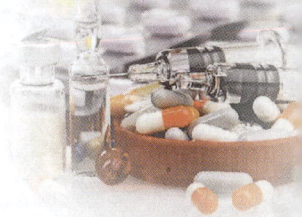

Drug name	Phenytoin sodium
Category	Anticonvulsant
Route	Intravenous, Oral
Strength	Inj (50 mg/mL ampoule); Syp or Susp (125 mg/5 mL, 30 mg/5 mL); Cap (30 mg, 100 mg, 300 mg); Tab (50 mg, 100 mg)
Brands	Dilantin (Inj, Tab, Syp), Epsolin (Inj, Tab), Eptoin (Inj, Cap, Syp, Tab)
Mechanism of action	Increases sodium efflux from neurons to stabilize the neuronal membrane and decrease hyperexcitability especially in motor cortex
Pharmacokinetics	*Half-life:* 22–25 hours mean. Steady-state therapeutic levels: 7–10 days. First excreted in bile, then reabsorbed from intestinal tract from where excreted in urine
Indications	Status epilepticus; Arrhythmias
Dosage as per indications	• *Loading dose:* 15–20 mg/kg by slow IV infusion at 25–50 mg/min • *Maintenance dose:* 5–10 mg/kg/day q 12 h IV/PO *Antiarrhythmic* • *Loading dose:* 1.25 mg/kg IV every 5 minutes. May repeat up to a loading dose of 15 mg/kg • *Maintenance dose:* 5–10 mg/kg/day orally or IV in 2–3 divided doses
Maximum dosage	300 mg/day
Dose adjustments	In renal and hepatic derangement
Adverse effects	Nystagmus, hypotension, Stevens–Johnson syndrome, rash, hepatitis, gingival hyperplasia, blood dyscrasia
Contraindications	Contraindicated in heart block or sinus bradycardia
Drug interactions	Antiepileptics, antibiotics

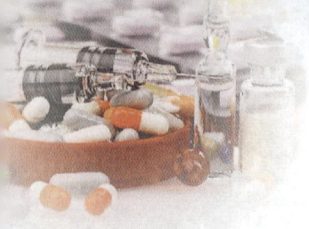

Physostigmine

Drug name	Physostigmine
Category	Reversible anticholinesterase
Route	Intravenous
Strength	Inj (2 mg/2 mL)
Brands	Eserine salicylate (Inj)
Mechanism of action	It has reversible anticholinesterase activity, which acts to increase the concentration of acetylcholine and reverse anticholinergic activity at central and peripheral sites as it crosses blood brain barrier
Pharmacokinetics	Effect noted within few minutes after the intravenous administration. Total duration of action: 45–60 minutes
Indications	Organophosphate poisoning
Dosage as per indications	0.02 mg/kg/dose every 5 minutes till desired effect is obtained or reached 2 mg of maximum dose
Maximum dosage	0.5 mg/dose
Dose adjustments	Not known
Adverse effects	Nausea, vomiting, bradycardia, salivation
Contraindications	Hypersensitivity
Drug interactions	Cholinergic drugs
Remarks	Avoid in asthma, cardiovascular disease, diabetes

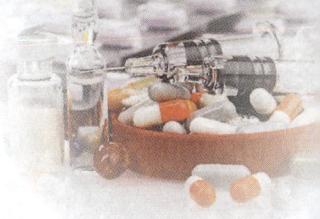

Pimozide

Drug name	Pimozide
Category	Antipsychotic
Route	Oral
Strength	Tab (2 mg, 4 mg)
Brands	Mozep (Tab), Orap (Tab), Pimodac (Tab)
Mechanism of action	Blocks dopaminergic receptors on neurons in the central nervous system to suppress motor and phonic tics in Tourette syndrome
Pharmacokinetics	Around 50% absorbed after oral administration, significant first pass metabolism, peak serum levels in 6–8 hours, metabolized extensively in liver, eliminated by kidneys. Elimination half-life: 55 hours
Indications	Tourette syndrome
Dosage as per indications	Initiate at 0.05 mg/kg as HS dose. Dose can be increased every third day to a maximum of 0.2 mg/kg but not more than 10 mg/day
Maximum dosage	10 mg/day
Dose adjustments	Needed in hepatic and renal derangement
Adverse effects	QT prolongation, tardive dyskinesia, neuroleptic malignant syndrome, extrapyramidal signs, increased risk of pituitary tumors
Contraindications	Hypersensitivity
Drug interactions	Drugs affecting CYP3A4 enzyme pathway
Remarks	*Not advised for:* • Any other types of tics, along with any other tics causing agents such as methylphenidate and amphetamines • In conditions or drugs causing long QT interval

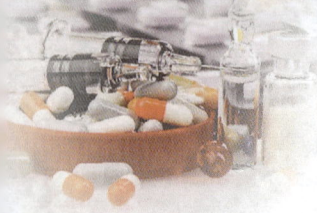

Piperacillin

Drug name	Piperacillin
Category	Antibiotic, Penicillin (Extended spectrum)
Route	Intravenous, Intramuscular
Strength	Inj (1 g, 2 g, 4 g vials)
Brands	Pipracil (Inj), Piplin (Inj), Pipralin (Inj)
Mechanism of action	Bactericidal, acts by inhibiting septum formation and cell wall synthesis
Pharmacokinetics	Peak plasma concentrations achieved rapidly after intravenous administration, almost in the same time as the infusion is completed. Approximately 30% bound to plasma proteins, are widely distributed into tissues and body fluids. Eliminated mainly via the kidney by glomerular filtration and tubular secretion. *Half-life:* Around 1 hour
Indications	Acts against gram-positive; Gram-negative bacteria
Dosage as per indications	100–300 mg/kg/day q 4–6 h
Maximum dosage	16 g/day
Dose adjustments	Renal derangement
Adverse effects	GI disturbances, rash, pruritus, headache, bleeding, SIS
Contraindications	Hypersensitivity
Drug interactions	Aminoglycosides, probenecid, vancomycin, heparin, methotrexate
Remarks	To keep a minimum gap of 2 hours between piperacillin and aminoglycoside administration

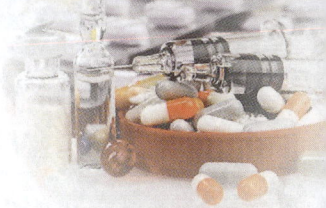

Piperacillin-tazobactam

Drug name	Piperacillin-tazobactam
Category	Antibiotic, Penicillin (Extended spectrum)
Route	Intravenous
Strength	Inj (4 g of Piperacillin with 500 mg of Tazobactam vial)
Brands	Piptaz (Inj), Tazact (Inj), Tazilin (Inj), Tazopen (Inj)
Mechanism of action	Bactericidal, acts by inhibiting septum formation and cell wall synthesis. Tazobactam is a β-lactamase inhibitor
Pharmacokinetics	Peak plasma concentrations of piperacillin and tazobactam achieved rapidly after intravenous administration. Both piperacillin and tazobactam are approximately 30% bound to plasma proteins, are widely distributed into tissues and body fluids. Both piperacillin and tazobactam are eliminated mainly via the kidney by glomerular filtration and tubular secretion. Piperacillin, tazobactam—*half-life*: 0.7–1.2 hours
Indications	Severe infections from gram-positive; Gram-negative bacteria
Dosage as per indications	300–400 mg/kg/day q 6–8 h. Dose based on piperacillin
Maximum dosage	16 g/day
Dose adjustments	Renal impairment, not needed in hepatic
Adverse effects	GI disturbances, rash, pruritus, headache, bleeding, Stevens-Johnson syndrome (SJS)
Contraindications	Hypersensitivity
Drug interactions	Aminoglycosides, probenecid, vancomycin, heparin, methotrexate
Remarks	To keep a minimum gap of 2 hours between piperacillin and aminoglycoside administration

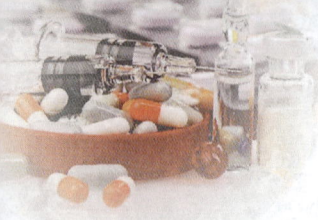

Piperazine

Drug name	Piperazine
Category	Antihelminthic
Route	Oral
Strength	Tab (500 mg); Elixir (750 mg/5 mL)
Brands	Avizin (Tab, Syp), Piperazine Citrate (Tab, Syp)
Mechanism of action	Anthelmintic, acts against roundworms and threadworms by paralysis of worms which are then dislodged from their position by movement of the gut and expelled in the feces
Pharmacokinetics	Not known
Indications	Ascariasis; *Enterobius* infection
Dosage as per indications	• *Ascariasis:* 75 mg/kg/day PO single dose on two consecutive nights • *Enterobius:* 65 mg/kg/day PO single dose × 7 days
Maximum dosage	*Ascariasis*: 3.5 g/day, *Enterobius*: 2.5 g/day
Dose adjustments	Liver and renal derangement
Adverse effects	Colicky pain, urticaria, bronchospasm. Seizures may get precipitated in children with epilepsy
Contraindications	Hypersensitivity
Drug interactions	Pyrantel pamoate

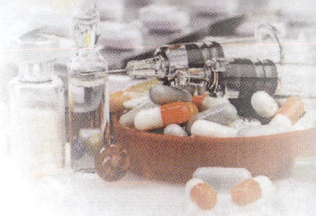

Piracetam

Drug name	Piracetam
Category	Miscellaneous
Route	Oral
Strength	Inj (200 mg); Tab (400 mg, 800 mg); Susp (500 mg/5 mL)
Brands	Alcetam, Cerecetam (Tab, Syp), Nootropil (Tab, Syp, Inj)
Mechanism of action	It increases membrane stability by binding to phospholipid heads. Stable membrane allows the membrane and transmembrane protein to exert their function
Pharmacokinetics	Rapidly and extensively absorbed following oral administration. Has very high bioavailability reaching nearly 100%. Most eliminated as unchanged in urine. *Half-life:* 5 hours
Indications	Learning disabilities; Sickle-cell vaso-occlusive crises
Dosage as per indications	30–160 mg/kg/day given in two to four divided doses oral. Intravenous route used rarely
Maximum dosage	Not known
Dose adjustments	In renal derangement, in hepatic derangement if accompanied with renal derangement
Adverse effects	Nervousness, hyperkinesia, weight gain
Contraindications	Hypersensitivity
Drug interactions	Not known
Remarks	Not used in end stage renal disease (ESRD), cerebral hemorrhage, Huntington's chorea

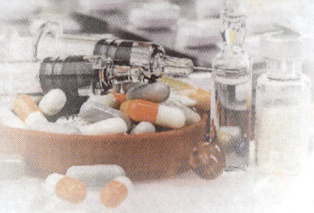

Piroxicam

Drug name	Piroxicam
Category	Nonsteroidal anti-inflammatory drug (NSAID)
Route	Oral, Topical (Gel)
Strength	Cap (20 mg)
Brands	Dolonex (Cap), Minicam (Cap), Pirox (Cap, Cream)
Mechanism of action	Inhibits prostaglandin synthesis leading to anti-inflammatory, analgesic, and antipyretic activities
Pharmacokinetics	• Well absorbed orally. Metabolism occurs by hydroxylation and conjugation • Excreted mainly in urine followed by feces
Indications	Analgesia
Dosage as per indications	0.2–0.3 mg/kg/24 h
Maximum dosage	15 mg/kg/24 h
Dose adjustments	Hepatic derangement, renal studies needed
Adverse effects	Diarrhea, ulcers, nausea, dizziness, depression, gastritis
Contraindications	History of urticaria/allergic reaction to any NSAIDs
Drug interactions	NSAIDs, aspirin, anticoagulants

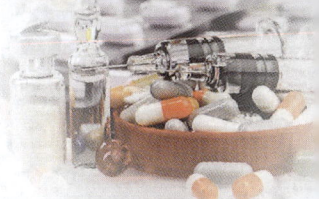

Polyethylene Glycol (PEG)

Drug name	Polyethylene glycol (PEG)
Category	Osmotic laxative
Route	Oral
Strength	Syp (13 g/25 mL); Sachet (13.8 g)
Brands	Movicol (Syp, Sachet), CremaPeg (Syp, Sachet)
Mechanism of action	Osmotic effect of polyethylene glycol 3,350, retains water in colon to produce watery stool usually within 4 hours
Pharmacokinetics	Poorly absorbed
Indications	Constipation
Dosage as per indications	• *PEG for disimpaction:* 25 mL/kg/h by mouth or nasogastric tube, 1.5–2 g/ kg/d in two divided doses for 3–6 d, depending upon clarity of rectal effluent • *PEG for maintenance:* 5–10 mL/kg/d or 0.4–0.8 g/kg/d
Maximum dosage	• 17 g per day for maintenance • 100 g per day for disimpaction
Dose adjustments	Diuretics
Adverse effects	Nausea, bloating, cramps, vomiting
Contraindications	Contraindicated in intestinal obstruction
Drug interactions	Not known

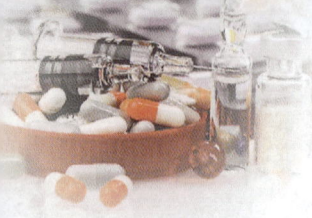

Polymyxin B

Drug name	Polymyxin B
Category	Antibiotic, Polypeptide
Route	Oral, Intravenous
Strength	Inj (500,000 IU per vial, 1 mg = 10,000 IU)
Brands	Aerosporin (Inj), Poly B (Inj), Oral preparation not available
Mechanism of action	Bactericidal, best against gram-negative bacilli, especially *Pseudomonas aeruginosa*. Does not work for *Proteus* and *Neisseria*. Acts by increasing the permeability of the bacterial cell membrane leading to cell death
Pharmacokinetics	Poorly absorbed from GI tract. Eliminated mainly from kidneys. Does not cross blood brain barrier
Indications	Severe/resistant gram-negative and *Pseudomonas* infections including sepsis; Meningitis and shunt infections
Dosage as per indications	• *For enteric infections:* 5–15 mg/kg/day q 8 h PO • *For systemic infections:* 1.5–2.5 mg/kg/day q 12 h IV • *For meningitis/ventriculitis:* 4 mg/kg/day q 8 h IV • *For ventriculitis/shunt infections:* Polymyxin may be additionally administered intrathecally or intraventricularly in a daily/alternate day dose of 2–5 mg • The exact duration of intraventricular therapy has not been defined
Maximum dosage	Not known
Dose adjustments	Renal disease
Adverse effects	Nephrotoxicity, drowsiness, dizziness, hypersensitivity, pain at injection site, neurotoxicity
Contraindications	Avoid use with other neuromuscular relaxants or blockers, nephrotoxic drugs
Drug interactions	Neuromuscular relaxants or blockers, nephrotoxic drugs

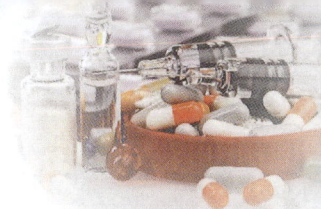

Potassium Chloride

Drug name	Potassium chloride
Category	Supplement
Route	Oral, Intravenous
Strength	Inj (1 mL/2 mEq); Syp (20 mEq/15 mL)
Brands	Potklor (Syp), Potasol (Syp), Kwin (Inj)
Mechanism of action	Involved in nerve impulse transmission, maintenance of intracellular tonicity; muscle contraction including cardiac, skeletal, and smooth muscle; and the maintenance of normal renal function
Pharmacokinetics	An active ion transport helps to maintain serum concentration of potassium between 3.5 and 5 mEq per liter. In stable conditions, the amount of potassium excreted in urine is equal to that absorbed from gut
Indications	For normal maintenance requirement in sick children; in children with hypokalemia
Dosage as per indications	*For hypokalemia:* • *Oral:* 1–4 mEq/kg/day in 3–4 divided doses • *IV:* 0.5–1 mEq/kg/dose administered as an infusion of 0.5 mEq/kg/h over 1–2 hours *As maintenance dose:* 2 mEq/kg/day incorporated in the parenteral nutrition solution when given intravenously
Maximum dosage	20 mEq/dose, rarely up to 40 mEq/dose Not to exceed 100 mEq/day
Dose adjustments	Renal derangement
Adverse effects	• *Oral:* GI upset, ulceration • *Intravenous:* Irritation, phlebitis, pain
Contraindications	Do not administer intravenous without dilution or rapidly as it may cause arrhythmias
Drug interactions	Drugs affecting potassium levels in body, for like furosemide, enalapril, digoxin
Remarks	• Oral administration should be diluted in water or juice • Max. IV infusion rate: 1 mEq/kg/hr • Max. peripheral IV solution concentration: 40 mEq/L

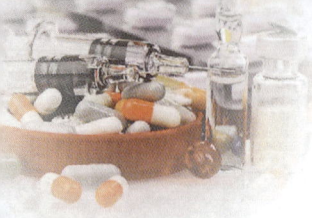

Pralidoxime

Drug name	Pralidoxime
Category	Antidote
Route	Intravenous
Strength	Inj (500 mg, 1g)
Brands	Aldopam (Inj), Neopam (Inj), Lyphe (Inj)
Mechanism of action	It reactivates peripheral cholinesterase which has been previously inactivated especially due to organophosphate poisoning. Due to peripheral action, does not act effectively for reversing respiratory depression
Pharmacokinetics	Short acting, minimum therapeutic obtained in about 16 minutes after IV administration. *Half-life:* 75 minutes
Indications	Organophosphate poisoning

Dosage as per indications	• *Loading dose:* 20–50 mg/kg over 15–30 minutes
	• *Followed by:*
	  – *Continuous infusion:* 10–20 mg/kg/h OR
	  – *Intermittent infusion:* A second dose of 20–50 mg/kg after 1 hour if muscle weakness unrelieved. Repeat dosing every 10–12 hours as needed

Maximum dosage	2,000 mg/dose as loading dose
Dose adjustments	In renal insufficiency
Adverse effects	Blurred vision, diplopia and impaired accommodation, dizziness, headache, drowsiness, nausea, tachycardia, increased systolic and diastolic blood pressure, hyperventilation, and muscular weakness, transient elevation of liver enzymes and creatinine kinase
Contraindications	Hypersensitivity
Drug interactions	Drugs with cholinergic and anticholinergic activity
Remarks	Not effective in carbamate toxicity

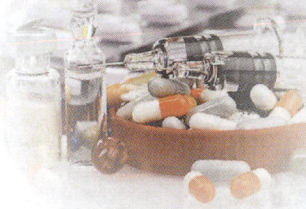

Praziquantel

Drug name	Praziquantel
Category	Antihelminthic
Route	Oral
Strength	Tab (500 mg, 600 mg)
Brands	Cysticide (Tab), Helminthex (Tab), Prazine (Tab)
Mechanism of action	Effects contractility of the helminth, increases permeability of cell membrane, causes vacuolization, disintegration
Pharmacokinetics	Rapid absorption after oral administration, maximum levels attained: 1–3 hours after intake, half-life: 40–90 minutes, mainly eliminated by kidneys as metabolites
Indications	Parasitic infections
Dosage as per indications	• *Neurocysticercosis:* 50 mg/kg/day q 8 h, oral × 15 day with steroids to counter the raised intracranial tension • *Tapeworm:* 5–10 mg/kg, single dose • *Schistosomiasis:* 20 mg/kg/dose PO 8–12 hourly × 1 day • *Liver fluke:* 25 mg/kg/dose q 8 h × 2 days • *Hymenolepis nana*: 25 mg/kg PO single dose (drug of choice) • *Fish tapeworm* (*Diphyllobothrium latum*): 5–10 mg/kg once
Maximum dosage	Not known
Dose adjustments	Both in hepatic and renal derangement
Adverse effects	Rash, headache, drowsiness, hyperglycemia
Contraindications	Ocular and intraventricular cysticercosis
Drug interactions	• Do not use with rifampicin • Other drugs affecting are P450 inducers, P450 inhibitors, dexamethasone

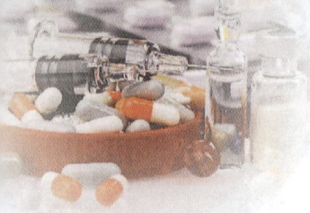

Prednisolone

Drug name	Prednisolone
Category	Corticosteroid
Route	Oral, Synthetic Adrenocortical Steroid Drug
Strength	Tab (5 mg, 10 mg, 20 mg); Syp (5 mg/5 mL)
Brands	Kidpred (Tab, Syp), Omnacortil (Tab, Syp), Predone (Tab, Syp), Wysolone (Tab)
Mechanism of action	Prednisolone mostly acts similar to endogenous glucocorticoid
Pharmacokinetics	Highly protein bound, half-life: 2–4 hours, metabolized in liver, eliminated in urine as sulfate and glucuronide conjugates
Indications	Nephrotic syndrome; Tubercular meningitis; Bronchial asthma; As anti-inflammatory in autoimmune; Collagen vascular disorders
Dosage as per indications	1–2 mg/kg/day q 6–12 h
Maximum dosage	60 mg/m^2
Dose adjustments	*Use with caution:* In renal and hepatic derangement
Adverse effects	Edema, hypertension, Cushing syndrome, peptic ulcer, hypothalamic pituitary-adrenal axis suppression
Contraindications	Infections
Drug interactions	NSAIDs, anticoagulants, antidiabetics, CYP3A4 inducer and inhibitor
Remarks	Avoid giving orally in empty stomach

Pregabalin

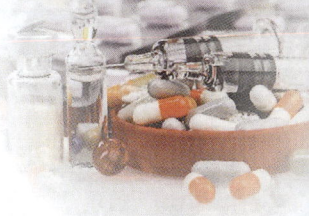

Drug name	Pregabalin
Category	Miscellaneous
Route	Oral
Strength	Tab (50 mg, 75 mg, 150 mg)
Brands	Gabamax (Tab), Gabasafe (Tab), Pregaba (Tab), Neuramed (Tab)
Mechanism of action	Binds to a subunit of voltage-gated calcium channels in CNS. It decreases neuropathic pain by affecting noradrenergic and serotonergic pathways in brainstem
Pharmacokinetics	Well absorbed when administered orally, high bioavailability, peak levels in 1.5 hours, poorly metabolized, eliminated largely by renal excretion, elimination *half-life:* 6 hours
Indications	Postherpetic neuralgia; For partial onset seizures; Neuropathic pain
Dosage as per indications	For children >4 years of age • *11–30 kg:* 3.5 mg/kg/day to max 14 mg/kg/day • *>30 kg:* 22.5 mg/kg/day to max 10 mg/kg/day or 600 mg/day
Maximum dosage	• *11–30 kg:* 14 mg/kg/day • *>30 kg:* 10 mg/kg/day or 600 mg/day
Dose adjustments	In renal derangement
Adverse effects	Increased weight, increased appetite, dizziness, peripheral edema, angioedema
Contraindications	Hypersensitivity
Drug interactions	Not known
Remarks	Taper gradually otherwise risk of seizures

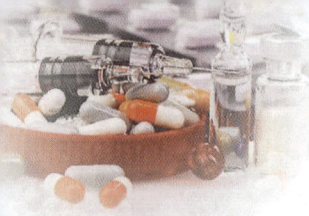

Primaquine

Drug name	Primaquine
Category	Antimalarial, 8-aminoquinoline
Route	Oral
Strength	Tab (2.5 mg, 7.5 mg, 15 mg)
Brands	Malirid (Tab), Primaquine (Tab), PMQ (Tab)
Mechanism of action	Acts to prevent relapse by eliminating exoerythrocytic infection in tissue, prevents erythrocytic form and active against gametocytes of *Plasmodium falciparum*
Pharmacokinetics	Well absorbed, half-life: 6 hours, poorly bound to protein, metabolized in liver, renal clearance <5%
Indications	Malaria
Dosage as per indications	• For radical cure in *Plasmodium vivax*: 0.25 mg/kg OD for 14 days • For gametocidal effect in *Plasmodium falciparum*: 0.75 mg/kg single dose
Maximum dosage	30 mg/day
Dose adjustments	Renal, hepatic derangement
Adverse effects	Nausea, vomiting, pain abdomen, visual disturbances, headache
Contraindications	Granulocytopenia, bone marrow suppression. Not to be used in infants
Drug interactions	Quinacrine
Remarks	• Use with caution in G6PD deficiency • Also used in pneumocystis infection

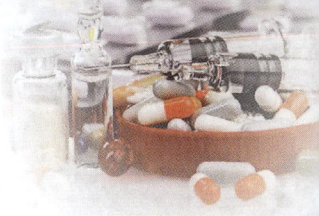

Probenecid

Drug name	Probenecid
Category	Uricosuric drug
Route	Oral
Strength	Tab (500 mg)
Brands	Bencid (Tab)
Mechanism of action	Inhibits tubular reabsorption of urates thereby increasing uric acid excretion
Pharmacokinetics	Metabolized in liver, around 80% bound to plasma proteins, half-life 6–12 hours
Indications	Hyperuricemia
Dosage as per indications	• *<45 kg:* 25 mg/kg (0.7 g/m^2) orally as single dose, followed by 10 mg/kg/dose 6 hourly • *>45 kg:* 500 mg 6 hourly
Maximum dosage	500 mg/dose
Dose adjustments	Use with caution in renal and hepatic derangement
Adverse effects	Nausea, vomiting, blood dyscrasia, convulsions, rash
Contraindications	Hypersensitivity, ESRD, blood dyscrasia
Drug interactions	Penicillin (prolongs levels), ketorolac, acyclovir
Remarks	Used in >2 years of age

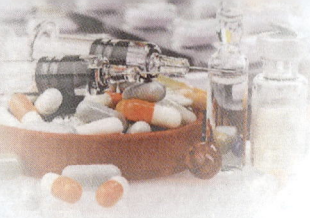

Procainamide Hydrochloride

Drug name	Procainamide hydrochloride
Category	Antiarrhythmic
Route	Intramuscular, Intravenous, Oral
Strength	Tab (250 mg, 375 mg, 500 mg); Inj (100 mg/mL, 500 mg/mL)
Brands	Pronestyl (Inj, Tab)
Mechanism of action	Increases the effective refractory period and reduces impulse conduction velocity of the atria, bundle of His-Purkinje system and ventricles of the heart
Pharmacokinetics	Effect starts in 15–60 minutes after intramuscular administration. Mostly distributes to highly perfused tissues. More than half is eliminated unchanged in an elimination half-life of 2.5–6 hours
Indications	Supraventricular; Ventricular arrhythmias
Dosage as per indications	• *IM:* 20–30 mg/kg/day q 4–6 h • *IV:* Load: 2–6 mg/kg/dose over 5 minutes • *Maintenance dose:* 20–80 µg/kg/min by continuous infusion • *Oral:* 20–30 mg/kg/day q 3–6 h
Maximum dosage	• *IV-loading:* 100 mg, maintenance: 2 g/day • *Oral/IM:* 4 g/day
Dose adjustments	Renal derangement
Adverse effects	Hypotension, atrioventricular block, arrhythmias, SLE-like syndrome, agranulocytosis
Contraindications	Complete heart block, SLE, myasthenia gravis, torsades de pointes
Drug interactions	Drugs prolonging QT interval, antiarrhythmics

Procaine Penicillin

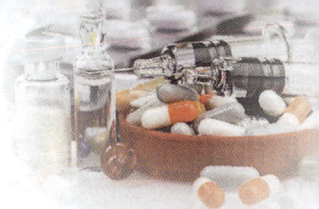

Drug name	Procaine penicillin
Category	Antibiotic, Penicillin
Route	Intramuscular
Strength	Inj (4 lakh units/vial)
Brands	Bistrepen (Inj), Cardiplegin (Inj)
Mechanism of action	It is a combination of procaine and penicillin. Acts by inhibiting cell wall synthesis
Pharmacokinetics	Not known
Indications	Mainly active against gram-positive infections; Syphilis; Anthrax
Dosage as per indications	• 25,000–50,000 units/kg/day single dose IM • Neonates 50,000 units/kg/day IM
Maximum dosage	Not known
Dose adjustments	Not needed in hepatic derangement
Adverse effects	Urticaria, hemolytic anemia, interstitial nephritis, Jarisch Herxheimer reaction may cause seizures
Contraindications	Hypersensitivity
Drug interactions	BCG vaccine
Remarks	• To be given only after test dose; give as intramuscular only • Never give IV as it may result in cardiac arrest and death

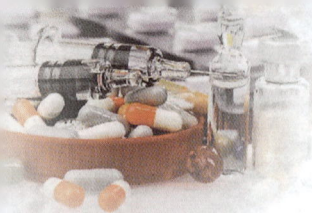

Prochlorperazine

Drug name	Prochlorperazine
Category	Antiemetic, Phenothiazine derivative
Route	Oral, Intramuscular
Strength	Tab (5 mg, 25 mg); Inj (12.5 mg/mL)
Brands	Stemetil (Inj, Tab), Emidoxyn (Tab)
Mechanism of action	Depresses the chemoreceptor trigger zone
Pharmacokinetics	*Onset of action:* 10–20 minutes, duration of action: 3–4 hours, well absorbed orally, metabolized in liver, excreted in feces and bile, half-life: 8–9 hours
Indications	Motion sickness; Vomiting
Dosage as per indications	For >2 years old or body weight >10 kg 0.4 mg/kg/day q 6–8 h oral. IM dose is half of oral dose
Maximum dosage	*Oral:* • 10–14 kg: 7.5 mg/day • 15–18 kg: 10 mg/day • 19–39 kg: 15 mg/day • >39 kg: up to 40 mg/day • >39 kg
Dose adjustments	In renal and hepatic derangement
Adverse effects	Extrapyramidal symptoms or orthostatic hypotension can occur
Contraindications	Hypersensitivity
Drug interactions	Anticoagulants, antihypertensives, phenytoin, propranolol
Remarks	Not for children <2 years

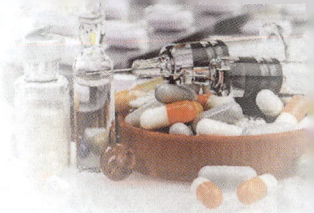

Promethazine Hydrochloride

Drug name	Promethazine hydrochloride
Category	Antihistamine, Antiemetic, Phenothiazine derivative
Route	Oral, Intramuscular, Per Rectal
Strength	Tab (10 mg, 25 mg); Elixir (5 mg/5 mL); Inj [2 mL (50 mg) ampoule]
Brands	Avomine (Tab), Phenergan (Amp, Tab, Elixir), Progene (Tab)
Mechanism of action	Acts on H1 receptor to block the histamine response. Also has sedative and antiemetic effects
Pharmacokinetics	Well absorbed from the gut. Effects starts in 20 minutes, lasting for 4–6 hours. Metabolized in liver and excreted in urine
Indications	Motion sickness; Antiemetic
Dosage as per indications	• *Motion sickness:* 0.5 mg/kg/dose q 12 h PO; first dose 30 minutes before starting • *Sedation/antiemetic:* 0.25–1 mg/kg/dose q 4–6 h, PO, IM, IV, or PR
Maximum dosage	25 mg/dose
Dose adjustments	Use with caution in liver disease
Adverse effects	Sedation, respiratory depression, blurred vision
Contraindications	Not recommended in children <2 years
Drug interactions	Sedatives and antihistaminics, topiramate, acetalopram
Remarks	Intravenous route is not recommended due to risk of severe tissue injury. If used should be diluted and given slowly

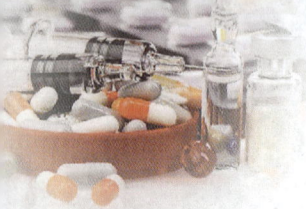

Propranolol

Drug name	Propranolol
Category	Beta-2 blocker
Route	Oral, Intravenous
Strength	Tab (10 mg); Inj (1 mg/mL ampoule)
Brands	Ciplar (Tab), Besprol (Tab), Inderal (Tab)
Mechanism of action	Acts to decrease cardiac output, inhibit renin release and decreases sympathetic nerve outflow from vasomotor centers in brain
Pharmacokinetics	Highly absorbed after oral intake. Has high first pass metabolism, only one-fourth drug reaches systemic circulation. Peak levels noted 1–4 hours after oral intake. Highly protein bound. Extensively metabolized, mostly eliminated via urine
Indications	Antihypertensive; Antiarrhythmic; Used to treat tremors; Infantile hemangiomas; Migraine; Cyanotic spells

Dosage as per indications	• *Supraventricular tachycardia:*
	  – *Oral:* 0.25 mg/kg/dose q 6–8 h
	  – *Intravenous:* 0.01–0.1 mg/kg/dose over 10–15 minutes, repeat q 6–8 h
	• *Thyrotoxicosis; neonates:* 0.5 mg/kg/dose orally q 6 h; children: 0.5–1 mg/kg/dose orally q 6 h
	• *Migraine prophylaxis:* 0.5–2 mg/kg/day orally q 6–8 h
	• *Hypertension:* Start at 0.5–1 mg/kg/day PO divided BID-QID, can increase weekly to a max of 8 mg/kg/day
	• *Tetralogy spells:*
	  – *IV:* 0.15–0.25 mg/kg/dose slow IV push
	  – *Oral:* 2–4 mg/kg/day divided 6 hourly
	• *Infantile hemangioma (see remarks):* Start in Infants from 0.6 mg/kg/dose twice a day orally, increase gradually over 1 month to 1.5–1.7 mg/kg/dose BID, drug to be given after feeds

Maximum dosage	• Not defined clearly
	• Most studies suggest
	  – *Oral:* 40–80 mg/day
	  – *IV:* 1 mg/dose in infants, 3 mg/dose in children

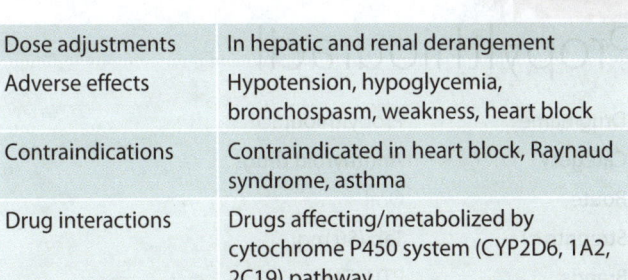

Dose adjustments	In hepatic and renal derangement
Adverse effects	Hypotension, hypoglycemia, bronchospasm, weakness, heart block
Contraindications	Contraindicated in heart block, Raynaud syndrome, asthma
Drug interactions	Drugs affecting/metabolized by cytochrome P450 system (CYP2D6, 1A2, 2C19) pathway

Propranolol

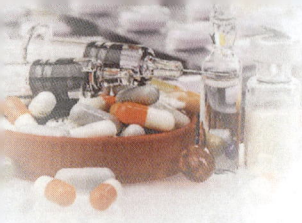

Propylthiouracil

Drug name	Propylthiouracil
Category	Antithyroid drugs
Route	Oral
Strength	Tab (50 mg)
Brands	PTU (Tab)
Mechanism of action	Inhibits the synthesis of thyroid hormones; inhibits conversion of thyroxine to triiodothyronine in peripheral tissues
Pharmacokinetics	Readily absorbed, extensively metabolized. One-third excreted in urine, within 24 hours
Indications	Intolerance to methimazole; Radioactive iodine therapy; Surgery not appropriate treatment
Dosage as per indications	*Loading:* • *6–10 years:* 50–100 mg/day divided 8 hourly • *>10 years:* 150–300 mg/day divided 8 hourly • *Maintenance:* One-third of loading dose 8–12 hourly
Maximum dosage	Not known
Dose adjustments	In renal and hepatic derangement
Adverse effects	Acute liver injury/liver failure, agranulocytosis, hypothyroidism, prolong prothrombin time
Contraindications	Hypersensitivity
Drug interactions	Digitalis, theophylline, anticoagulants
Remarks	Not a preferred drug in children, used only in rare conditions

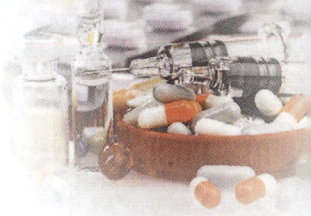

Protamine

Drug name	Protamine
Category	Antidote
Route	Intravenous
Strength	Inj (10 mg, 50 mg)
Brands	Neoprota, Newtain (Inj)
Mechanism of action	Protamine has an anticoagulant effect when used separately but when given in the presence of heparin, a stable complex is formed disrupting anticoagulant activity of both the drugs
Pharmacokinetics	Rapid onset of action after IV administration, neutralization occurs within 5 minutes, the complexes once formed are either metabolized by liver or broken down by fibrinolysin
Indications	Heparin overdose
Dosage as per indications	• Each mg of protamine sulfate (dried), neutralizes 100 USP heparin units • Given as slow intravenous injection over 10 minutes, maximum 50 mg • Protamine dose decreases with time as heparin disappears rapidly from circulation. Dose should be monitored by PT/APTT-INR values
Maximum dosage	50 mg total dose
Dose adjustments	Not needed in liver derangement
Adverse effects	Anaphylaxis, anaphylactoid reactions, hypotension, bradycardia, dyspnea, nausea, vomiting, dyspnea, pulmonary edema
Contraindications	Hypersensitivity
Drug interactions	Anticoagulant drugs

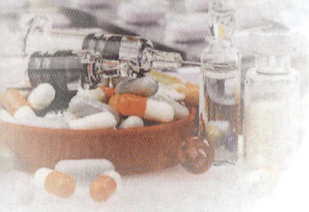

Pseudoephedrine

Drug name	Pseudoephedrine
Category	Decongestant
Route	Oral
Strength	Tab (60 mg); Syp (30 mg/5 mL)
Brands	Pseudoephedrine (Tab), Sudafed (Syp)
Mechanism of action	Agonist of alpha- and beta-adrenergic receptors but inhibits norepinephrine, dopamine, and serotonin transporters
Pharmacokinetics	Low protein binding, poorly metabolized, eliminated mainly unchanged from kidneys, elimination half-life 6 hours
Indications	Allergic rhinitis; Common cold; Vasomotor rhinitis
Dosage as per indications	• *2–12 years:* 4 mg/kg/day in 4 divided doses • *>12 years:* 60 mg/dose 6–8 hourly
Maximum dosage	Not known
Dose adjustments	Not needed, use with caution in renal derangement
Adverse effects	Headache, dizziness, insomnia, tremors, tachycardia, dry mouth
Contraindications	Hypersensitivity
Drug interactions	MAO inhibitors, amphetamines, sympathomimetic

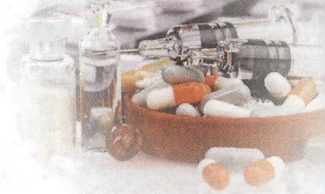

Pyrantel Pamoate

Drug name	Pyrantel pamoate
Category	Antihelminthic
Route	Oral
Strength	Tab (250 mg); Susp (250 mg/5 mL)
Brands	Expent (Tab, Syp), Nemocid (Tab, Syp), Pymolar (Tab), Pyraleb (Syp)
Mechanism of action	Depolarizing neuromuscular-blocking agent, activates nicotine receptor, releases acetylcholine and inhibits cholinesterase leading to excessive depolarization and spastic paralysis in the organism
Pharmacokinetics	Poorly absorbed, peak levels in 1–3 hours, partially metabolized in liver and excreted in feces
Indications	Parasitic infections; Ascariasis; Hookworm infestation
Dosage as per indications	11 mg/kg single dose, repeat after 2 weeks; hookworm: 11 mg/kg/dose, once daily × 3 days
Maximum dosage	1 g/dose
Dose adjustments	Required in liver disease
Adverse effects	Increased liver enzymes, abdominal cramps, rash
Contraindications	Hypersensitivity
Drug interactions	Not known

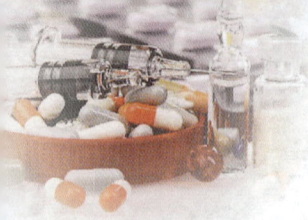

Pyridostigmine

Drug name	Pyridostigmine
Category	Cholinesterase inhibitor
Route	Oral
Strength	Tab (30 mg, 60 mg, 120 mg)
Brands	Pyrido (Tab), Gravitor (Tab)
Mechanism of action	Acetylcholinesterase inhibitors, increases acetylcholine levels, acts similar as neostigmine with less toxicity
Pharmacokinetics	Poorly absorbed when administered orally, bioavailability 10–20%, primarily renally eliminated, half-life 0.5–1 hour
Indications	Myasthenia gravis; Congenital myasthenic syndromes
Dosage as per indications	*Oral:* • *Neonate:* 5 mg every 4–6 hourly • *Children:* 7 mg/kg/day divided 4 hourly *Inj:* 0.05–0.15 mg/kg IV/IM 4–6 hourly
Maximum dosage	10 mg/dose
Dose adjustments	In renal derangement
Adverse effects	Cholinergic crisis
Contraindications	Hypersensitivity
Drug interactions	Atropine, succinylcholine, neomycin, streptomycin

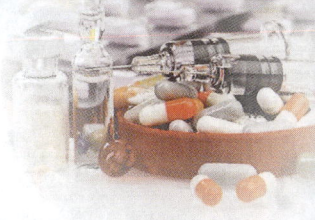

Pyridoxine

Drug name	Pyridoxine
Category	Vitamin B_6
Route	Intravenous, Intramuscular, Oral
Strength	Tab (25 mg, 50 mg, 100 mg); Inj (100 mg/mL)
Brands	Pyricontin (Tab), Ingavit B6 (Tab), B long (Tab) Pyridoxine hydrochloride (Inj)
Mechanism of action	Acts as coenzymes in metabolism of fat, protein, and carbohydrate
Pharmacokinetics	Half-life 15–20 days; degraded to 4-pyridoxic acid in liver, the metabolite is excreted in urine
Indications	Pyridoxine-dependent seizures; Pyridoxine deficiency; INH intoxication; Drug-induced neuritis
Dosage as per indications	• *For pyridoxine-dependent seizures:* Loading 50–100 mg PO/IV followed by 50–100 mg/24 h PO • *Drug-induced neuritis:* 1 mg/kg/24 h daily • *Dietary deficiency:* 5–15 mg/24 h for 3–4 weeks then half dose daily
Maximum dosage	Not known
Dose adjustments	Not known
Adverse effects	Increased liver enzymes, decreased serum folic acid levels. Large intravenous doses can cause seizure
Contraindications	Hypersensitivity
Drug interactions	Not known

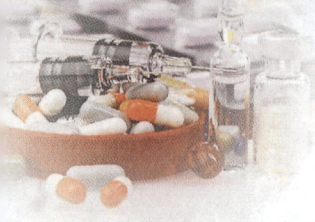

Pyrimethamine-Sulfadoxine

Drug name	Pyrimethamine-sulfadoxine
Category	Antiparasitic
Route	Oral
Strength	Tab (25 mg Pyrimethamine + 500 mg Sulfadoxine); Syp (12.5 mg Pyrimethamine + 250 mg Sulfadoxine/5 mL)
Brands	Rimodar Forte (Tab), Malin (Syp), Malasulf Forte (Tab)
Mechanism of action	• *Pyrimethamine:* Inhibits dihydrofolate reductase, acts selectively against *Plasmodia* (schizonticidal form in blood and tissue) and *Toxoplasma gondii* • Sulfadoxine inhibits the activity of dihydropteroate synthase
Pharmacokinetics	Well absorbed orally, peak serum levels: 2–6 hours after intake. Highly protein bound, slowly eliminated; elimination half-life: 96–100 hours for pyrimethamine; 200 hours for sulfadoxine; eliminated via kidneys
Indications	Toxoplasmosis; Chloroquine-resistant uncomplicated *Plasmodium falciparum* malaria
Dosage as per indications	• 1.25 mg/kg pyrimethamine/25 mg/kg sulfadoxine as single dose with artesunate for treatment of chloroquine resistant uncomplicated *P. falciparum* malaria • Toxoplasmosis (administered with sulfadiazine and leucovorin) *Congenital:* Loading: 2 mg/kg/24 h PO div q12 h for 2 days Maintenance: 1 mg/kg/24 h PO OD for 2–6 months f/b 1 mg/kg/24 h thrice per week to complete 12 months therapy. *Child:* Loading: 2 mg/kg/24 h PO div BD for 3 days Maintenance: 1 mg/kg/24 h PO div OD-BD for 4 weeks

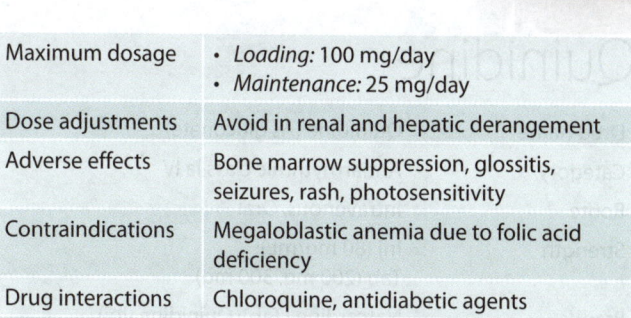

Maximum dosage	• *Loading:* 100 mg/day • *Maintenance:* 25 mg/day
Dose adjustments	Avoid in renal and hepatic derangement
Adverse effects	Bone marrow suppression, glossitis, seizures, rash, photosensitivity
Contraindications	Megaloblastic anemia due to folic acid deficiency
Drug interactions	Chloroquine, antidiabetic agents
Remarks	Always give folinic acid along

Pyrimethamine-Sulfadoxine

339

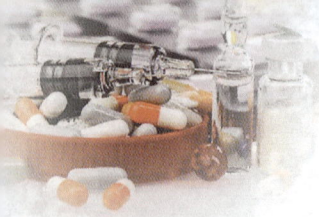

Quinidine

Drug name	Quinidine (As gluconate)
Category	Antiarrhythmic class Ia IV
Route	Intravenous, Oral
Strength	Inj (80 mg/mL); Tab (200 mg, 300 mg)
Brands	Natcardine (Tab), Quinidine (Inj)
Mechanism of action	• Acts on sodium channels in Purkinje fibers to produce antiarrhythmic action • Has intraerythrocytic schizonticide action, and gametocidal effect on *Plasmodium vivax* and *P. malariae*, when used in malaria
Pharmacokinetics	High bioavailability when taken orally, peak serum levels: 3–5 hours after intake, high protein bound, elimination half-life 3–4 hours, elimination mainly by renal route
Indications	Arrhythmia; Malaria
Dosage as per indications	*Antiarrhythmic:* • IV (as gluconate) 2–10 mg/kg/dose q 3–6 h • PO (as sulfate) 15–60 mg/kg/day q 6 h *Antimalarial:* • *Loading dose:* 10 mg/kg/dose IV over 1–2 hours • *Maintenance dose:* 0.02 mg/kg/min IV as continuous infusion
Maximum dosage	Max loading dose: 600 mg
Dose adjustments	In renal and hepatic derangement
Adverse effects	GI symptoms, hypotension, rash, TTP, heart block
Contraindications	Hypersensitivity
Drug interactions	May cause an increase in digoxin levels. May potentiate neuromuscular blockade
Remarks	• Test dose 2 mg/kg IM/PO (max 200 mg) should be done to look for idiosyncratic reaction • Once on maintenance therapy, shift to oral as soon as possible • Dose to be reduced by 30–50% if IV therapy required for >48 hours

Quinine Dihydrochloride

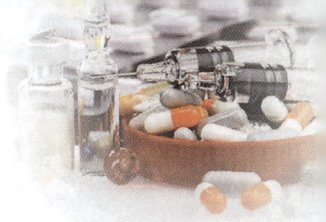

Drug name	Quinine dihydrochloride
Category	Antimalarial
Route	Intravenous, Intramuscular
Strength	Inj (300 mg/mL ampoule)
Brands	Quinlup (Inj), Quin-9 (Inj), Cinkona (Inj), Qinarsol (Inj)
Mechanism of action	Acts on schizonticides by inhibiting protein synthesis leading to prevention of DNA replication and transcription to RNA; also exerts gametocytocidal effect on *P. vivax* and *P. malariae*
Pharmacokinetics	Highly protein bound; metabolized in the liver eliminated in the urine. The elimination half-life: 11 hours
Indications	Severe malaria; Chloroquine-resistant falciparum malaria
Dosage as per indications	• Intravenous 20 mg/kg salt diluted in normal saline or 5% dextrose in a concentration of 1 mg/mL, given as a loading dose over 4 h; followed by 10 mg/kg/dose as infusion over 4 h every 8 h for 7–10 days • Shift to oral therapy as soon as possible
Maximum dosage	Loading 1.4 g, maintenance 0.7 g/dose
Dose adjustments	In liver disease
Adverse effects	Hypoglycemia, hypotension, cinchonism
Contraindications	Hypersensitivity, prolong QT interval, G6PD deficiency
Drug interactions	Anticoagulants, neuromuscular blocking drugs, antiarrhythmics, diuretics
Remarks	Do not give rapidly or as bolus

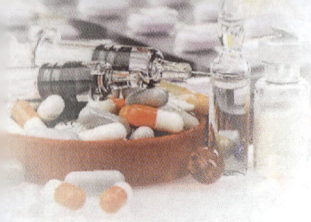

Quinine Sulfate

Drug name	Quinine sulfate
Category	Antimalarial
Route	Oral
Strength	Tab (150, 300 mg salt)
Brands	Calquin, Quin-9, Cinkona (Tab)
Mechanism of action	Inhibits nucleic acid synthesis, protein synthesis, and glycolysis in *Plasmodium falciparum* and can bind with hemozoin in parasitized erythrocytes. Quinine sulfate acts primarily on the blood schizont form of *P. falciparum*. It is not gametocidal and has little effect on the sporozoite or pre-erythrocytic forms
Pharmacokinetics	High oral bioavailability, moderately protein bound, poor CSF penetration, metabolized in liver by P450 enzyme, excretion via kidney, increases with alkaline urine
Indications	For uncomplicated chloroquine resistant *P. falciparum* infections
Dosage as per indications	• Oral 10 mg/kg/dose of salt every 8 h × 7 days • Used in combination with tetracycline (40 mg/kg/day q 6 h × 10 days), or clindamycin (20–40 mg/kg/day q 8 h × 3 days) or Pyrimethamine (0.75 mg/kg/day q 12 h × 3 days), or sulfadiazine (150 mg/kg/day q 8 h × 6 days) to prevent drug resistance
Maximum dosage	600 mg/dose
Dose adjustments	Renal and hepatic impairment
Adverse effects	Tinnitus, cinchonism, blurred vision, GI discomfort, nausea, vomiting
Contraindications	Hypersensitivity, prolong QT interval, G6PD deficiency
Drug interactions	Antiarrhythmic drugs, those affecting QT interval, rifampicin
Remarks	Do not crush the tablet. Do not eat on empty stomach

Quinupristin/Dalfopristin

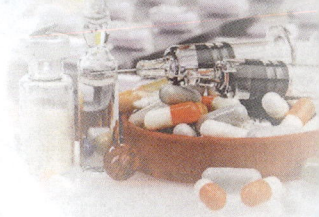

Drug name	Quinupristin/Dalfopristin
Category	Macrolide-lincosamide streptogramin antibacterial antibiotic
Route	Intravenous
Strength	Inj (500 mg/vial)
Brands	Synercid (Inj)
Mechanism of action	Quinupristin and dalfopristin act on bacterial ribosome. Dalfopristin inhibit the early phase of protein synthesis while quinupristin inhibits the late phase of protein synthesis
Pharmacokinetics	Both the components undergo conjugation. The elimination half-life of quinupristin and dalfopristin is 50 min and 40 min respectively. Both the drugs and their metabolites are mainly excreted through renal route. Fecal excretion constitutes the main elimination route for both parent drugs and their metabolites
Indications	Vancomycin-resistant *Staphylococcus aureus*; Vancomycin-resistant *Enterococcus faecium* infections
Dosage as per indications	7.5 mg/kg IV infusion in 5% dextrose 8–12 hourly for 7–14 days
Maximum dosage	Not known
Dose adjustments	Not required in renal, studies in hepatic derangement are insufficient
Adverse effects	Pain and swelling at infusion site, nausea, diarrhea, vomiting, rash, headache, pruritus, myalgia, arthralgia
Contraindications	Not recommended for children below 16 years age, contraindicated in case of hypersensitivity to the drug
Drug interactions	Drugs affecting P450 enzyme or leading to prolong QT interval
Remarks	Do not dilute in normal saline

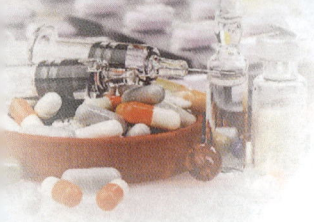

Rabeprazole

Drug name	Rabeprazole
Category	Proton pump inhibitor
Route	Oral
Strength	Tab (10 mg, 20 mg); Inj (20 mg)
Brands	Aciraz (Tab, Inj), Cyra (Tab, Inj), Dazol (Tab, Inj)
Mechanism of action	Inhibits gastric $H^+:K^+$ ATPase pump thus decreasing the secretion from gastric mucosa
Pharmacokinetics	Converted to active form, sulfenamide, in gastric mucosa. Well absorbed when taken orally, around 50% bioavailability, metabolized in liver, eliminated from urine. Half-life 1–2 hours
Indications	Gastric ulcer; *Helicobacter pylori* infection
Dosage as per indications	*Gastritis/gastric ulcer:* 20 mg OD oral *H. pylori* infection: 1.5–2.5 mg/kg/day in two divided doses PO as part of 3-drug regime
Maximum dosage	20 mg/day
Dose adjustments	Caution needed in severe hepatic derangement. Not needed in renal or mild to moderate hepatic involvement
Adverse effects	Bone fracture, hypomagnesemia, risk of bleeding when used with warfarin
Contraindications	Hypersensitivity
Drug interactions	Cyclosporine, warfarin, methotrexate
Remarks	Not preferred in <12 years

Rabies Human Monoclonal Antibody

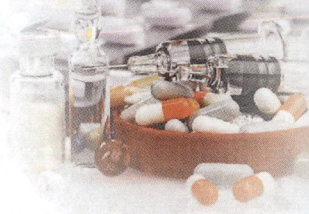

Drug name	Rabies human monoclonal antibody (Recombinant)
Category	rDNA monoclonal antibody
Route	Intramuscular, Local wound site, Intradermal
Strength	Inj (100 IU, 250 IU)
Brands	Rabishield (Inj)
Mechanism of action	Rabies monoclonal antibodies produced through recombinant DNA technology provides immediate passive immunity
Pharmacokinetics	Not known
Indications	As postexposure prophylaxis
Dosage as per indications	3.33 IU/kg, maximum to be given at the site of bite, rest to be given intramuscular
Maximum dosage	Not known
Dose adjustments	Not known
Adverse effects	Injection site pain, redness, and swelling, headache, muscle pain
Contraindications	No absolute contraindication, risk-benefit ratio to be assessed in hypersensitivity
Drug interactions	Not known

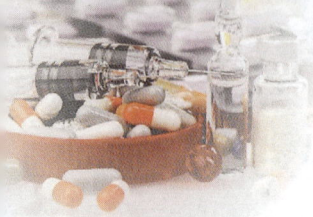

Rabies Immunoglobulin (RIG)

Drug name	Rabies immunoglobulin (RIG)
Category	Immunoglobulin (Human)
Route	Intramuscular
Strength	Inj (150 U/mL vial)
Brands	Favirab (Inj), Imogam (Inj), Pars (Inj)
Mechanism of action	Human rabies immunoglobulin contains mainly immunoglobulin G (IgG) with a specifically high content of antibodies against rabies virus
Pharmacokinetics	After an intramuscular dose, the drug is available in body's circulation after 2–3 days with a half-life of 3–4 weeks, though the half-life may vary in different individuals
Indications	Postexposure prophylaxis
Dosage as per indications	Given to all category III exposures. 20 IU/kg, infiltrate in local site as much as possible, rest to be given IM in gluteal region
Maximum dosage	20 IU/kg
Dose adjustments	None
Adverse effects	Headache, fever, chills, nausea, vomiting, itching, rash, allergic reaction, or Inj site reactions
Contraindications	Hypersensitivity
Drug interactions	Live vaccines
Remarks	• If the patient presents between 1 and 7 days, give the entire dose IM. Administer rabies vaccine simultaneously • *Caution:* To be given within 24 hours of bite. Perform prior intradermal testing for hypersensitivity

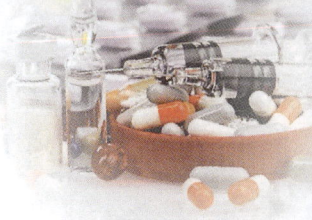

Racecadotril

Drug name	Racecadotril
Category	Antidiarrheal
Route	Oral
Strength	Cap (10 mg, 30 mg, 100 mg); Sachet (10 mg, 30 mg, 100 mg, 300 mg, 1 g, 3 g)
Brands	Lomorest (Cap, Sachet), Racotil (Cap, Sachet), Redotil (Cap, Sachet)
Mechanism of action	Inhibits enkephalinase, thereby increasing the availability of endogenous enkephalins causing decreased intestinal secretion
Pharmacokinetics	Rapid and fast absorption after oral administration, further metabolized to its active metabolite thiorphan. Effect noted within 30 minutes with peak levels obtained 1 hour after administration. Half-life 3 hours
Indications	Noninfective poorly responding secretory diarrhea
Dosage as per indications	1.5 mg/kg/dose 8 hourly PO
Maximum dosage	Not known
Dose adjustments	Not known
Adverse effects	Headache, hypokalemia
Contraindications	Hypersensitivity
Drug interactions	Not known
Remarks	Not used routinely in children with diarrhea

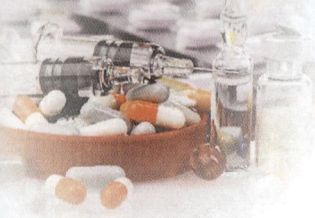

Ramipril

Drug name	Ramipril
Category	Antihypertensive
Route	Oral
Strength	Tab (1.25 mg, 2.5 mg, 5 mg, 10 mg)
Brands	Cardace (Tab), Ramistar, Ramace, Ramipres
Mechanism of action	Inhibits angiotensin-converting enzyme (ACE) leading to decreased angiotensin II levels. This causes decreased vasopressor effect
Pharmacokinetics	Around 50% absorbed when administered orally, peak levels in 1 hour, metabolized to 6 times more potent form ramiprilat; half-life is 2–4 hours for initial binding to ACE. Elimination half-life is bi-peaked, one representing clearance of free ramiprilat (9–18 hours) and other represents the ramiprilat/ACE complex clearance (*Half-life:* >2 days)
Indications	Hypertension
Dosage as per indications	Initial dose 2.5 mg/day in 1–2 divided doses, can be gradually increased every 15–20 days till 20 mg/day or if the desired effect achieved, whichever is less
Maximum dosage	20 mg/day
Dose adjustments	In renal impairment
Adverse effects	Headache, dizziness, fatigue, and cough, Angioedema, hypotension, hyperkalemia
Contraindications	Hypersensitivity, angioedema, severe renal impairment
Drug interactions	Diuretics, antihypertensives, NSAIDs
Remarks	Not an Approved Drug in children yet

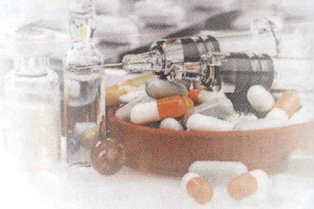

Ranitidine

Drug name	Ranitidine
Category	Histamine-2-blocker
Route	Intravenous, Oral
Strength	Inj (50 mg/2 mL); Cap (150 mg, 300 mg); Syp (15 mg/mL)
Brands	Aciloc (Inj, Tab), Histac (Inj, Tab), Rantac (Inj, Tab), Zinetac (Inj, Tab)
Mechanism of action	Reversible inhibitor at H2-receptors
Pharmacokinetics	Rapid and almost complete absorption after IV and IM administration. Eliminated in urine as N-oxide with elimination half-life 2–2.5 hours
Indications	Gastritis; Gastric ulcer
Dosage as per indications	*Antiulcer:* • Intravenous 1–2 mg/kg/day q 12 h • Oral 2–4 mg/kg/day q 12 h
Maximum dosage	*Oral:* 300 mg/day; IV: 50 mg/dose
Dose adjustments	Dose adjustment in severe renal disease
Adverse effects	Headache, drowsiness, arthralgia, fatigue
Contraindications	Hypersensitivity
Drug interactions	Warfarin, procainamide, ketoconazole, midazolam

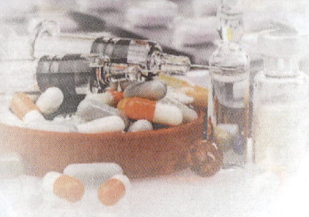

Rasburicase

Drug name	Rasburicase
Category	Recombinant urate oxidase
Route	Intravenous
Strength	Inj (3 mL, 10 mL vials)
Brands	Elitek (Inj)
Mechanism of action	Catalyzes enzymatic oxidation of poorly soluble uric acid into an inactive and more soluble metabolite (allantoin)
Pharmacokinetics	Not much known. *Terminal half-life:* 15–23 hours
Indications	Used for treating hyperuricemia in tumor lysis syndrome; Rhabdomyolysis with kidney failure; Gout
Dosage as per indications	0.2 mg/kg IV infused over 30 minutes q 12–24 h for up to 5 days
Maximum dosage	Not known
Dose adjustments	None
Adverse effects	Anaphylaxis, methemoglobinemia in G6PD deficient persons
Contraindications	Contraindicated in G6PD deficiency
Drug interactions	None

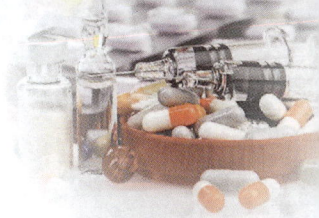

Remdesivir

Drug name	Remdesivir
Category	Antiviral drug, Nucleotide analog
Route	Intravenous
Strength	Inj (100 mg)
Brands	Covifor, Cipremi (Inj)
Mechanism of action	It is an adenosine nucleotide prodrug which inhibits SARS-CoV-2 RNA-dependent RNA polymerase, needed for viral replication
Pharmacokinetics	90% plasma protein bound, extensively metabolized, primarily excreted in urine, elimination half-life 1 hour
Indications	SARS COV-2 infections
Dosage as per indications	• *3.5–40 kg:* 5 mg/kg IV on day 1 followed by 2.5 mg/kg/day IV for 5 days once a day • *40 kg:* 200 mg IV on day 1 followed by 100 mg IV from day 2–5 once a day
Maximum dosage	• *Loading:* 200 mg/dose • *Maintenance:* 100 mg/dose
Dose adjustments	Renal impairment, hepatic impairment not known
Adverse effects	Hypersensitivity, transaminitis, hyperuricemia
Contraindications	Contraindicated in severe hepatic dysfunction, severe renal impairment
Drug interactions	Hydroxychloroquine

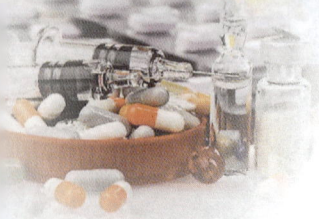

Respiratory Syncytial Virus (RSV) IG

Drug name	Respiratory syncytial virus (RSV) IG
Category	Immunoglobulin
Route	Intravenous
Strength	Vial (50 mg/mL)
Brands	RespiGam (Inj)
Mechanism of action	Recombinant humanized monoclonal antibody, binds to RSV envelope fusion protein (RSV F) preventing membrane fusion process and cell-to-cell fusion of RSV-infected cells
Pharmacokinetics	Mean half-life 20 hours. Bioavailability after IM injection around 70%
Indications	Prophylaxis against RSV in preterm babies
Dosage as per indications	May administer prophylactically in preterm infants (<32 weeks) who do not have BPD. For those ≤28 weeks, consider till 12 months of age and for those with gestational age 29–32 weeks, may give RSV IG until 6 months of age. 750 mg/kg IV every 30 days during RSV season
Maximum dosage	Not known
Dose adjustments	Not known
Adverse effects	Fever, respiratory distress, vomiting, wheezing
Contraindications	IgA deficiency and cyanotic heart disease
Drug interactions	Live vaccines not to be given
Remarks	Initiate RSV IG within 6 months before RSV season

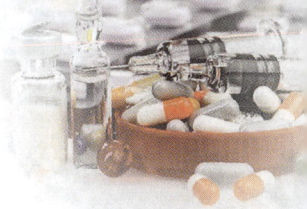

Ribavirin

Drug name	Ribavirin
Category	Antiviral drug
Route	Oral
Strength	Cap (100 mg, 200 mg); Syp (50 mg/5 mL)
Brands	Virazide (Cap, Syp), Ribavin (Cap, Syp)
Mechanism of action	Acts by direct antiviral activity, increased mutation frequency and inhibits HCV polymerase
Pharmacokinetics	Rapid and extensive absorption after oral intake. Metabolized via phosphorylation. Mainly excreted via urine. Terminal half-life 120–170 hours
Indications	HCV infection
Dosage as per indications	• <25 kg: 7.5 mg/kg/dose BID • 25–36 kg: 200 mg BID • 37–49 kg: 200 mg in morning and 400 mg in evening (12 hourly) • 50–61 kg: 400 mg BID • >61–75 kg: 400 mg in morning and 600 mg in evening (12 hourly) • >75 kg: 600 mg BID
Maximum dosage	Not known
Dose adjustments	In renal and hepatic impairment
Adverse effects	Anemia, psychiatric disturbances
Contraindications	Pregnancy, hepatitis, heart disease, severe renal disease
Drug interactions	NRTIs, azathioprine

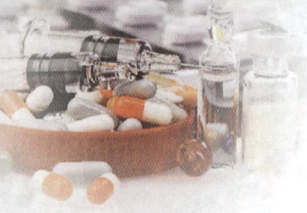

Riboflavin

Drug name	Riboflavin
Category	Vitamin B$_2$
Route	Oral
Strength	Available as multivitamin combination
Brands	Folwin, A to Z, Becadex (Tab, Syp)
Mechanism of action	Works as coenzymes for flavin mononucleotide and flavin adenine dinucleotide
Pharmacokinetics	Predominantly absorbed in the proximal small intestine, excess amount not absorbed or absorbed and excreted in urine
Indications	Ariboflavinosis; Cheilitis/stomatitis
Dosage as per indications	• *Daily requirement:* 0.1–2 mg/day • *Deficiency state:* 2.5–10 mg/day 8–12 hourly, up to 30 mg in children >12 years
Maximum dosage	Not known
Dose adjustments	Not known
Adverse effects	Nausea, gastritis
Contraindications	Hypersensitivity
Drug interactions	Not known

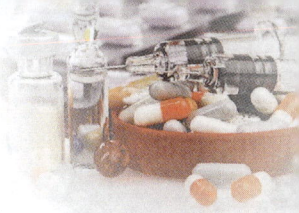

Rifampicin

Drug name	Rifampicin
Category	Antibiotic, Antitubercular
Route	Oral
Strength	Cap (150 mg, 300 mg, 450 mg); Syp (20 mg/mL)
Brands	R-Cin (Cap, Syp), Rimactane (Cap, Syp), Rimpacin (Cap)
Mechanism of action	Inhibits DNA-dependent RNA polymerase activity in susceptible bacteria, especially *Mycobacterium tuberculosis*, without affecting mammalian enzyme
Pharmacokinetics	Well absorbed after oral administration, undergoes deacetylation while being metabolized and eliminated by bile, detected in bile for 6 hours. Also one-third of drug eliminated in urine as unchanged drug
Indications	Tuberculosis; Meningococcal prophylaxis

Dosage as per indications	• *TB:* 10–15 mg/kg/day
	• *Meningococcal prophylaxis:*
	  >1 month of age: 10 mg/kg/dose 12 hourly for 48 hours
	  Neonates: 5 mg/kg/dose 12 hourly for 48 hours

Maximum dosage	600–1200 mg/day
Dose adjustments	Needed in liver derangement, not needed in renal derangement
Adverse effects	Nausea, vomiting, abdominal pain, increased liver enzymes, brownish-red or orange discoloration of the skin, urine and other body secretion
Contraindications	Hypersensitivity
Drug interactions	Anticonvulsants, digoxin, antiarrhythmics, anticoagulants, phenobarbitone
Remarks	Risk of hepatocellular toxicity in patients on ritonavir-saquinavir combination

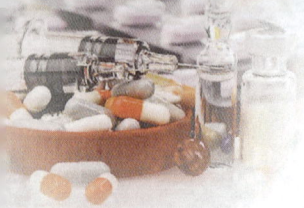

Ritonavir (RTV)

Drug name	Ritonavir (RTV)
Category	Antiretroviral, Protease inhibitor
Route	Oral
Strength	Sol (80 mg/mL); Tab (100 mg)
Brands	Ritomax (Tab), Ritomune (Tab)
Mechanism of action	Acts as an enhancer of other protease inhibitors (PIs)
Pharmacokinetics	Peak levels in 2–4 hours, poorly metabolized, excreted mainly in feces
Indications	HIV infection/AIDS
Dosage as per indications	350–400 mg per m^2 twice a day; Start at doses of 250 mg/m^2; Increase gradually
Maximum dosage	600 mg/dose
Dose adjustments	Not recommended in severe hepatic derangement, no dose adjustment in mild to moderate dysfunction
Adverse effects	Nausea, vomiting, diarrhea, taste alteration, paresthesia, hypertriglyceridemia, pancreatitis, hepatitis, hyperglycemia, and rash
Contraindications	Hypersensitivity
Drug interactions	CYP3A4 inhibitors or inducers

Rituximab

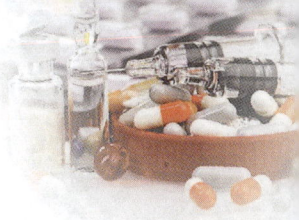

Drug name	Rituximab
Category	Monoclonal antibody against CD20
Route	Intravenous
Strength	Inj (10 mg/mL, 10 mL or 50 mL vials)
Brands	Rituxan (Inj)
Mechanism of action	Binds CD20 antigen on pre-B and mature B lymphocytes, and most cells of B-cell non-Hodgkin's lymphomas (NHL)
Pharmacokinetics	Not much known. Elimination half-life varies from 18 to 22 days
Indications	Used in non-Hodgkin lymphoma, immune diseases (Wegener granulomatosis; Microscopic polyangiitis; Rheumatoid arthritis, autoimmune hemolytic anemia); Steroid-resistant nephrotic syndrome
Dosage as per indications	Largely vary in each condition and protocol being used, 375 mg/m^2/week is the most commonly used dose
Maximum dosage	Not known
Dose adjustments	Not studied
Adverse effects	Severe mucocutaneous reaction, hepatitis B reactivation, progressive multifocal leukoencephalopathy (PML)
Contraindications	Hypersensitivity
Drug interactions	Cisplatin
Remarks	Administer as IV infusion. Do not administer as IV push or bolus

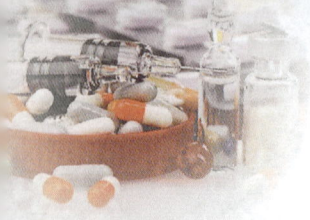

Rizatriptan Benzoate

Drug name	Rizatriptan benzoate
Category	Serotonin agonist
Route	Oral
Strength	Tab (5 mg, 10 mg)
Brands	Rizact, Rizora, Rizatan (Tab)
Mechanism of action	Serotonin (5-HT) 1B/1D receptor agonist, binds to their receptors present on intracranial blood vessels and sensory nerves of the trigeminal system
Pharmacokinetics	Well absorbed when taken orally. Metabolized by oxidative deamination by monoamine oxidase-A (MAO-A). Peak plasma levels in 60–90 minutes, eliminated in urine, half-life 2–3 hours
Indications	Migraine without aura for children >6 years of age
Dosage as per indications	• <40 kg: 5 mg single dose • >40 kg: 10 mg single dose
Maximum dosage	30 mg/day in adults
Dose adjustments	In moderate liver dysfunction
Adverse effects	Fatigue, dizziness, sleepiness
Contraindications	Hypersensitivity
Drug interactions	HT1 agonist or ergotamine-containing medication, MAO inhibitors
Remarks	Avoid in ischemic heart disease, stroke, Ischemic bowel disease, severe hypertension, on 5-HT1 agonist or ergotamine-containing medication, MAO inhibitors

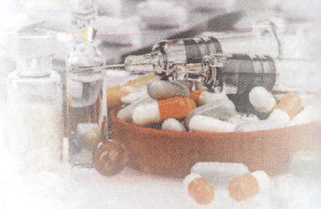

Roxithromycin

Drug name	Roxithromycin
Category	Antibiotic, Macrolide
Route	Oral
Strength	Tab (50 mg, 150 mg); Syp (50 mg/5 mL)
Brands	Acitrom (Tab), Altrox (Tab), Arbid (Tab), Roxid (Tab)
Mechanism of action	Binds to bacterial 50S ribosome to inhibit protein synthesis
Pharmacokinetics	Rapid absorption after oral intake, highly protein bound, metabolized in liver, excreted in urine and feces, half-life 12 hours
Indications	Respiratory tract; Urinary; Soft tissue infections
Dosage as per indications	5–8 mg/kg/day q 12 h
Maximum dosage	Not known
Dose adjustments	In hepatic derangement
Adverse effects	GI disturbance, vertigo, candidiasis, tinnitus with warfarin increases risk for bleeding
Contraindications	Hypersensitivity
Drug interactions	Cyclosporine

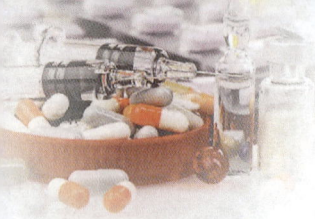

Salbutamol (Albuterol)

Drug name	Salbutamol (Albuterol)
Category	Bronchodilator, β2 adrenergic agonist
Route	Oral, Inhalational
Strength	Syp (2 mg/5 mL); Tab (2 mg, 4 mg, 8 mg); Nebulizing Sol (5 mg/mL, 2.5 mg/3 mL); MDI (100 µg/puff)
Brands	Asthalin (Syp, MDI, Neb sol), Asthacure (Syp), Ventolin (MDI, Syp)
Mechanism of action	Acts on beta 2 receptors and activates adenyl cyclase to increase cyclic AMP. Cyclic AMP inhibits myosin phosphorylation and decreases intracellular calcium by inhibiting protein kinase. All these lead to muscle relaxation
Pharmacokinetics	MDI has poor systemic absorption, terminal half-life around 4–5 hours
Indications	Bronchial Asthma; Wheezy illness; Hyperkalemia
Dosage as per indications	*Asthma:* • *Oral:* 0.1–0.2 mg/kg/dose 2–3 times/day • *Nebulization:* 0.15 mg/kg/dose; min 1.25 mg; max 3 mg • *Acute exacerbation:* 2–4 puffs by MDI every 20 min followed by 2 puffs every 4–6 h *Hyperkalemia:* Salbutamol given as nebulization in the above dose
Maximum dosage	3 mg/dose for nebulization; 800 mcg/day as MDI; 4 mg/dose as oral
Dose adjustments	Not known
Adverse effects	Tachycardia, tremors, hypokalemia, palpitations, nervousness, insomnia, headache, nausea. Systemic side effects are dose related
Contraindications	Hypersensitivity
Drug interactions	Sympathomimetic drugs, digoxin, MAO, TCA
Remarks	Use of spacers may enhance the efficacy of inhaled salbutamol. Use cautiously with monitoring of cardiac side effects and serum potassium levels

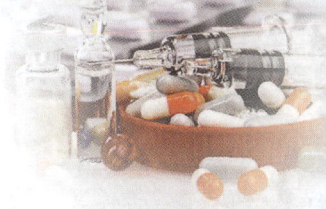

Salmeterol (MDI)

Drug name	Salmeterol (MDI)
Category	Bronchodilator, β2 adrenergic agonist (Long-acting)
Route	Inhalational
Strength	Usually available in combination with fluticasone (MDI 25 µg and 50 µg; 50 µg and 100 µg)
Brands	Airtec SF, Esiflo, Serobid, Salmeter (MDI)
Mechanism of action	Acts on beta 2 receptors and activates adenyl cyclase to increase cyclic AMP. Cyclic AMP inhibits myosin phosphorylation and decreases intracellular calcium by inhibiting protein kinase. All these lead to muscle relaxation
Pharmacokinetics	*Onset:* 10–20 minutes, peak effect: 3 hours. Systemic absorption is very low after inhalation. Salmeterol base is extensively metabolized by hydroxylation, with subsequent elimination predominantly in the feces
Indications	Asthma
Dosage as per indications	MDI (25 µg/puff): 50–100 µg/day
Maximum dosage	Not known
Dose adjustments	Not known
Adverse effects	Tachycardia, tremors, hypokalemia, palpitations, arrhythmias, hypertension, nervousness, insomnia, headache, and nausea. Should not be used in treatment of acute asthma
Contraindications	Not to be used as monotherapy. Not to be used in children <4 years
Drug interactions	Avoid concomitant usage with ketoconazole, clarithromycin, itraconazole, and protease inhibitors due to added cardiac adverse effects, e.g., QTc prolongation, tachycardia

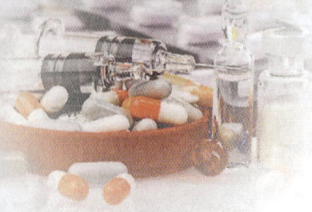

Saquinavir (SQV)

Drug name	Saquinavir (SQV)
Category	Antiretroviral, Protease inhibitor
Route	Oral
Strength	Tab (500 mg)
Brands	Invirase, Saquin (Tab)
Mechanism of action	Inhibits HIV protease
Pharmacokinetics	Not much known. Poorly absorbed with high first pass metabolism when given alone. Highly protein bound, metabolized in liver, excreted in feces and urine
Indications	HIV infection/AIDS
Dosage as per indications	Dosing based on body weight and in combination with ritonavir • *5–15 kg:* SQV 50 mg/kg + RTV 3 mg/kg BD • *15–40 kg:* SQV 50 mg/kg + RTV 2.5 mg/kg BD • *≥40 kg:* SQV 50 mg/kg + RTV 100 mg BD
Maximum dosage	Not known
Dose adjustments	Not known
Adverse effects	Liver dysfunction, cardiac rhythm disturbances
Contraindications	Hypersensitivity
Drug interactions	Rifampin, terfenadine, cisapride, astemizole, midazolam
Remarks	Avoid in children

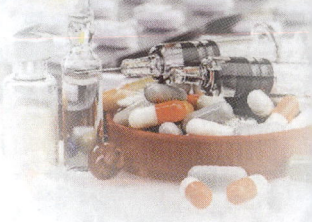

Sevelamer

Drug name	Sevelamer
Category	Phosphate binder
Route	Oral
Strength	Tab (400 mg, 800 mg)
Brands	Renagel, Renvela (Tab)
Mechanism of action	Nonabsorbable. It has multiple amines which bind with phosphate molecules through ionic and hydrogen bonding, and decrease phosphate absorption
Pharmacokinetics	No systemic absorption. Reduces absorption of fat soluble vitamins by binding to bile acids and thus hampering fat absorption
Indications	Chronic kidney disease; Tumor lysis syndrome
Dosage as per indications	Dosage in children is not established. 400 mg given orally every 8 hours in children >6 years
Maximum dosage	Not known
Dose adjustments	Not known
Adverse effects	Hypotension, hypertension, nausea, vomiting, constipation
Contraindications	Bowel obstruction
Drug interactions	Mycophenolate, ciprofloxacin, thyroxine
Remarks	When taken with meals, it binds to dietary phosphate and prevents its absorption

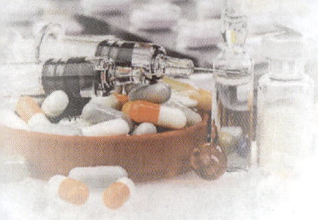

Sildenafil

Drug name	Sildenafil
Category	Phosphodiesterase inhibitor
Route	Oral, Intravenous
Strength	Tab (50 mg)
Brands	Viagra (Tab), Vigore (Tab), Manforce (Tab)
Mechanism of action	It enhances the effect of NO by inhibiting phosphodiesterase type 5 (PDE5), degradation of cGMP in the corpus cavernosum and causes vasodilation
Pharmacokinetics	Rapidly absorbed after oral administration, <50% bioavailability, metabolized and eliminated by CYP3A4 enzyme in liver, with terminal half-lives of 4 hours
Indications	Persistent Pulmonary Hypertension of Newborn (PPHN)

Dosage as per indications	• *Newborn:* Oral: 0.5–3 mg/kg/dose 6–12 hourly IV: loading: 0.4 mg/kg/dose IV over 3 hours followed by a continuous infusion of 1.6 mg/kg/24 h for up to 7 days
	• *Child:* Oral: 0.25–2 mg/kg/dose Q 6 h
	  – ≥8–20 kg: 10 mg TID
	  – >20–45 kg: 20 mg TID
	  – >45 kg: 40 mg TID

Maximum dosage	Not known
Dose adjustments	Hepatic derangement and severe renal impairment
Adverse effects	Headache, fever, vomiting, diarrhea, hypotension
Contraindications	Contraindicated with nitrates
Drug interactions	Ritonavir, CYP3A4 inhibitor, alpha blocker, antihypertensives

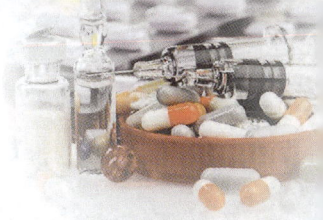

Simethicone

Drug name	Simethicone
Category	Miscellaneous
Route	Oral
Strength	Strip (62.5 mg); Cap (140 mg)
Brands	Gasofilm (Strip, Cap), Flatubust (Cap)
Mechanism of action	Forms a film on the surface of stomach due to its low surface tension property, forms gas bubbles which expels out
Pharmacokinetics	Not absorbed following oral administration, has no effect on gastric secretion, eliminated unchanged in feces
Indications	Gastritis
Dosage as per indications	• *<2 years:* 20 mg PO after meals QID/SOS • *2–12 years:* 40 mg PO QID/SOS • *>12 years; and adult:* 40–250 mg PO PRN
Maximum dosage	• <12 years: Max 240 mg/24 h • >12 years: 500 mg/24 h
Dose adjustments	Not known
Adverse effects	Not known
Contraindications	Hypersensitivity
Drug interactions	Not known
Remarks	Avoid carbonated beverages

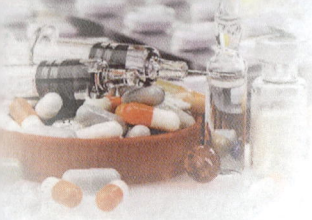

Sodium Benzoate/ Sodium Phenylacetate

Drug name	Sodium benzoate/sodium phenylacetate
Category	Miscellaneous
Route	Intravenous
Strength	Inj Sol 10–10%: 1 mL = 100 mg Sodium Benzoate and 100 mg Sodium Phenylacetate
Brands	Ammonul (Inj)
Mechanism of action	Removes glutamine and glycine thereby facilitating excretion of waste nitrogen
Pharmacokinetics	Benzoate forms hippurate whereas phenylacetate is converted to phenylacetylglutamine, the rate of formation and elimination of hippurate is more than phenylacetylglutamine
Indications	Hyperammonemia
Dosage as per indications	• *Loading dose:* Arginine hydrochloride 600 mg/kg in combination with sodium phenylacetate 250 mg/kg and sodium benzoate 250 mg/kg as an IV infusion over 90–120 minutes • *Maintenance dose:* Arginine hydrochloride 600 mg/kg in combination with sodium phenylacetate 250 mg/kg and sodium benzoate 250 mg/kg as an IV infusion over 24 hours
Maximum dosage	Not known
Dose adjustments	In hepatic and renal derangement
Adverse effects	Hypotension, hypokalemia, metabolic acidosis, cerebral edema, seizures, anemia, disseminated intravascular coagulation
Contraindications	Hypersensitivity
Drug interactions	Valproate, probenecid, penicillin
Remarks	Should be administered through a central line. To be diluted in 10% dextrose

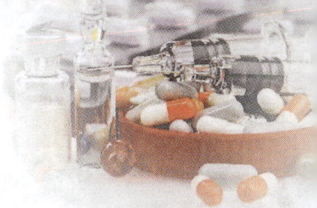

Sodium Bicarbonate

Drug name	Sodium bicarbonate
Category	Miscellaneous
Route	Intravenous
Strength	Amp (7.5%, 10 mL); Contains (0.9 mEq/mL)
Brands	Nodosis (Inj), Nabico (Inj), Sodanet (Inj)
Mechanism of action	Increases plasma bicarbonate, increases blood pH and reverses clinical manifestations of acidosis by buffering excess hydrogen ion concentration
Pharmacokinetics	Not known
Indications	Metabolic acidosis; Hyperkalemia
Dosage as per indications	1–2 mEq/kg/dose IV or calculate as base deficit × weight × 0.6 = mEq or mL of 7.5% solution of sodium bicarbonate (total correction)
Maximum dosage	Rate of administration should not be >8 mEq/kg/day
Dose adjustments	In renal derangement
Adverse effects	May cause hypernatremia, hypokalemia, hypomagnesemia, hypocalcemia, hyperreflexia, edema, and tissue necrosis (extravasation)
Contraindications	Loosing chloride by vomiting or from continuous gastrointestinal suction, and in patients receiving diuretics
Drug interactions	Do not mix with calcium, dobutamine, or norepinephrine
Remarks	To be diluted in distilled water only in a dilution of 1:6 (1 part sodium bicarbonate and 6 parts of distilled water) and given as IV infusion; Half the correction is given stat followed by the remaining in divided doses over the next 12–24 hours. Repeat blood gas as necessary. In neonates, it may be given as 1:3 dilution in emergent situations

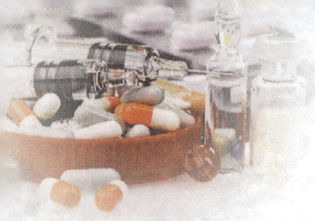

Sodium Nitroprusside

Drug name	Sodium nitroprusside
Category	Vasodilator
Route	Intravenous
Strength	Inj (25 mg/mL, 2 mL ampoule)
Brands	Niside (Inj), Nipride (Inj), Pruside (Inj), Sonide (Inj)
Mechanism of action	It combines with oxyhemoglobin to produce methemoglobin, cyanide, and nitric oxide (NO). NO with the help of guanylate cyclase produce cGMP that reduces intracellular calcium concentrations in vascular smooth muscles. This leads to relaxation of vascular smooth muscle and dilatation of peripheral vessels.
Pharmacokinetics	Rapidly distributed, half-life: 2 minutes. Onset of action is 2 min with a 1–10 min duration of effect
Indications	Hypertensive emergency
Dosage as per indications	50 mg is dissolved in 1 liter of 5% dextrose to provide a concentration of 50 µg/mL. Start at 0.5–3 µg/kg/min as continuous intravenous infusion. May increase up to 3–4 µg/kg/min
Maximum dosage	10 µg/kg/min
Dose adjustments	Dose adjustment needed in renal and hepatic derangement
Adverse effects	It gets converted to cyanide nonenzymatic mechanically and further to thiocyanate. Cyanide may result in methemoglobinemia and metabolic acidosis. Thiocyanate can cause seizures and psychosis
Contraindications	Do not use in coarctation of aorta, arteriovenous shunts, raised intracranial tension, liver failure, and congestive heart failure
Drug interactions	Not known
Remarks	It should not be used beyond 72 h.

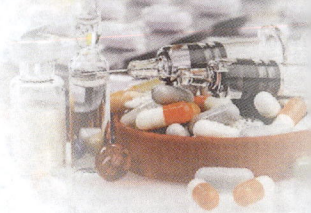

Sodium Picosulfate

Drug name	Sodium picosulfate
Category	Stimulant laxative
Route	Oral
Strength	5 mg/5 mL, 100 mL Sol bottles
Brands	Dulcolax, Pico, Picolax (Sol)
Mechanism of action	Converted to [bis-(p-hydroxy-phenyl)-pyridyl-2-methane] BHPM by colonic bacteria, the resultant metabolite stimulates peristalsis in colon
Pharmacokinetics	Peak levels attained in 7 hours, elimination half-life: 7 hours, converted in glucuronide form and eliminated via urine
Indications	Constipation
Dosage as per indications	• *1 month to <4 years:* 0.25 mg/kg • *4–10 years:* 2.5–5 mg • *>10 years:* 5–10 mg
Maximum dosage	<10 years: 5 mg; >10 years: 10 mg
Dose adjustments	In renal insufficiency
Adverse effects	Vomiting, nausea, headache
Contraindications	Hypersensitivity
Drug interactions	Tetracycline and fluoroquinolone antibiotics, iron, digoxin, chlorpromazine, penicillamine, drugs affecting fluid and electrolytes like diuretics
Remarks	Generally, taken as bedtime dose

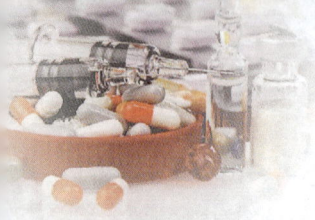

Somatropin

Drug name	Somatropin
Category	Growth hormone agonist
Route	Subcutaneous
Strength	Inj (5 mg, 10 mg, 15 mg)
Brands	Norditropin, Nordilet (Inj)
Mechanism of action	Binds to GH receptor located on the target cells. As there is intracellular signal transduction effects are mediated by IGF-1 and by local action
Pharmacokinetics	The drug stimulates linear growth, cell growth, skeletal growth, organ growth, protein synthesis, lipolysis and increased synthesis of collagen. *Half-life:* 7–10 hours
Indications	Growth failure due to growth hormone deficiency (GHD); Short stature in Noonan syndrome; Turner syndrome, small for gestational age (SGA) babies with failed catch-up growth by 4 years
Dosage as per indications	• Growth hormone deficiency, 0.18–0.3 mg/kg/week divided into 6–7 daily doses subcutaneous till accepted height or epiphyseal fusion • *Turner/Noonan syndrome/SGA:* 0.36 mg/kg/week divided into 6–7 daily doses subcutaneous
Maximum dosage	Not known
Dose adjustments	Not known
Adverse effects	Rash, lipoatrophy. headaches, hypothyroidism, hypoadrenalism, slipped capital femoral epiphysis
Contraindications	Acute illness, malignancy, Prader–Willi syndrome, diabetes, closed epiphysis, hypersensitivity
Drug interactions	Estrogen, insulin oral hypoglycemics, drugs affected by P450 enzyme system

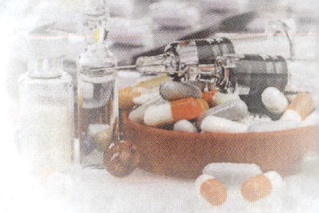

Spironolactone

Drug name	Spironolactone
Category	Potassium sparing diuretic
Route	Oral
Strength	Tab (25 mg, 100 mg)
Brands	Aldactone, Lactone (Tab)
Mechanism of action	Binds to receptors on aldosterone-dependent sodium-potassium exchange site in the distal convoluted renal tubule, leading to antialdosterone effect
Pharmacokinetics	*Half-life:* 1.4 hours. Highly protein bound, rapidly metabolized, eliminated mainly by kidneys followed by bile
Indications	Ascites; Heart failure
Dosage as per indications	2–3 mg/kg/day q 8–24 h, PO
Maximum dosage	Not known
Dose adjustments	Renal and hepatic insufficiency
Adverse effects	Hyperkalemia, GI disturbance, rash, lethargy, dizziness, gynecomastia
Contraindications	Addison disease, renal failure, hyperkalemia
Drug interactions	NSAIDs, lithium. Avoid concomitant use with ACE inhibitors, angiotensin II antagonists, aldosterone blockers and other potassium sparing diuretics as hyperkalemia may occur. May potentiate ganglionic blockers and other antihypertensives
Remarks	It is coadministered with thiazides

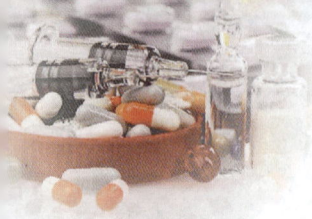

Stavudine (d4T)

Drug name	Stavudine (d4T)
Category	Antiretroviral, Nucleoside reverse transcriptase inhibitor (NRTI)
Route	Oral
Strength	Cap (15 mg, 20 mg, 30 mg, 40 mg); Oral sol (1 mg/mL)
Brands	Stavir, Virostav, Stadine (Cap)
Mechanism of action	Nucleoside reverse transcriptase inhibitor
Pharmacokinetics	Rapidly absorbed, peak levels in 1 hour, eliminated via kidneys and endogenous pathways
Indications	HIV infection/AIDS
Dosage as per indications	1 mg/kg/dose BID
Maximum dosage	Daily dose of 80 mg
Dose adjustments	In renal impairment
Adverse effects	Headache, gastrointestinal discomfort, and rash. Peripheral neuropathy, pancreatitis, lactic acidosis, and raised liver enzymes may occur
Contraindications	Hypersensitivity
Drug interactions	Zidovudine

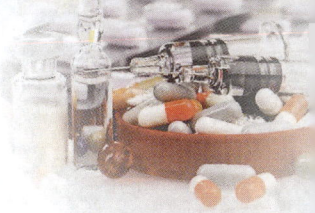

Streptomycin

Drug name	Streptomycin
Category	Aminoglycoside
Route	Intramuscular
Strength	Inj (500 mg, 750 mg, 1 g vials)
Brands	Ambistryn, Cipstryn, Streptomycin (Inj)
Mechanism of action	Bactericidal, acts by inhibiting normal protein synthesis
Pharmacokinetics	Not absorbed orally hence given only parenterally. Distributed in all tissues except brain. Rapidly eliminated via kidney through glomerular filtration
Indications	Antituberculous therapy. Also used for treating brucellosis; Tularemia; Plague; Rat bite fever
Dosage as per indications	20–40 mg/kg/day once daily IM
Maximum dosage	1 g/day
Dose adjustments	Renal insufficiency
Adverse effects	Myocarditis, ototoxicity, nephrotoxicity, serum sickness, CNS depression, neurological problems
Contraindications	Aminoglycoside and sulfite hypersensitivity
Drug interactions	Neuromuscular blocking agents
Remarks	It needs to be used with caution in patients receiving neuromuscular blocking agents, those with vertigo, tinnitus, and neuromuscular disorders. It is a painful injection and hence may be mixed with lignocaine injection. Given by deep IM injection

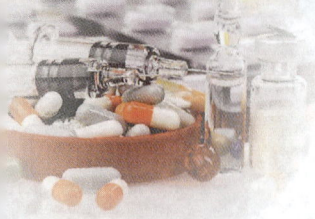

Sucralfate

Drug name	Sucralfate
Category	Antiulcer agent
Route	Oral
Strength	Susp (100 mg/mL); Tab (1 g)
Brands	Alfate (Syp), Sucral (Tab, Syp), Sucrafil (Tab, Syp)
Mechanism of action	Combines with the ulcer exudates to form a complex which binds to the ulcer site. It also inhibits pepsin activity in gastric juice
Pharmacokinetics	Only minimally absorbed from the gastrointestinal tract
Indications	Duodenal/gastric ulcer; Stomatitis
Dosage as per indications	• *Duodenal/gastric ulcer:* 40–80 mg/kg/day q 6 h • *Stomatitis:* Swish and swallow 5–10 mL
Maximum dosage	2,000 mg/day
Dose adjustments	Renal impairment
Adverse effects	Vertigo, dry mouth, constipation; Aluminum containing antacids when given alongside can potentiate aluminum toxicity especially in patients with renal failure
Contraindications	Hypersensitivity
Drug interactions	Digoxin, fluoroquinolone L-thyroxine, phenytoin, ranitidine, fat-soluble vitamins, omeprazole, and oral anticoagulants. Keep a gap of 2 hours between administrations
Remarks	Administer it empty stomach (1 hour before meals) or before bedtime. It needs an acidic medium to be effective by forming a protective polymer coating over the damaged GI mucosa

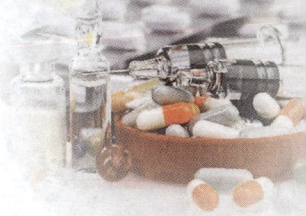

Sumatriptan

Drug name	Sumatriptan
Category	Selective serotonin agonist
Route	Oral
Strength	Tab (25 mg, 50 mg, 100 mg); Susp (5 mg/mL)
Brands	Headset (Comb tab), Migratan (Tab), Suminat (Tab), Sumitrex (Tab)
Mechanism of action	Binds to 5-HT1B/1D receptors to have agonistic effect leading to constriction of intracranial blood vessels and decreased activity of sensory branch of trigeminal nerve, and inhibition of proinflammatory neuropeptide release
Pharmacokinetics	Increased absorption with food, low protein binding, elimination half-life: 2.5 hours
Indications	Migraine
Dosage as per indications	Adolescents and adults: 25 mg, may repeat 2 hours if required
Maximum dosage	200 mg/day. Max single dose: 100 mg/dose
Dose adjustments	Hepatic impairment
Adverse effects	When given with SSRIs it may cause life-threatening serotonin syndrome, weakness, hyperreflexia, and incoordination. Use carefully in hepatic and renal disease
Contraindications	Contraindicated with concomitant administration of MAO inhibitors (or if used within the previous 2 weeks), vasoconstrictive agents and ergotamine derivatives
Drug interactions	MAO inhibitors (or if used within the previous 2 weeks), vasoconstrictive agents and ergotamine derivatives

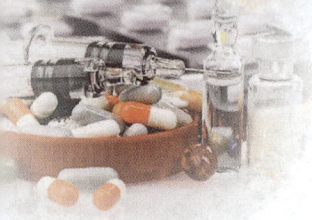

Surfactant

Drug name	Surfactant
Category	Miscellaneous/Pulmonary surfactant
Route	Intratracheal
Strength	Bovine extract (phospholipid: 100 mg/4 mL; 4 mL, 8 mL vials); calf extract (phospholipid: 35 mg/mL, 3 mL, 6 mL vials); poractant alpha (phospholipid: 120 mg/1.5 mL; 1.5 mL, 3 mL vials)
Brands	Survanta (bovine lung extract), Infasurf (calf lung extract), Curosurf (porcine lung extract)
Mechanism of action	It lowers the surface tension of the alveoli thus preventing alveoli to collapse at the end of expiration and also decreases the inspiratory pressure required to open the alveoli during inspiration
Pharmacokinetics	Not known
Indications	Hyaline membrane disease
Dosage as per indications	- *Survanta:* 4 mL/kg/dose; can be repeated after 6 hours - *Infasurf:* 3 mL/kg/dose, can be repeated in 12 hours - *Curosurf:* 2.5 mL/kg/dose. May administer 2 more doses 1.25 mL/kg/dose at 12 hourly intervals as needed.
Maximum dosage	Survanta: Max 4 doses, Infasurf: 3 doses, Curosurf: 3 doses (total of 5 mL/kg)
Dose adjustments	Not known
Adverse effects	Transient bradycardia, desaturation, hypotension, pallor CO_2 retention, tube block, apnea
Contraindications	Hypersensitivity
Drug interactions	Not known
Remarks	- Do not shake - All surfactants to be give within 48 hours of birth - Warm by standing at room temperature for 20 minutes

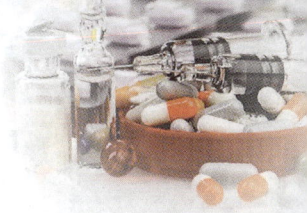

Tacrolimus

Drug name	Tacrolimus
Category	Antibiotic
Route	Oral, Intravenous
Strength	Inj (0.5 mg, 1, 5 mg); Cap (0.5 mg, 1, 5 mg); Oint (0.03%)
Brands	Biomus (Cap, Oint), Prograf (Cap, Oint), Pangraf (Cap, Oint)
Mechanism of action	Inhibits T-lymphocyte activation, acts via binding to intracellular protein FKB-12. The complex formation inhibits calcineurin activity and inhibition of T-lymphocyte activation
Pharmacokinetics	Poor absorption when taken orally. Highly protein bound. Extensively metabolized by P450 enzyme
Indications	As immunosuppresant in post-transplant patients; Steroid resistant nephrotic syndrome
Dosage as per indications	• *IV:* 0.05–0.15 mg/kg/day by continuous infusion • *PO:* 0.15–0.3 mg/kg/day q 12 h
Maximum dosage	Not known
Dose adjustments	Renal, hepatic insufficiency
Adverse effects	Tremor, headache, insomnia, diarrhea, nausea, hypertension, renal dysfunction, and bleeding
Contraindications	Hypersensitivity
Drug interactions	CYP3A4 inducers and inhibitors (Macrolide antibiotics and antifungals)
Remarks	Monitor trough levels. Steady state levels may take 2–5 days of continuous dosing. Therapy should be started 6 hours or more after transplantation

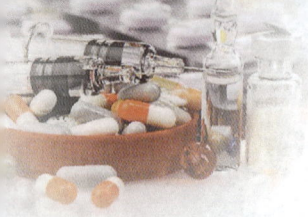

Teicoplanin

Drug name	Teicoplanin
Category	Antibiotic, Glycopeptide
Route	Intravenous
Strength	Inj (200 mg, 400 mg vials)
Brands	Platico, Targocid, Ticocin, T-Planin, Teicoplanin (Inj)
Mechanism of action	Bactericidal, inhibits cell wall synthesis at a site different from that affected by beta-lactams
Pharmacokinetics	Poor oral absorption hence administered parenterally. High bioavailability when given parenterally; 40% eliminated in active form
Indications	For treating infections caused by gram-positive bacteria; Including methicillin-resistant *Staphylococcus aureus*; *Enterococcus faecalis*
Dosage as per indications	10 mg/kg/dose q 12 h for three doses followed by 10 mg/kg/dose 24 h IV
Maximum dosage	400 mg/dose
Dose adjustments	In renal impairment
Adverse effects	Fever, chills, allergic reactions, GI disturbances, headache, dizziness, "red-man" syndrome, disturbances in liver enzymes, renal impairment, ototoxicity, blood dyscrasias. Rarely Stevens–Johnson syndrome and toxic epidermal necrolysis may occur
Contraindications	Hypersensitivity
Drug interactions	Other nephrotoxic drugs

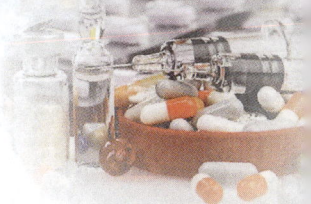

Terbinafine Hydrochloride

Drug name	Terbinafine hydrochloride
Category	Antifungal
Route	Oral
Strength	Tab (125 mg, 250 mg); Cream 1%
Brands	Derbina (Tab, Cream), Exifine (Tab, Cream), Fungotek (Tab, Cream)
Mechanism of action	Inhibits ergosterol biosynthesis required in formation of fungal cell membrane by inhibiting squalene epoxidase enzyme. This leads to increased membrane permeability causing cell death
Pharmacokinetics	Well absorbed, nearly 50% bioavailability, highly bound to plasma proteins, half-life: 36 hours, mostly eliminated in urine
Indications	Used for >4 years
Dosage as per indications	• *<25 kg:* 125 mg/day OD • *25–35 kg:* 187 mg/day OD • *>35 kg:* 250 mg/day OD
Maximum dosage	250 mg/day
Dose adjustments	In renal and hepatic dysfunction
Adverse effects	Rash, liver derangement, headache, taste disturbance, pain abdomen, diarrhea
Contraindications	Hypersensitivity
Drug interactions	Rifampicin, cimetidine, fluconazole, cyclosporine

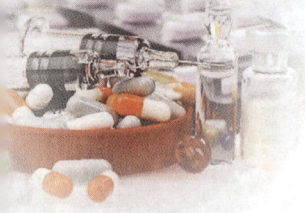

Terbutaline

Drug name	Terbutaline
Category	Inhaled bronchodilator, β2 agonist
Route	Oral, Intravenous, Subcutaneous
Strength	Syp (1.5 mg/mL); Inj (0.5 mg/mL ampoule); Tab (2.5 mg, 5 mg); MDI 250 (μg/puff); Nebulizing sol (10 mg/mL)
Brands	Bricanyl (Syp), Tetrasma (Tab, Syp)
Mechanism of action	Acts on beta 2 receptors and activates adenyl cyclase to increase cyclic AMP. Cyclic AMP inhibits myosin phosphorylation and decreases intracellular calcium by inhibiting protein kinase. All these lead to muscle relaxation
Pharmacokinetics	Effect noted within 5 minutes of subcutaneous Inj, peak within 30–60 minutes, elimination half-life around 4 hours, eliminated mainly via kidney
Indications	Asthma
Dosage as per indications	• *Oral:* 0.05 mg/kg/dose 3 times/day; SC: 0.005–0.01 mg/kg/dose, (0.01–0.02 mL/kg/dose) up to 4 times/day. Inhale 1–2 puffs of 250 μg q 6–8 h • *Nebulization:* 2.5 mg in children below 20 kg and 5 mg in children >20 kg
Maximum dosage	Oral: • 5 mg/day in children <12 years • 7.5 mg/day in children in 12–15 years • 15 mg/day in 15–18 years
Dose adjustments	Use cautiously in renal failure
Adverse effects	Tachycardia, arrhythmias, flushing, headache, tremors, hypokalemia
Contraindications	Hypersensitivity
Drug interactions	Arrhythmogenic drugs, drugs affecting potassium levels in body
Remarks	Excessive use can cause paradoxical bronchoconstriction; discontinue use, if seen

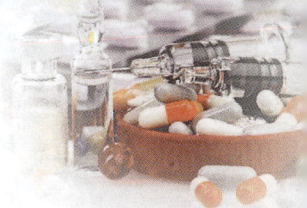

Tetanus Immunoglobulin (TIG)

Drug name	Tetanus immunoglobulin (TIG)
Category	Immunoglobulin (Human)
Route	Intramuscular, Local, Intrathecal
Strength	Inj (250 IU, 500 IU vials)
Brands	Igantet (Inj), Tetglob (Inj)
Mechanism of action	Provides passive immunity in form of antibodies against tetanus toxin
Pharmacokinetics	*Peak levels:* 2 days after administration, half-life (IgG): 23 days
Indications	Tetanus
Dosage as per indications	• *Prophylaxis:* 250 IU IM (500 IU if heavy contamination or >24 hours elapsed) • *Treatment:* 30–300 IU/kg IM; intrathecal 250–500 IU single dose
Maximum dosage	500 IU total dose
Dose adjustments	Not known
Adverse effects	Local site reactions (pain, redness), flu-like symptoms, hypersensitivity
Contraindications	Hypersensitivity
Drug interactions	Live vaccines
Remarks	Avoid in persons with selected IgA deficiency

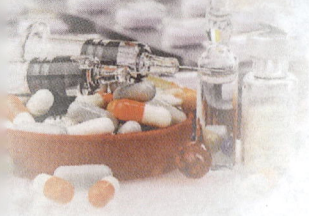

Tetracycline Hydrochloride

Drug name	Tetracycline hydrochloride
Category	Antibiotic
Route	Oral
Strength	Tab (250 mg)
Brands	Achromycin (Tab), Hostacycline (Tab)
Mechanism of action	Bacteriostatic, acts by inhibiting protein synthesis. Effective against both gram-negative and gram-positive organisms
Pharmacokinetics	Well absorbed, bound to plasma proteins in varying amount, concentrated in liver and bile, excreted in the urine and feces
Indications	Gram-positive; Gram-negative infections
Dosage as per indications	25–50 mg/kg/day divided 6-hourly PO
Maximum dosage	3 g/day
Dose adjustments	In renal derangement
Adverse effects	Tooth and enamel discoloration, increase BUN, fibula growth retardation in preterm, nausea, vomiting, diarrhea, glossitis, black hairy tongue, poor appetite
Contraindications	Hypersensitivity
Drug interactions	Anticoagulants, penicillin, antacids

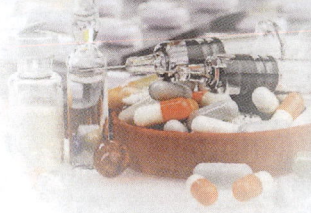

Theophylline

Drug name	Theophylline
Category	Bronchodilator, Methylxanthine
Route	Oral
Strength	Tab (100 mg, 150 mg, 200 mg, 250 mg, 400 mg, 600 mg); Syp (80 mg/15 mL, 50 mg/5 mL)
Brands	Deriphyllin (Comb Tab, Inj), Unicontin (Tab), TR Phyllin (Tab, Syp)
Mechanism of action	Acts to relax smooth muscle and suppress airway hyperresponsiveness by the inhibition of phosphodiesterase (PDE III/IV)
Pharmacokinetics	Rapid and complete absorption after oral administration, 40% bound to plasma protein, metabolized primarily in liver, mostly eliminated by kidneys, half-life: 8 hours
Indications	Acute asthma

Dosage as per indications	*Neonatal apnea:*
	• Loading: 5 mg/kg/dose PO
	• Maintenance: 3–6 mg/kg/day divided TID-QID
	
	Acute asthma:
	• Loading dose: A single 5 mg/kg/dose produces a serum concentration of 10 mcg/mL theophylline levels:
	• Maintenance:
	  – *Preterm:* 1–1.5 mg/kg/dose BD
	  – *Infant:* [(0.2 × age in weeks) + 5] × (kg body weight)/day in 3–4 divided doses
	    - *>1 year/<45 kg:* 12–14 mg/kg/day in 4 divided doses
	    - *>45 kg:* 300 mg/day in 4 divided doses

Maximum dosage	• *<45 kg but >1 year:* 300 mg/day • *>45 kg:* 600 mg/day
Dose adjustments	Hepatic insufficiency, not needed in renal insufficiency

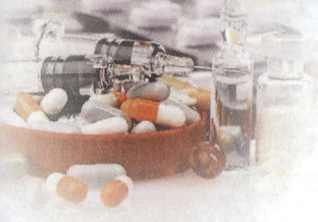

Theophylline

Adverse effects	Nausea, vomiting, abdominal pain, GERD, nervousness, arrhythmia, seizure, and anorexia
Contraindications	Hypersensitivity
Drug interactions	Its levels may be decreased by phenytoin, carbamazepine, phenobarbitone, and rifampicin
Remarks	Serum therapeutic levels to be maintained between 5 and 15 mcg/mL

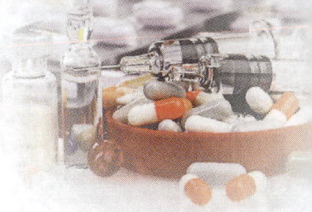

Thiabendazole

Drug name	Thiabendazole
Category	Antihelminthic
Route	Oral
Strength	Tab (500 mg); Susp (500 mg/5 mL)
Brands	Mintezol (not available in India)
Mechanism of action	Inhibit fumarate reductase in helminths
Pharmacokinetics	Rapidly absorbed after oral intake, peak levels: 1–2 hours after oral administration, metabolized as glucuronide and sulfate conjugate which are eliminated via kidney
Indications	Strongyloidiasis; Visceral/cutaneous larva migrans; Trichinosis; Fungicidal
Dosage as per indications	50 mg/kg/day q 12 h *Duration of therapy:* • *For strongyloides, intestinal nematodes:* 2 days • *Visceral larva migrans:* 5–7 days • *Trichinosis:* 2–4 days • *Cutaneous larva migrans:* 2–5 days
Maximum dosage	3 g/day
Dose adjustments	In renal and hepatic dysfunction, careful monitoring needed
Adverse effects	Drowsiness, dizziness, blurred vision, high blood sugar, decreased appetite, diarrhea
Contraindications	Hypersensitivity
Drug interactions	Theophylline
Remarks	Take thiabendazole after meals. Chew thoroughly before swallowing.

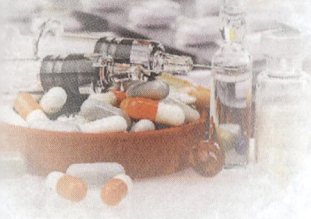

Thiamine

Drug name	Thiamine
Category	Vitamin B$_1$
Route	Oral, Intravenous
Strength	Inj (200 mg); Tab (100 mg)
Brands	Berin (Tab), Thiamin (Inj), Thymine (Tab)
Mechanism of action	Acts as coenzyme, after combining with ATP, in decarboxylation of pyruvic acid and alpha-keto acids during carbohydrate metabolism
Pharmacokinetics	Highly protein bound, metabolized in liver
Indications	Beriberi; Maple syrup urine disease; Respiratory chain defects
Dosage as per indications	• *Children up to 18 years:* 0.1–1 mg/day PO • *MSUD:* 100 mg/day PO • *Beriberi:* (IV/IM)—10–25 mg/day; oral—10–50 mg/day for 2 weeks, followed by 5–10 mg/day for 1 month oral
Maximum dosage	Not known
Dose adjustments	Not known
Adverse effects	Urticaria, pruritus, restlessness, pulmonary edema, GI hemorrhage
Contraindications	Hypersensitivity
Drug interactions	Neuromuscular drugs

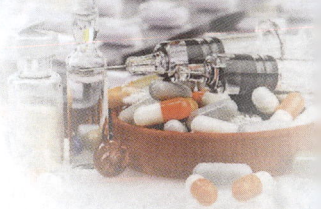

Thiopental

Drug name	Thiopental
Category	Thiobarbiturate, Anesthetic
Route	Intravenous
Strength	Inj (250 mg, 500 mg, 1 g)
Brands	Thiosol (Inj), Pentone (Inj), Pentothal (Inj), Thipen (Inj)
Mechanism of action	Ultrashort acting, depresses central nervous system to produce hypnosis and anesthesia, but not analgesia
Pharmacokinetics	Highly protein bound, elimination half-life: 3–8 hours. Metabolized in liver, degraded in the liver, and eliminated in urine
Indications	Uncontrolled status epilepticus
Dosage as per indications	Loading dose 5–10 mg/kg IV over 2–5 min followed by 2–10 mg/kg/h continuous drip for uncontrolled status epilepticus
Maximum dosage	Not known
Dose adjustments	Renal and hepatic insufficiency
Adverse effects	Patient to be mechanically ventilated. Cough, sneezing, hiccups, drowsiness. Thiopental can cause severe drowsiness or dizziness, which may last for several hours
Contraindications	Hypersensitivity
Drug interactions	CNS depressants, MAO inhibitors

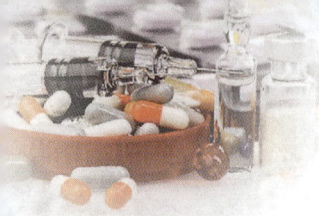

Ticarcillin Disodium/Clavulanate

Drug name	Ticarcillin disodium/Clavulanate
Category	Antibiotic, Extended spectrum penicillin
Route	Intravenous, Intramuscular
Strength	Inj (1 g, 3 g, 5 g vials)
Brands	Timentin (Inj)
Mechanism of action	• Ticarcillin is bactericidal, susceptible to β-lactamases. It acts by inhibiting bacterial cell wall synthesis • *Clavulanic acid:* It is a β-lactamase inhibitor, which inactivates β-lactamase enzymes
Pharmacokinetics	The mean serum half-life is 4 hours in neonates and 1 hour in infant and children. Around two-thirds of ticarcillin and 40% of clavulanic acid are eliminated unchanged in urine during the first 6 hours
Indications	Beta-lactamase producing gram-positive, anaerobic and gram-negative bacteria including *Pseudomonas*
Dosage as per indications	200–300 mg/kg/day q 4–6 h
Maximum dosage	>60 kg: 3 g/dose
Dose adjustments	Renal insufficiency
Adverse effects	Bleeding, hypernatremia, hypokalemia, allergy, deranged hepatic transaminases
Contraindications	Avoid, if hypersensitivity to penicillin
Drug interactions	Aminoglycosides, probenecid, oral contraceptives
Remarks	Avoid use in children

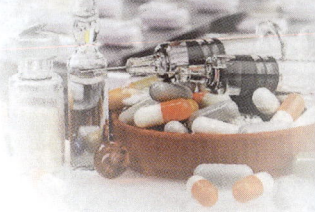

Tigecycline

Drug name	Tigecycline (not yet approved in <18 years)
Category	Antibiotic
Route	Intravenous
Strength	Inj (50 mg)
Brands	Tigez, Tygacil (Inj)
Mechanism of action	Binds to the 30S ribosomal subunit to inhibit protein translation in bacteria by blocking entry of aminoacyl-tRNA molecules into the A site of the ribosome
Pharmacokinetics	High protein binding, poorly metabolized, excreted in 2:1 ratio in feces/bile versus urine
Indications	Severe resistant infections: by gram-positive, gram-negative and anaerobic bacteria
Dosage as per indications	In children >8 years: 1.2 mg/kg/dose 12 hourly IV
Maximum dosage	50 mg/dose
Dose adjustments	Severe hepatic impairment
Adverse effects	Nausea, vomiting, diarrhea, abdominal pain, pancreatitis, headache, and increased SGPT
Contraindications	Hypersensitivity
Drug interactions	Warfarin, oral contraceptives

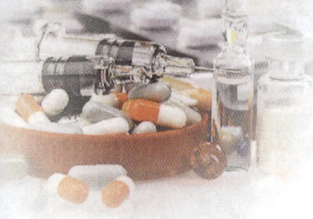

Tinidazole

Drug name	Tinidazole
Category	Antiprotozoal, Antibacterial
Route	Oral
Strength	Tab (300 mg, 500 mg, 1 g)
Brands	Enidazol (Tab), Fasigyn (Tab), Tiniba (Tab)
Mechanism of action	Mechanism of action against *Giardia* and *Entamoeba* species not known, the activity against *Trichomonas* is due to free nitro radicals generated after reduction by cell extracts of *Trichomonas*
Pharmacokinetics	Rapidly and completely absorbed after oral administration. Half-life: 12–14 hours. Metabolized in liver, biotransformed mainly by CYP3A4, excreted by liver and kidneys, poorly protein bound
Indications	Giardiasis; Amebiasis
Dosage as per indications	• *Giardiasis:* 50 mg/kg (up to 2 g) single dose • *Intestinal amebiasis:* 50 mg/kg/day for 3 days • *Amebic liver abscess:* 50/mg/kg/day for 3–5 days
Maximum dosage	2 g/day
Dose adjustments	Cautious use in liver derangement, not needed in renal dysfunction
Adverse effects	Seizures and neuropathy, transient neutropenia, nausea, weakness, malaise, vomiting, anorexia, headache
Contraindications	Hypersensitivity
Drug interactions	Warfarin, phenytoin, cyclosporine, tacrolimus, drugs affecting CYP3A4
Remarks	For children 3 years and above

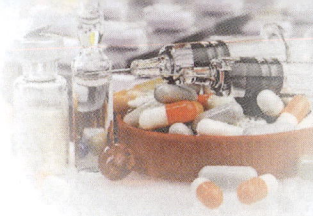

Tiotropium

Drug name	Tiotropium
Category	Long-acting antimuscarinic agent
Route	Inhalational
Strength	Rotacap (9 µg, 18 µg)
Brands	Tiate, Tiova (Rotacap)
Mechanism of action	Acts on M3 muscarinic receptors located in smooth muscles of airways
Pharmacokinetics	Not much known. Terminal half-life on inhalation around 2 days. As it is inhalational not much is absorbed in systemic circulation
Indications	Asthma
Dosage as per indications	2.5 µg once a day
Maximum dosage	Not known
Dose adjustments	Use with caution in moderate to severe renal dysfunction
Adverse effects	Dry mouth, sinusitis, pharyngitis, chest pain, rhinitis
Contraindications	Hypersensitivity
Drug interactions	Potassium chloride, anticholinergic drugs
Remarks	Used for children >6 years of age; not used as rescue medicine

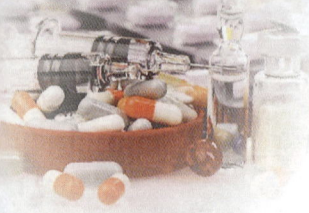

Tobramycin

Drug name	Tobramycin
Category	Antibiotic (Aminoglycoside)
Route	Intravenous, Intramuscular, Eye drops
Strength	Inj (20 mg, 40 mg, 80 mg in 2 mL vial)
Brands	Tobacin, TMC, Tobex, Tobracin (Inj)
Mechanism of action	Bactericidal, acts by inhibiting bacterial protein synthesis
Pharmacokinetics	Poor oral absorption whereas rapid absorption after IM dose. Peak levels: 30–90 minutes. Eliminated by kidneys via glomerular filtration. Serum half-life: 2 hours
Indications	Gram-negative; Some gram-positive infections
Dosage as per indications	6–7.5 mg/kg/day q 8–12 h IV, IM
Maximum dosage	Not known
Dose adjustments	Renal insufficiency
Adverse effects	Nephrotoxicity, hearing loss, diarrhea, headache, allergy, myelotoxicity
Contraindications	Avoid in patients with myasthenia gravis or Parkinson disease
Drug interactions	Furosemide
Remarks	Ototoxicity potentiated on concomitant use with furosemide

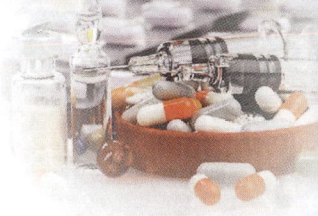

Tocopherol

Drug name	Tocopherol
Category	Vitamin E
Route	Oral
Strength	Cap (200 mg, 400 mg); Drops (50 mg/mL)
Brands	BioE (Cap), Evion (Cap, Drops), Vit-E (Cap)
Mechanism of action	It is a radical scavenge, acting as an antioxidant for lipid bilayers
Pharmacokinetics	Presence of fat is essential for absorption, bioavailability 35%, highly bound to lipoprotein, metabolized in liver, undergoes hydroxylation followed by beta oxidation, eliminated in feces, half-life 2.5–3 hours
Indications	Premature babies with very low birth weight; Fat malabsorption; Abetalipoproteinemia

Dosage as per indications	1 unit Vit E = 1 mg alpha tocopherol
	• *Recommended daily allowance:*
	  – <6 months: 4 mg/day
	  – 6–12 months: 5 mg/day
	  – 1–3 years: 65 mg/day
	  – 4–8 years: 75 mg/day
	  – 9–13 years: 11 mg/day
	  – >13 years: 15 mg/day
	• *Cholestasis:*
	  – Preterm: 25–50 mg/day
	  – Infant: 50 mg/day
	  – 1–8 years: 50–200 mg/day
	  – >8 years: 200–400 mg/day

Maximum dosage	• 1–3 years: 200 mg/day • 4–8 years: 300 mg/day • 8–13 years: 600 mg/day • >14 years: 800 mg/day
Dose adjustments	Not needed in hepatic dysfunction
Adverse effects	Bleeding/hemorrhage, contact dermatitis, dizziness, headache, fatigue
Contraindications	Hypersensitivity
Drug interactions	Warfarin, niacin, cyclosporine

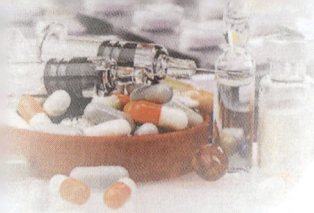

Tolazoline Hydrochloride

Drug name	Tolazoline hydrochloride
Category	Alpha-adrenergic blocking drug
Route	Intravenous
Strength	Inj (100 mg, 200 mg)
Brands	Not readily available in India
Mechanism of action	Acts as vasodilator, increases cardiac output, decreases total peripheral resistance, relaxes vascular smooth muscle
Pharmacokinetics	Not much known, excreted in urine, half-life 3–10 hours
Indications	Hypertension
Dosage as per indications	• *Loading:* 1–2 mg/kg over 10 min IV • *Maintenance:* 1–2 mg/kg/hour as continuous infusion
Maximum dosage	>5 mg/kg/h not effective
Dose adjustments	In renal derangement, not needed in liver derangement
Adverse effects	Transient tachycardia, sweating, fasciculation
Contraindications	Cardiotoxic accumulation in renal failure
Drug interactions	Adrenergic drugs like epinephrine and norepinephrine

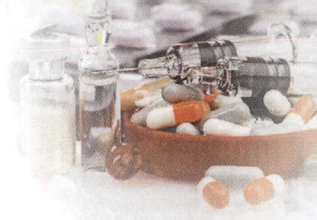

Topiramate

Drug name	Topiramate
Category	Anticonvulsant
Route	Oral
Strength	Tab (25 mg, 50 mg, 100 mg)
Brands	Epitop, Nuramate, Topamed, Topival (Tab)
Mechanism of action	Blocks voltage-dependent sodium channels, increases GABA activity, antagonize glutamate receptor, and inhibits the carbonic anhydrase enzyme
Pharmacokinetics	Rapid absorption after oral intake, high bioavailability, peak levels: 2 hours after intake, moderately metabolized and eliminated in urine
Indications	• Seizures (partial onset seizures; primary generalized tonic-clonic; Lennox–Gastaut syndrome) • May be used as monotherapy or add-on therapy
Dosage as per indications	*Children >2 years:* 1–3 mg/kg/24 h oral HS; increase by 1–3 mg/kg/day q 12 h in next 1–2 weeks till 5–10 mg/kg/day
Maximum dosage	• <11 kg: 250 mg/day • 12–22 kg: 300 mg/day • >23 kg: 350 mg/day
Dose adjustments	Renal and hepatic insufficiency
Adverse effects	Ocular side effects, oligohidrosis, hyperthermia, metabolic acidosis, suicidal tendency, neuropsychiatric disturbances
Contraindications	Glaucoma
Drug interactions	Sodium valproate
Remarks	Concomitant administration of topiramate and valproic acid has been associated with hyperammonemia

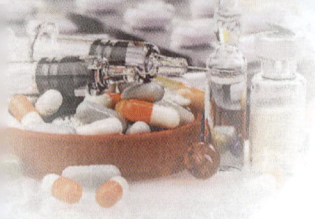

Tramadol

Drug name	Tramadol
Category	Narcotic analgesic
Route	Oral, Inj
Strength	Inj (50 mg, 100 mg vials)
Brands	Tramazac (Inj, Tab), Contramal (Inj, Tab), Supridol, (Inj, Tab)
Mechanism of action	Binds to µ-opioid receptors, inhibits norepinephrine and serotonin re-uptake
Pharmacokinetics	Well absorbed when taken orally (75% after 1 hour), extensively metabolized by CYP2D6 and CYP3A4. Eliminated via kidney and liver
Indications	Analgesia
Dosage as per indications	• *Initial dose:* 25 mg orally once daily, may titrate in 25 mg increments every 3 days to reach a dose of 25 mg four times a day; thereafter increase by 50 mg as tolerated every 3 days to reach a dose of 50 mg four times a day • *Maintenance dose:* After titration, 50–100 mg orally as needed for pain every 4–6 hours
Maximum dosage	400 mg per day
Dose adjustments	In hepatic and renal derangement
Adverse effects	Pruritus, agitation, anxiety, constipation, diarrhea, dry mouth, hallucination, nausea, tremor, vomiting, and diaphoresis
Contraindications	Hypersensitivity
Drug interactions	CNS depressant
Remarks	Avoid in children

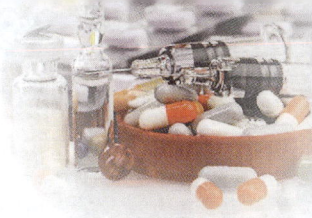

Triamcinolone

Drug name	Triamcinolone
Category	Steroid
Route	Intramuscular, Oral, Inhalational, Intra-articular
Strength	Tab (4 mg); Inj (10 mg, 40 mg); Cream (0.1%)
Brands	Kenacort (Tab, Inj), Tricort (Tab, Inj), Ledercort (cream)
Mechanism of action	Decreases prostaglandin and leukotriene synthesis by inhibiting phospholipase A2 on cell membranes. It also reverses vascular dilation and decreases permeability, preventing macrophage and leukocyte migration thereby providing an anti-inflammatory response
Pharmacokinetics	Not much known. Around 70% protein bound, half-life around 2.5–3 hours, mostly eliminated through renal route
Indications	Inflammatory dermatosis; Severe allergic conditions; Inflammatory joint disease
Dosage as per indications	• *Anti-inflammatory/antiallergic:* Child and adolescent (IM): 0.11–1.6 mg/kg/day divided in 3–4 doses • *Dermatosis:* – *Intralesional:* (≥12 years) up to 1 mg/site at intervals of 7 or more days. – *Topical:* 0.025–0.5% BID-TID thin layer application
Maximum dosage	Not known
Dose adjustments	Use cautiously in liver defragment
Adverse effects	As other steroids
Contraindications	Hypersensitivity, infections
Drug interactions	Amphotericin, aspirin, barbiturates, phenytoin

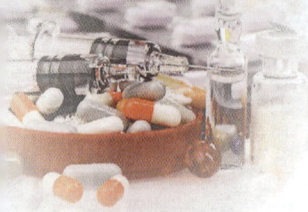

Triamterene

Drug name	Triamterene
Category	Potassium-sparing diuretic, Antihypertensive
Route	Oral
Strength	Tab (50 mg Triamterene + 25 mg Benzthiazide)
Brands	Ditide (Tab)
Mechanism of action	Acts on the distal renal tubule; to inhibit the reabsorption of sodium in exchange for potassium and hydrogen ions
Pharmacokinetics	*Well absorbed, onset of diuresis:* 1 hour, peaks at 2–3 hours and tapers off during the subsequent 7–9 hours
Indications	Diuresis; Hypertension; Ascites
Dosage as per indications	1–4 mg/kg/day q 12 h, PO
Maximum dosage	300 mg/day
Dose adjustments	In hepatic and renal insufficiency
Adverse effects	Depletion of sodium, folic acid and calcium, nausea, vomiting, diarrhea, headache, dizziness, fatigue, dry mouth, palpitations
Contraindications	Renal failure, hyperkalemia
Drug interactions	ACE inhibitors, NSAIDs, lithium

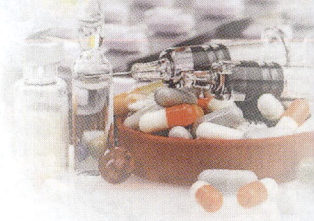

Triclofos Sodium

Drug name	Triclofos sodium
Category	Sedative
Route	Oral
Strength	Syp (500 mg/5 mL)
Brands	Tricloryl, Pedichloryl (Syp)
Mechanism of action	Limited data available; melatonin agonist, has sleep inducing and anxiolytic action
Pharmacokinetics	Not known
Indications	Sedation
Dosage as per indications	25–50 mg/kg/dose
Maximum dosage	Not known; up to 100 mg/kg tried
Dose adjustments	Avoid in renal and hepatic derangement
Adverse effects	Disorientation, dizziness, vertigo, headache, gastritis
Contraindications	Hypersensitivity
Drug interactions	Anticoagulants, furosemide, CNS depressants
Remarks	Not used in renal and hepatic derangement, cardiac disease and severe gastritis

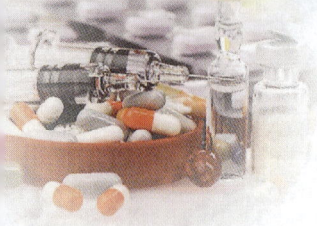

Trifluoperazine Hydrochloride

Drug name	Trifluoperazine hydrochloride
Category	Phenothiazine
Route	Oral
Strength	Tab (10 mg)
Brands	Neocalm, Trazine (Tab)
Mechanism of action	• Blocks postsynaptic mesolimbic dopaminergic D1 and D2 receptors in the brain • Depress hypothalamic and hypophyseal hormones release • Depress the reticular activating system
Pharmacokinetics	Not much known. Half-life: 10–20 hours, metabolized in liver
Indications	Anxiety; Schizophrenia
Dosage as per indications	6–12 years: 1 mg once or twice a day, >12 years: 2–5 mg 12 hourly PO
Maximum dosage	6–12 years: 15 mg/day; >12 years: 40 mg/day
Dose adjustments	Not used in hepatic damage
Adverse effects	Dry mouth, extrapyramidal symptoms, convulsions, constipation
Contraindications	Hypersensitivity
Drug interactions	Citalopram, metoprolol
Remarks	Not used in <6 years old, depressed bone marrow function, liver damage

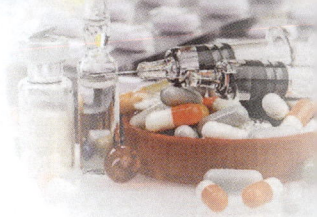

Trimethoprim Sulfamethoxazole

Drug name	Trimethoprim sulfamethoxazole
Category	Antibiotic, Sulfonamide
Route	Oral
Strength	Syp (Trimethoprim 40 mg and Sulfamethoxazole 200 mg/5 mL); Tab (Trimethoprim 20 mg/80 mg Sulfamethoxazole 100 mg/400 mg)
Brands	Septran (Syp, Tab), Bactrim (Syp, Tab)
Mechanism of action	Sulfamethoxazole inhibits formation of dihydrofolic acid in bacteria by competing with para-aminobenzoic acid (PABA). Trimethoprim binds to dihydrofolate reductase to inhibit conversion of dihydrofolic acid to tetrahydrofolic acid
Pharmacokinetics	Rapidly absorbed on oral intake. Peak concentration: 1–4 hours after oral administration. The mean serum half-lives of sulfamethoxazole and trimethoprim are 10 and 8 hours respectively
Indications	UTI; Typhoid fever; Respiratory tract infection
Dosage as per indications	• 5–8 mg/kg/day of trimethoprim q 12 h • 20–50 mg/kg/d of sulfamethoxazole q 12 h • *For typhoid fever:* 10 mg/kg/d q 12 h of trimethoprim • *For Pneumocystis carinii pneumonia:* 20 mg/kg/d q 6–8 h of trimethoprim
Maximum dosage	960 mg/day (trimethoprim component)
Dose adjustments	Renal insufficiency
Adverse effects	Bleeding, rash, abdominal pain, fever, sore throat, cough, diarrhea
Contraindications	Contraindicated, if allergic to any ingredient in sulfamethoxazole/trimethoprim or to any other sulfonamide. Avoid in G6PD deficiency
Drug interactions	Warfarin, phenytoin, digoxin, NSAIDs

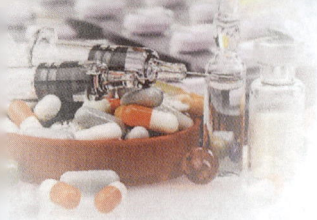

Triprolidine Hydrochloride

Drug name	Triprolidine hydrochloride
Category	Antihistaminic
Route	Oral
Strength	Tab (25 mg)
Brands	Triprolidine Hcl (Tab)
Mechanism of action	First-generation histamine H1 antagonist
Pharmacokinetics	Rapid absorption, 4–6 hours half-life, metabolized in liver
Indications	Allergic rhinitis
Dosage as per indications	• 6–12 years: 1.25 mg PO • >12 years: 2.5 mg PO every 4–6 hourly
Maximum dosage	• 6-12 years: 5 mg/day • >12 years: 10 mg/dose
Dose adjustments	Not known
Adverse effects	Drowsiness, headache, nausea, vomiting, decreased coordination
Contraindications	Hypersensitivity
Drug interactions	Triprolidine, cyclopentolate, CNS depressants

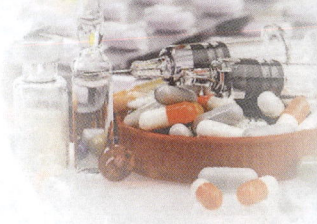

Triptorelin

Drug name	Triptorelin
Category	GnRH agonist
Route	Intramuscular
Strength	Inj (0.5 mg)
Brands	Decapeptyl, Tryplog
Mechanism of action	Leads to transient rise of follicle-stimulating hormone (FSH), luteinizing hormone (LH), estradiol, and testosterone followed by consistent decrease in FSH and LH, and significant reduction of testicular steroidogenesis, the suppressive effect generally takes 2–4 weeks of therapy
Pharmacokinetics	Well absorbed, poorly bound to plasma protein, eliminated by kidneys and liver
Indications	Precocious puberty
Dosage as per indications	22.5 mg IM once every 24 weeks
Maximum dosage	Not known
Dose adjustments	In hepatic derangement
Adverse effects	Hot flushes, pain redness at injection site, nasopharyngitis, torsades de pointes
Contraindications	Hypersensitivity
Drug interactions	Amiodarone, anagrelide, antidiabetic
Remarks	Used in children >2 years

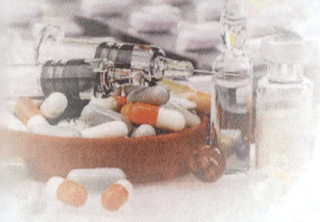

Ursodeoxycholic Acid (Ursodiol)

Drug name	Ursodeoxycholic acid (Ursodiol)
Category	Cholelitholytic drug
Route	Oral
Strength	Tab (150 mg, 250 mg, 300 mg)
Brands	Udiliv, Ursodil, Ursocol, Urso, Udihep (Tab)
Mechanism of action	It acts by increasing the hydrophilic component of bile acid, inhibits liver cell apoptosis, protects bile duct epithelial cells and stimulates bile secretion
Pharmacokinetics	Following oral administration, most of the drug is absorbed by passive diffusion, almost 2/3rd bound to plasma proteins, conjugated in liver, eliminated in feces. Half-life 3–6 days
Indications	Cholestasis
Dosage as per indications	10–15 mg/kg/day q 8 h
Maximum dosage	Not known
Dose adjustments	Not known
Adverse effects	Deranged liver enzymes, arthralgia, GI upset
Contraindications	Contraindicated in bile stones, calcified cholesterol stones
Drug interactions	Cholestyramine, colestipol, estrogen, oral contraceptives, clofibrate

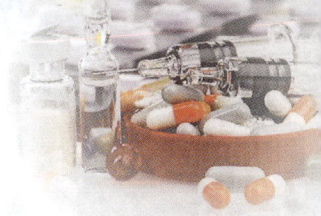

Valganciclovir

Drug name	Valganciclovir
Category	Antiviral
Route	Oral
Strength	Tablet (450 mg)
Brands	Valgan (Tab), Valcip (Tab)
Mechanism of action	It attaches to DNA by acting as guanosine analogue. As a result DNA reading gets disturbed resulting termination of CMV replication
Pharmacokinetics	It is a prodrug of ganciclovir. It is converted to ganciclovir by hepatic and intestinal esterases. Well absorbed orally, poorly bound to plasma proteins, metabolized in liver and intestine. Mainly eliminated by renal route
Indications	Cytomegalovirus (CMV) infection treatment; Prophylaxis
Dosage as per indications	*Neonate:* • *CMV infection:* 16 mg/kg per dose orally every 12 hours for at least 6 weeks Child: CMV prophylaxis in transplant: 7 × BSA × CrCl once PO *Adolescents:* • *CMV prophylaxis:* 900 mg PO once daily CMV retinitis: Induction therapy—900 mg PO BID × 21 days with food; Maintenance therapy—900 mg PO once daily with food
Maximum dosage	900 mg/dose
Dose adjustments	In renal derangement, not studied in hepatic derangement
Adverse effects	Headache, insomnia, peripheral neuropathy, neutropenia, anemia, thrombocytopenia
Contraindications	Contraindicated with hypersensitivity to valganciclovir/ganciclovir ANC <500 mm^3; platelets <25,000 mm^3; hemoglobin <8 g/dL; hemodialysis
Drug interactions	Zidovudine, didanosine, mycophenolate

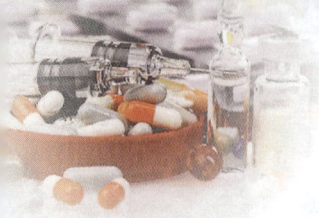

Valproate

Drug name	Valproate
Category	Broad-spectrum anticonvulsant
Route	Oral, Intravenous
Strength	Syp (200 mg/5 mL); Tab (200 mg, 300 mg, 500 mg); Inj (100 mg/mL)
Brands	Sodium Encorate (Inj, Syp, Tab), Epilex (Syp, Tab), Valprin (Inj, Syp, Tab), Torvate (Inj, Syp, Tab)
Mechanism of action	Increased brain concentrations of gamma-aminobutyric acid (GABA) by reducing GABA metabolism
Pharmacokinetics	Has high bioavailability when taken orally. Metabolized via liver conjugation and mitochondrial beta oxidation. Mean terminal half-life around 16 hours. The plasma protein binding of valproate is concentration dependent
Indications	Seizures
Dosage as per indications	*Initial dose:* 10–15 mg/kg/day q 8–12 h; increase by 5–10 mg/kg every week
Maximum dosage	60 mg/kg/day
Dose adjustments	In hepatic derangement
Adverse effects	Hepatotoxicity, abdominal pain, alopecia, nausea, Reye's like syndrome, thrombocytopenia, teratogenic
Contraindications	Hypersensitivity, IEM (MELAS), hepatic failure
Drug interactions	Hepatic enzyme inducing drugs
Remarks	Therapeutic levels 50–100 µg/mL

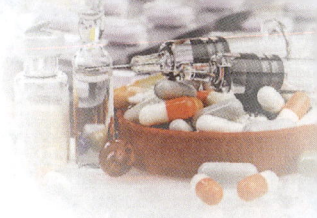

Vancomycin Hydrochloride

Drug name	Vancomycin hydrochloride
Category	Antibiotic
Route	Intravenous, Oral
Strength	Inj (500 mg, 1 g vials); Cap (125 mg)
Brands	Cytovan, Celovan, Vancorin, Vancomate (Inj)
Mechanism of action	Acts by inhibiting cell-wall biosynthesis, altering bacterial-cell-membrane permeability and RNA synthesis
Pharmacokinetics	Mean elimination half-life is 4–6 hours. Nearly half is protein bound. Almost three-fourths is excreted in urine by glomerular filtration
Indications	Penicillin-resistant staphylococcal infections; MRSA
Dosage as per indications	• *Staphylococcal sepsis:* 10 mg/kg/dose q 6 h IV infusion • *Meningitis:* 15 mg/kg/dose q 6 h IV infusion • *Antibiotic-associated pseudomembranous enterocolitis:* 40–50 mg/kg/day q 6–8 h PO
Maximum dosage	3 g/day or 750 mg/dose
Dose adjustments	Renal insufficiency
Adverse effects	Nephrotoxicity, ototoxicity, red-man syndrome (flushing, hypotension, erythema), urticaria, thrombophlebitis, blood dyscrasia (neutropenia and thrombocytopenia), eosinophilia
Contraindications	Hypersensitivity
Drug interactions	Nephrotoxic drugs like loop diuretics, aminoglycosides, amphotericin B, colistin and polymyxin B
Remarks	Monitor renal functions, blood counts, and auditory functions

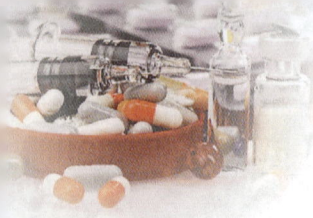

Varicella-Zoster Immunoglobulin (VZIG)

Drug name	Varicella-zoster immunoglobulin (VZIG)
Category	IVIG
Route	Intramuscular
Strength	Inj (125 U per vial)
Brands	Vartiect-CP, Varilix, Okavax (Inj)
Mechanism of action	Used in nonimmune individuals exposed to varicella zoster, acts by providing passive immunity
Pharmacokinetics	Not much known. The mean peak concentration noted around fifth day of administration
Indications	Prophylaxis for varicella
Dosage as per indications	Prophylaxis of neonates of mother developing varicella 5 days before to 2 days after pregnancy, postnatally exposed preterm infants (≥28 weeks) of susceptible mothers, and exposed immunocompromised children. 125 U for each 10 kg body weight IM, max 625 U, min 125 U
Maximum dosage	625 U total single dose
Dose adjustments	Not known
Adverse effects	Local erythema and pain, gastrointestinal symptoms, malaise, headache, rash, chest pain, dyspnea, tremor, dizziness, glossitis, buccal ulceration, facial edema, arthralgia
Contraindications	Hypersensitivity
Drug interactions	Live vaccines
Remarks	Give IM within 48 hours or at least 96 hours of exposure

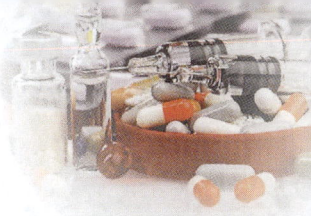

Vasopressin

Drug name	Vasopressin
Category	Antidiuretic hormone
Route	Intravenous, Subcutaneous
Strength	Inj (20 U/mL)
Brands	Cpressin, Vascel, Pitressin (Inj)
Mechanism of action	Acts on vascular smooth muscles by binding to V1 receptors. This causes release of calcium leading to vasoconstriction. The antidiuretic action occurs through adenyl cyclase on V2 receptors
Pharmacokinetics	Poorly bound to plasma proteins. Mostly metabolized and excreted via urine. Half-life: 10 minutes
Indications	Diabetes insipidus; Bleeding esophageal varices; Catecholamine refractory shock
Dosage as per indications	• *Diabetes insipidus:* 2.5–10 U/dose q 6–12 h SC or IV • *Bleeding esophageal varices:* 0.33 U/kg IV infusion followed by 0.2 U/1.73 m^2/min • *Catecholamine refractory shock:* 0.3–2 U/kg/min
Maximum dosage	Not known
Dose adjustments	Not known
Adverse effects	Water intoxication and hyponatremia, abdominal cramps, feeling of constant movement of self or surroundings, pale skin, throbbing headache, dizziness, sweating, trembling, or shaking of the hands or feet, bronchospasm
Contraindications	Contraindicated in heart failure, asthma, epilepsy
Drug interactions	Catecholamine, Indomethacin

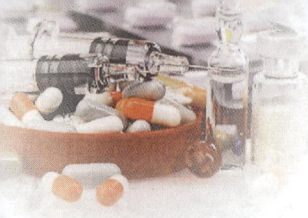

Vecuronium

Drug name	Vecuronium
Category	Neuromuscular blocking agent
Route	Intravenous
Strength	Inj (4 mg, 10 mg, 20 mg)
Brands	Vecuron, Norcuron (Inj)
Mechanism of action	It is a nondepolarizing neuromuscular blocking agent and acts by competing for cholinergic receptors at the motor endplate
Pharmacokinetics	Onset of action: 1–3 minutes. Duration: 30–40 minutes. Higher dose and frequency needed in children. Time to onset is inversely proportional to the dose whereas duration of maximum effect is directly proportional. More than 50% is bound to plasma protein. Average half-life after single IV dose is 4 minutes
Indications	Intubation; Ventilation
Dosage as per indications	• *Newborn:* Initial—0.1 mg/kg/dose; maintenance—0.03–0.15 mg/kg/dose IV Q1–2 h • *Infants: Initial*—0.08–0.1 mg/kg/dose IV; maintenance—0.05–0.1 mg/kg/dose IV Q1 h continuous infusion—0.06–0.09 mg/kg/h IV • *>1 year–adult:* Initial—0.08–0.1 mg/kg/dose IV; maintenance—0.05–0.1 mg/kg/dose IV Q1 h continuous infusion—0.09–0.15 mg/kg/h IV
Maximum dosage	Not known
Dose adjustments	Hepatic and renal insufficiency
Adverse effects	Arrhythmias, rash, and bronchospasm
Contraindications	Hypersensitivity
Drug interactions	Other neuromuscular blocking agents, aminoglycosides
Remarks	Antidote: Neostigmine or edrophonium

Verapamil

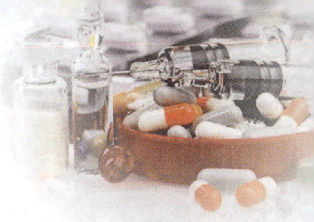

Drug name	Verapamil
Category	Antihypertensive
Route	Oral, Intravenous
Strength	Tab (40 mg, 80 mg, 120 mg); Inj (5 mg/2 mL)
Brands	Calaptin (Tab), Vepramil (Inj), Celovera (Inj)
Mechanism of action	Causes dilatation of main coronary arteries and arterioles. Also inhibits coronary artery spasm, decreases total peripheral systemic resistance
Pharmacokinetics	Highly absorbed after oral intake. 20–30% bioavailability. Highly protein bound. Extensively metabolized in liver. Mainly excreted via urine. Peak levels 1–2 hours after oral intake
Indications	Hypertension
Dosage as per indications	• *Infants:* 0.1–0.2 mg/kg IV over 2–3 min using continuous ECG monitoring. May repeat after 30 min • *Children:* 0.1–0.3 mg/kg/dose IV PO 1–2 mg/kg/dose q 6–8 h
Maximum dosage	*Initial dose:* 5 mg, repeat doses: 10 mg
Dose adjustments	Renal and hepatic insufficiency
Adverse effects	Bradycardia, AV block, heart failure, hypotension, constipation, flushing, nausea
Contraindications	Hypersensitivity, cardiogenic shock, severe CHF, sick-sinus syndrome, or AV block
Drug interactions	Beta adrenergic blocking agents, disopyramide, HMG-CoA reductase inhibitors
Remarks	Avoid IV use in neonates and young infants due to apnea, bradycardia, and hypotension. Antidote calcium gluconate

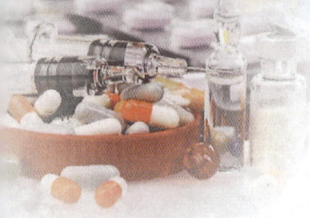

Vigabatrin

Drug name	Vigabatrin
Category	Adjunctive anticonvulsant drug
Route	Oral
Strength	Tab (500 mg)
Brands	Sabril (Tab)
Mechanism of action	Causes irreversible inhibition of enzyme γ-aminobutyric acid transaminase (GABA-T), thereby decreasing the metabolism of GABA
Pharmacokinetics	Near complete absorption when taken orally. Poorly protein bound, poorly metabolized. Elimination is mainly via renal excretion. Half-life: 5–10 hours, increases with increasing age
Indications	For resistant partial seizures; Infantile spasms; Especially useful in children with tuberous sclerosis; Lennox–Gastaut syndrome
Dosage as per indications	20–40 mg/kg/day, maintenance 80–100 mg/kg/day q 8–12 h
Maximum dosage	<60 kg: 2,000 mg/day; >60 kg: 3,000 mg/day
Dose adjustments	In renal impairment
Adverse effects	Visual disturbances, arthralgia, confusion, depression, weight gain, cough, increase in seizures
Contraindications	Hypersensitivity
Drug interactions	Phenytoin, clonazepam, oral contraceptives
Remarks	Use the lowest possible dose for the shortest duration. Avoid use of vigabatrin for >3 months

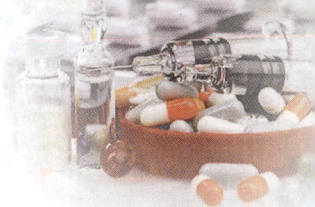

Vincristine Sulfate

Drug name	Vincristine sulfate
Category	Vinca alkaloid (Anti-cancer drug)
Route	Intravenous
Strength	Inj (1 mg/mL)
Brands	Oncocristin, Vinlon (Inj)
Mechanism of action	It inhibits microtubule formation in mitotic spindle, leads to arrest of dividing cells at the metaphase stage
Pharmacokinetics	Terminal half-life has a wide variation from as low as 19 hours to up to 155 hours. Elimination is mainly via hepatic metabolism by cytochrome P450 isoenzymes
Indications	Acute lymphoblastic leukemia; Hodgkin disease; Neuroblastoma; Non-Hodgkin lymphoma; Acute myeloid leukemia
Dosage as per indications	1.4–1.5 mg/m^2 IV once weekly
Maximum dosage	2 mg/dose
Dose adjustments	Hepatic
Adverse effects	Peripheral neuropathy and other neurological symptoms (convulsions, ileus, constipation, ptosis, hoarseness, blindness, optic neuropathy, weakness in limbs, jaw pain), leukopenia, azoospermia, hyperuricemia, vomiting, diarrhea, SIADH
Contraindications	Never give intrathecally
Drug interactions	Phenytoin, itraconazole, antineoplastic drugs
Remarks	Monitor for side effects and neurological symptoms, may warrant dose reduction or substitution with vinblastine

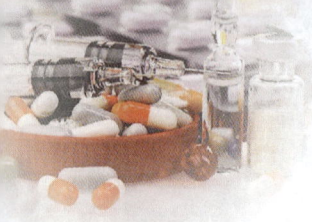

Vitamin A

Drug name	Vitamin A
Category	Vitamin B$_2$
Route	Oral, Intramuscular
Strength	Inj (50,000 IU/2 mL); Cap (25,000, 50,000 IU); Drops (1.5 L/mL)
Brands	Aquasol (Inj, Cap), Vitamin A (Drops, Cap)
Mechanism of action	Retinal is needed for rhodopsin formation as retinal combines with opsin. Rhodopsin is needed for visual dark adaptation. Vitamin A is also needed for growth and epithelial cell integrity
Pharmacokinetics	It is readily absorbed from the gut on oral intake in the presence of bile salts, pancreatic lipase, and dietary fat. It is stored in Kupffer cells of the liver. Metabolized in liver, eliminated in feces and urine
Indications	As routine supplementation; As treatment of xerophthalmia
Dosage as per indications	• 1 IU of vitamin A = 0.3 µg of retinol • WHO recommended treatment of xerophthalmia: oral—50,000 IU (<6 months of age), 100,000 IU (6–12 months of age) and 200,000 IU (>12 months of age) daily for 2 days followed by an additional dose after 2 weeks. In measles, above mentioned doses once daily for 2 days, irrespective of vitamin A status • *As part of National Immunization Program:* – 9 months: 1 lakh IU oral – 16–18 months, then 6 monthly till 5 years: 2 lakh IU oral • *Cholestasis:* 5,000–25,000 IU/day oral
Maximum dosage	Not known
Dose adjustments	Not required
Adverse effects	Raised intracranial tension, headache, nausea, irritability, vomiting
Contraindications	Hypersensitivity
Drug interactions	Cholestyramine, neomycin

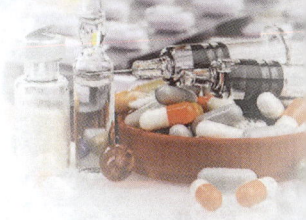

Vitamin K

Drug name	Vitamin K
Category	Vitamin
Route	Oral, Intravenous, Intramuscular
Strength	Inj (10 mg)
Brands	Kapilin (Inj)
Mechanism of action	Cofactor for enzyme required for post-translational carboxylation of inactive hepatic precursors of factors II, VII, IX, and X
Pharmacokinetics	Adequately absorbed from the gut in presence of bile salts, which is further stored in liver and used rapidly. Not much is known on metabolism and excretion
Indications	Hemorrhagic disease of newborn; Prolong prothrombin time/INR; Liver disease
Dosage as per indications	• *Prophylaxis (hemorrhagic disease of newborn):* 1 mg IM single dose in term newborns >1.5 kg birth weight, 0.5 mg IM single dose in babies weighing <1.5 kg • *Therapeutic* 2.5–10 mg/dose IV/IM • *Cholestasis:* 2–5 mg IM/IV/SC 4 weekly or 2.5 mg twice a week up to 5 mg/day
Maximum dosage	10 mg/dose
Dose adjustments	Not known
Adverse effects	Hemolysis
Contraindications	Hypersensitivity
Drug interactions	Not known

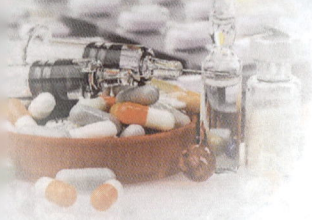

Voriconazole

Drug name	Voriconazole
Category	Triazole antifungal drug
Route	Intravenous, Oral
Strength	Inj (200 mg/vial); Tab (50 mg and 200 mg)
Brands	Vorier (Tab, Inj), Voritrol (Tab, Inj), Vorizol (TAB, inj)
Mechanism of action	It inhibits fungal cytochrome P450-mediated 14 alpha-lanosterol demethylation, needed for fungal ergosterol biosynthesis
Pharmacokinetics	High bioavailability. Maximum plasma levels: 1–2 hours after oral intake. There is extensive distribution into tissues. Plasma protein binding is around 60%. Elimination is via hepatic metabolism
Indications	Aspergillosis; Invasive candidemia; Fungal infections due to emerging pathogens like *Fusarium* species in immunocompromised patients
Dosage as per indications	<2 years: 9 mg/kg/dose 12 hourly IV/PO 2 to <12 years/12–14 years and <50 kg: • *Loading:* 9 mg/kg/dose 12 hourly IV for 2 doses • *Maintenance:* IV: 8 mg/kg/dose 12 hourly (given for at least 5–7 days); PO: 9 mg/kg/dose 12 hourly ≥15 years/12–14 years and ≥50 kg: • *Loading:* 6 mg/kg/dose IV 12 hourly × 2 doses • *Maintenance:* IV: 4 mg/kg/dose 12 hourly; PO: 200 mg 12 hourly
Maximum dosage	350 mg/dose
Dose adjustments	Required in renal and hepatic derangment
Adverse effects	Transient visual disturbances, hepatotoxicity, fever, rash, nausea, vomiting, abdominal pain, diarrhea, headache, peripheral edema, and rarely cardiac arrhythmias

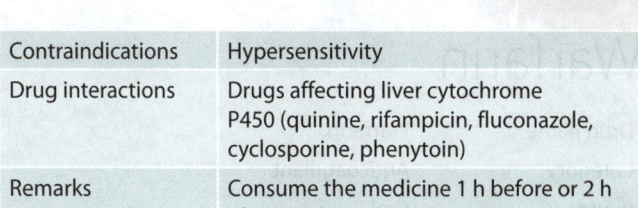

Contraindications	Hypersensitivity
Drug interactions	Drugs affecting liver cytochrome P450 (quinine, rifampicin, fluconazole, cyclosporine, phenytoin)
Remarks	Consume the medicine 1 h before or 2 h after meals

Voriconazole

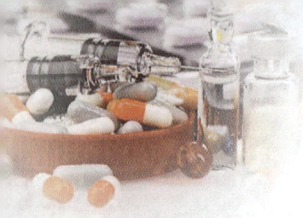

Warfarin

Drug name	Warfarin
Category	Anticoagulant
Route	Oral
Strength	Tab (1 mg, 2 mg, 2.5 mg, 3 mg, 4 mg, 5 mg, 6 mg, 7.5 mg, 10 mg)
Brands	Warf, Sofarin (Tab)
Mechanism of action	Inhibits synthesis of vitamin K-dependent clotting factors, proteins C and S. Warfarin inhibits C1 subunit of vitamin K epoxide reductase (VKORC1) enzyme complex, leading to decreased regeneration of vitamin K_1 epoxide, thus inhibiting coagulation cascade
Pharmacokinetics	Anticoagulant effect is noted from 24 hours extending up to 96 hours. It is completely absorbed after oral administration, peak levels found after first 4 hours. Most of the drug is bound to plasma proteins. It is metabolized by hepatic cytochrome P450 (CYP450) microsomal enzymes. The terminal half-life is around 1 week
Indications	Anti-coagulation; Post-transplant
Dosage as per indications	• Initial dose 0.2 mg/kg PO × 2 days, In liver dysfunction 0.1 mg/kg/dose PO × 2 days • *Maintenance:* Children—0.1 mg/kg/24 h, infants—0.3 mg/kg/24 h
Maximum dosage	10 mg/dose
Dose adjustments	In hepatic impairment, not needed in renal impairment
Adverse effects	Fever, nausea, vomiting, diarrhea, skin lesions, and bleeding
Contraindications	Contraindicated in severe liver or kidney disease, uncontrolled bleeding, GI ulcers, and malignant hypertension.
Drug interactions	Inhibitors and inducers of CYP2C9, 1A2, or 3A4, and NSAIDs
Remarks	Therapeutic range 1.5–2 times normal. Antidote is vitamin K and fresh frozen plasma

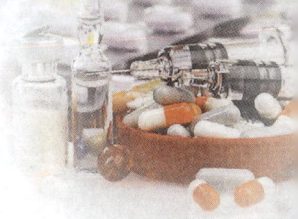

Zalcitabine (ddC)

Drug name	Zalcitabine (ddC)
Category	Antiretroviral drug
Route	Oral
Strength	Cap (0.375 mg, 0.75 mg)
Brands	Hivid (Cap)
Mechanism of action	Nucleoside reverse transcriptase inhibitor, inhibits the activity of the HIV-reverse transcriptase
Pharmacokinetics	High bioavailability, poorly metabolized, mainly eliminated unchanged via renal route, elimination half-life 2 hours
Indications	HIV infection/AIDS
Dosage as per indications	0.01 mg/kg/dose TID
Maximum dosage	Not known
Dose adjustments	Adjust dose in renal disease
Adverse effects	Peripheral neuropathy, headache, malaise, gastrointestinal disturbances, lactic acidosis
Contraindications	Hypersensitivity
Drug interactions	Zidovudine, probenecid, cimetidine
Remarks	Use cautiously in patients with liver disease, pancreatitis, or severe myelosuppression

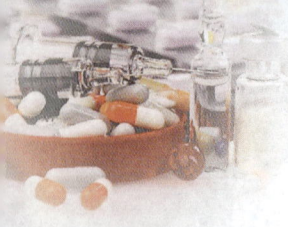

Zafirlukast

Drug name	Zafirlukast
Category	Antiallergic
Route	Oral
Strength	Tab (20 mg)
Brands	Zuvair (Tab)
Mechanism of action	Competitive receptor antagonist of leukotriene D4 and E4 (LTD4 and LTE4)
Pharmacokinetics	Rapidly absorbed after oral administration, peak levels noted 3 hours after oral administration, highly bound to plasma proteins, extensively metabolized to hydroxylated metabolites and excreted in the feces
Indications	Asthma; Allergic rhinitis
Dosage as per indications	• *6–11 years:* 10 mg/dose 12 hourly PO • *>12 years:* 20 mg/dose 12 hourly PO
Maximum dosage	Not known
Dose adjustments	Not known
Adverse effects	Hepatotoxicity, prolong prothrombin time, neuropsychiatry event, eosinophilia
Contraindications	Hypersensitivity
Drug interactions	Theophylline, aspirin, fluconazole, erythromycin
Remarks	Used above 5 years of age

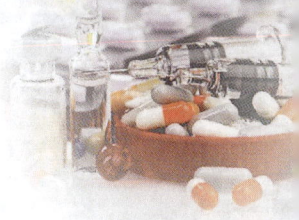

Zanamivir

Drug name	Zanamivir
Category	Antiflu drug, Neuraminidase blocking drug
Route	Inhaled
Strength	Rotadisk (5 mg)
Brands	Relenza Rotadisk (Blister for oral inhalation: 5 mg; Rotadisk with Diskhaler)
Mechanism of action	Antiviral drug with main activity against influenza virus
Pharmacokinetics	Serum half-life after inhalation varies from 2.5–5 hours. Between 5 and 15% is absorbed systemically and eliminated by renal filtration
Indications	For treating and preventing influenza A and B in children >7 years and adults
Dosage as per indications	• Two inhalations 2 hours apart (5 mg/inhalation) 12 hours apart) for 5 days. For better results treatment should be started as soon as symptoms develop • The recommended dose for prevention of influenza in a household setting is 10 mg once daily for 10 days. The recommended dose for preventing influenza in a community setting is 10 mg once daily for 28 days
Maximum dosage	Not known
Dose adjustments	In renal impairment
Adverse effects	Headache, nausea, diarrhea, cough, dizziness, bronchospasm
Contraindications	Hypersensitivity
Drug interactions	Do not give live influenza vaccine till 2 weeks
Remarks	It may interfere with efficacy of flu vaccine. Do not vaccinate 2 weeks before or 2 days after taking zanamivir

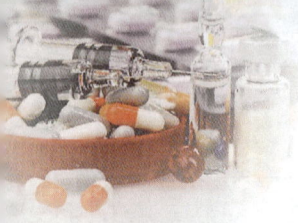

Zidovudine (AZT/ZDV)

Drug name	Zidovudine (AZT/ZDV)
Category	Antiretroviral drug
Route	Oral, Intravenous
Strength	Cap (100 mg); Liquid (50 mg/5 mL); Inj (10 mg/mL)
Brands	Zidovir (Tab, Syp), Zidine (Tab), Viro Z (Tab)
Mechanism of action	Nucleoside reverse transcriptase inhibitor
Pharmacokinetics	Rapid absorption after oral administration, peak levels in 1 hour, metabolized in liver and eliminated via renal route
Indications	HIV infection/AIDS

Dosage as per indications	• Daily dose 360 mg/m^2 to maximum 600 mg.
	• Weight-based dosing:
	  – 4–9 kg: 12 mg/kg BD
	  – 9–30 kg: 9 mg/kg BD
	  – ≥30 kg: 300 mg BD
	• Neonate 2 mg/kg/dose QID PO or 1.5 mg/kg/dose QID IV over 60 min. Begin within 12 hours of birth and continue until 6 weeks of age

Maximum dosage	600 mg/day
Dose adjustments	In renal impairment
Adverse effects	Anemia, neutropenia, headache, vomiting, neuropathy, anorexia, vomiting, hepatitis, lactic acidosis, myopathy
Contraindications	Hypersensitivity
Drug interactions	Do not use in combination with stavudine. Do not administer intramuscular Retrovir
Remarks	Available also in combination with lamivudine as Combivir (Tab: 300 mg AZT + 150 mg 3TC)

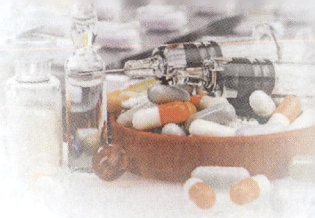

Zinc Sulfate

Drug name	Zinc sulfate
Category	Miscellaneous
Route	Oral
Strength	Syp (10 mg/5 mL); Tab (20 mg); Cap (20 mg); Drops (20 mg/mL)
Brands	Zioral (Syp, Drops, Tab), Zn 20 (Syp, Tab), Z and D (Drops)
Mechanism of action	It is a gut protective agent, works as a cofactor of various enzymes, coordinator of protein structural folding, catalyst of essential biochemical reactions and also signaling mediator
Pharmacokinetics	Zinc is absorbed from the gastrointestinal tract, predominantly concentrated in hair, eyes, bones and reproductive organs (male) and in lesser amount in liver, kidney and muscle and erythrocytes. Nearly 50% is bound to albumin
Indications	Acute diarrhea; Acrodermatitis enteropathica; Wilson disease
Dosage as per indications	• *Acute diarrhea 6 weeks to 6 months:* 10 mg PO × 14 days 6 months to 5 years 20 mg PO × 14 days • *Acrodermatitis enteropathica:* 6 mg/kg/day • *Wilson Disease:* >10 years 75 mg/day up to 150 mg/day tried
Maximum dosage	Not known
Dose adjustments	Not known
Adverse effects	Nausea, vomiting, leukopenia. Excessive zinc intake may cause copper deficiency
Contraindications	Hypersensitivity
Drug interactions	Quinolone, tetracycline, cephalexin
Remarks	Therapeutic levels 70–130 µg/d

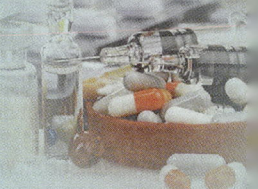

Index

A

Abacavir 1
Acebutolol 146
Acetalopram 329
Acetaminophen 146, 150
Acetazolamide 2, 150
Acetylsalicylic acid 3
Acyclovir 5, 259, 325
Adefovir 141
   dipivoxil 7
Adenosine 8, 19, 61, 125
Adjunctive anticonvulsant drug 412
Adrenaline 9
Adrenergic agonist 206, 276
Adrenergic drugs 394
Albendazole 11, 213
Albumin 13
Albuterol 360
Alcohol 246
Alfacalcidol 14
Alkylating drug 60
Allopurinol 15, 19, 28, 29, 45, 299-301
Alpha-adrenergic
   agonist, central 101
   blocking drug 394
Alpha-blocker 364
Alprostadil 16
Aluminum hydroxide 38, 148
Amantadine 17, 187
Amikacin 18
Aminoglycoside 80, 97, 141, 165, 167, 171, 202, 265, 267, 292, 299, 300, 312, 313, 373, 388, 392, 407, 410
   antibiotic 18, 297
Aminophylline 19, 135, 247
Aminoquinolines 23
Amiodarone 20, 211, 264, 403
Amitriptyline 10, 21
Amlodipine 22, 233
Ammonium desiccant 265
Amodiaquine 23
Amoxicillin 24
Amoxicillin-clavulanic acid 25
Amphetamine 26, 38, 334

Amphotericin 18, 165, 397
   B 27, 407
Ampicillin 28, 29, 90, 293
Amrinone 30
   infusions 30
   solutions 30
Anagrelide 403
Anakinra 147
Anesthetic drug 103, 183, 217, 292, 387
Angiotensin-converting enzyme inhibitors 15, 65, 178, 398
Anidulafungin 31
Antacids 14, 46, 75, 81, 90, 137, 154, 211, 216, 242, 252, 258, 259, 275, 286, 382
Antiallergic drug 205, 215, 420
Antiangiogenic drug 53
Antiarrhythmic drug 8, 20, 41, 122, 125, 129, 206, 212, 219, 247, 326, 341, 342, 355
Antibacterial drug 118, 390
Antibiotic 24, 25, 28, 29, 46, 47, 51, 67, 72, 74-78, 80-86, 89, 96-98, 102, 108, 134, 152, 154, 170, 171, 190, 202, 216, 220, 221, 234, 252, 258, 261, 267, 273, 277, 280, 292, 301, 309, 313, 318, 327, 355, 377, 378, 382, 388, 389, 392, 401, 407
   bacteriostatic 136
Anti-cancer drug 413
Anticholinergic activity 44, 320
Anticholinergic drug 17, 44, 92, 103, 122, 187, 196, 266, 391
Anticholinesterase agent 266
Anticoagulant drug 3, 24, 25, 29, 51, 72-74, 77, 78, 84, 85, 89, 95, 98, 121, 143, 180, 231, 237, 246, 252, 263, 271, 285, 288, 316, 322, 328, 332, 333, 341, 355, 382, 399, 418
Anticonvulsant drug 66, 150, 168, 209, 211, 219, 226, 242, 249, 355, 395

Antidepressant drug 21, 128, 161, 186, 191, 223
Antidiabetic drug 41, 91, 184, 194, 216, 222, 322, 339, 403
Antidiarrheal drugs 347
Antidiuretic hormone 409
Antidote 241, 260, 333
 flumazenil 119
Antiemetic drug 93, 132, 173, 244, 328, 329
Antiepileptic drug 99, 100, 115, 136, 150, 214, 218, 264, 288, 290, 308, 309
Antiflu drug 421
Antifungal drug 27, 31, 71, 156, 157, 175, 200, 248, 278, 293, 302, 379
Antihelminthic drug 11, 124, 201, 213, 230, 246, 269, 321, 335, 385
Antihistamine 87, 92, 186, 187
Antihistaminic drug 39, 107, 114, 126, 128, 155, 225, 329, 402
Antihyperglycemic drug 235
Antihypertensive drug 22, 42, 65, 70, 91, 101, 120, 183, 146, 183, 184, 193, 222, 227, 253, 274, 328, 348, 398, 411
Antihypoglycemic agent 120, 172
Anti-IgE antibody 283
Anti-inflammatory drug 243
Antileishmanial drug 251
Antimalarial drug 23, 35, 37, 90, 232
Antimetabolite 157
Antimigraine 144
Antimuscarinic drugs 138
 long-acting 391
Antimyasthenic drug 139
Antineoplastic drugs 27, 413
Antiparasitic drug 271, 338
Antiplatelet agent 3
Antiprotozoal 390
Antipsychotic 122, 176, 187, 272, 281
Antipyretic agent 3
Antiretroviral drug 1, 40, 109, 123, 131, 140, 141, 192, 208, 224, 236, 280, 285, 294, 356, 362, 372, 419, 422
Anti-RhD immunoglobulin 32
Antisnake venom serum 33
Antispasmodic drug 122, 138
Antithymocyte globulin 34
Antithyroid drug 68, 237, 332
Antitubercular drug 50, 64, 105, 148, 149, 355
Antituberculous drug 197
Antitussive 117
Antiuric acid 15
Antiviral drug 5, 7, 17, 165, 169, 211, 213, 264, 268, 271, 351, 353, 405
Appetite stimulant 107
Arrhythmogenic drugs 236, 380
Artemether 35
Arterial vasodilator 183
Artesunate 37
Ascorbate 154
Ascorbic acid 38
Aspirin 3, 244, 316, 397, 420
Astemizole 39, 140, 192, 264, 362
Atazanavir 40
Atenolol 41
Atomoxetine 42
Atorvastatin 43
Atracurium 220
Atropine 336
 sulfate 44
Azathioprine 15, 45, 147, 353
Azelastine 99
Azithromycin 46, 114, 215
Azole 156
 antifungals 22, 99, 123
Aztreonam 47

B

Baclofen 48
Bactericidal 18
Bacteriostatic agents 76
Barbiturates 94, 203, 296, 397
BCG vaccine 327
Beclomethasone dipropionate 49
Bedaquiline 50
Benzathine penicillin 51
Benzimidazole 230
Benzodiazepine 66, 99, 100, 119, 128, 138, 214, 249, 272, 303
 antidote for 159
Benzyl penicillin 52
Beta-1 receptor blocker 245
Beta-1 selective adrenergic blocker 146
Beta-2 adrenergic agonist 360, 361
 long-acting 164
Beta-2 agonist 217, 380
 inhaled long-acting 57
Beta-2 blocker 330

Beta-adrenergic
 agents 187
 blocking drugs 237, 411
Beta-agonist 19
Beta-antagonist 19
Beta-blocker 10, 41, 58, 68, 70, 101, 130, 164, 172, 270, 279
Beta-lactam 80
Bevacizumab 53
Biguanide 235
Bisacodyl 54
Bleomycin 55
Broad-spectrum
 anticonvulsant 406
Bronchodilator 19, 196, 217, 228, 360, 361, 383
Budesonide 56, 57
Bumetanide 59
Busulfan 60
Butyrophenones group 176

C

Caffeine 96
 citrate 61
Calcipotriene 63
Calcium 279, 367
 antagonist 206
 carbonate 62
 channel blocker 22, 99, 125, 160, 270, 290
 gluconate 63
 injections 84
 supplement 62
Capreomycin 64
Captopril 65, 145
Carbamazepine 66, 93, 100, 106, 116, 197, 281, 384
Carbapenem 134, 234
 antibiotic 190
Carbenicillin 67
Carbimazole 68
Carbonic anhydrase 235
 inhibitor 2
Carboplatin 145
Carboxypenicillin 67
Cardiac glycosides 19, 59, 63, 193, 207, 218, 228
Cardiovascular bipyridine 30
Carnitine 69
Carvedilol 70
Caspofungin acetate 71
Catecholamine 409
 depleting drugs 245
Cefaclor 72
Cefadroxil 73
Cefazolin sodium 74

Cefdinir 75
Cefepime 76
Cefixime 77
Cefoperazone-sulbactam 78
Cefotaxime 79
Cefoxitin 80
Cefpodoxime 151, 275
 proxetil 81
Cefprozil 82
Ceftazidime 83
Ceftriaxone 63
 sodium 84
Cefuroxime axetil 85
Cephalexin 86, 423
Cephalosporin 18, 72, 74-86, 97
 antibiotic 73
Cetirizine dihydrochloride 87
Chelating agent 110, 111, 113, 127, 137
Chemotherapeutic drug 55
Chickenpox 5
Chloral hydrate 88
Chlorambucil 166
Chloramphenicol 89, 166
Chlordiazepoxide 166
Chloroquine 68, 339
 phosphate 90
Chlorothiazide 91
Chlorpheniramine maleate 92
Chlorpromazine 93, 369
Cholecalciferol 94
Cholelitholytic drug 404
Cholestyramine 86, 95, 404, 414
Cholinergic drug 139, 266, 310, 320
Cholinesterase inhibitor 336
Cidofovir 165
Cilastatin 152
Cimetidine 6, 12, 39, 90, 99, 215, 225, 287, 298, 379, 419
Ciprofloxacin 39, 96, 123, 154, 363
Cisapride 140, 362
Cisplatin 18, 357
Citalopram 400
Clarithromycin 22, 97, 144
Clavulanate 388
Clindamycin 98
Clobazam 99
Clofibrate 404
Clonazepam 100, 412
Clonidine hydrochloride 101
Cloxacillin 102
CNS
 depressants 99, 126, 272, 399, 402
 stimulants 17
Codeine phosphate 103
Colchicine 240

Colestipol 404
Colistimethate sodium 104
Colistin 104, 407
Colloid 13
Corticosteroid 91, 162, 184, 322
    metabolism of 116
Corticotropin 4
Coumarin
    anticoagulants 175, 242
    derivatives 15
Cyclic lipopeptide 108
Cyclic polypeptide antibacterial
    agent 104
Cyclopentolate 402
Cyclophosphamide 147
Cycloserine 105, 149
Cyclosporine 18, 43, 106, 136,
    147, 175, 216, 244, 259,
    261, 279, 298, 344, 359,
    379, 390, 393, 417
CYP3A4 cytochrome P450
    enzyme 209
CYP3A4 enzyme 305
    drugs affecting 200
CYP3A4 inducers 50, 112, 224,
    286, 377
CYP3A4 inhibitors 22, 36, 43, 50,
    162, 356, 364
CYP3A4 pathway 56, 58
CYP450 3A4 inhibitors 144
Cyproheptadine hydrochloride 107
Cytarabine 157
Cytochrome P450 285
    system 331
Cytotoxic chemotherapy 60

D

Dalfopristin 343
Daptomycin 108
Darunavir 109
Decongestant 191, 334
Deferasirox 110
Deferiprone 111
Deferoxamine 38
Deflazacort 112
Dehydropeptidase inhibitor 190
Desferrioxamine 113
Desloratadine 114
Desmopressin 115
Dexamethasone 12, 116, 321
Dextromethorphan 117
Diaminodiphenyl sulfone 118
Diazepam 119, 197, 203, 281
Diazoxide 120
Diclofenac 121
Dicoumarol 178

Dicyclomine 122
Didanosine 123, 169, 405
Diethylcarbamazine 124
Digitalis 27, 41, 68, 271, 332
Digoxin 14, 43, 46, 55, 125, 146,
    158, 210, 211, 216, 258,
    294, 319, 355, 360, 369,
    374, 401
Diltiazem 22, 70
Dimenhydrinate 126
Dimercaprol 127
Diphenhydramine 128
Diphenylmethane derivatives
    group 54
Direct vasodilator 253
Disopyramide 129, 411
Disulfiram 246
Diuretics 2, 4, 14, 15, 58, 65, 94,
    91, 142, 161, 171, 193, 222,
    223, 229, 282, 341, 348
Dobutamine 130, 367
Dofetilide 131
Dolutegravir 131
Domperidone 132, 187
Dopamine 133
    agonist 242, 281
Doripenem 134
Doxapram 135
Doxycycline 73, 136, 220
D-penicillamine 137
Droperidol 220
Drotaverine 138

E

Echinocandin 31, 71, 248
Edrophonium 139
Efavirenz 23, 140
Electrolytes 369
Emtricitabine 141
Enalapril 319
    maleate 142
Enoxaparin 9, 120, 143, 180, 394
Equine 34
Ergot derivatives 46, 192
Ergotamine tartrate 144
Erythromycin 22, 39, 106, 114,
    144, 155, 156, 215, 225,
    227, 420
Erythropoiesis, glycoprotein
    hormone for 145
Erythropoietin 145
Esmolol hydrochloride 146
Estrogen 370, 404
Etanercept 147
Ethambutol 148
Ethanol 296

Ethionamide 105, 149, 294
Ethosuximide 66, 150
Extended spectrum penicillin 388

F

Famotidine 151
Faropenem 152
Fentanyl 153, 274
Ferrous sulfate 154
Fexofenadine hydrochloride 155
Fluconazole 106, 156, 227, 379, 420
Flucytosine 27, 157
Fludrocortisone acetate 158
Flumazenil 159
Flunarizine 160
Fluoroquinolone 96, 170, 280
    antibiotics 369
    L-thyroxine 374
Fluoxetine 93, 161
Fluticasone propionate 162
Fluvoxamine 233, 247, 281
Folic acid 163
Formoterol 57
    fumarate 164
Foscarnet 165, 298
Fosphenytoin 163, 166
Fumarate 154
Furosemide 82, 152, 167, 319, 392, 399

G

Gabapentin 168, 233
Ganciclovir 123, 169
Gatifloxacin 170
Gentamicin sulfate 171
Glucagon hydrochloride 172
Glucocorticoid 112, 116
Glucocorticoid 57
Gluconate 154
Glycopeptide 378
    antibiotic drug 55
Granisetron 173
Granulocyte colony-stimulating factor 174
Griseofulvin 175
Growth factor 174
Growth hormone agonist 370
Guanethidine 253

H

H1 antagonist 39
H2 blockers 81
H2 receptor antagonist 151
Haloperidol 93, 176, 223
Heparin 312, 313
    sodium 178

Hepatic enzyme
    inducers 160
    inducing drugs 406
Hepatitis B immunoglobulin 181
Histamine-2-blocker 349
Hormone 4, 212
Hydralazine hydrochloride 183
Hydrochlorothiazide 184
Hydrocortisone sodium succinate 185
Hydroxychloroquine 351
Hydroxyzine hydrochloride 186
Hyoscine butylbromide 187
Hypercalcemia, drugs causing 63
Hypnotics 205
Hypoglycemia, drugs causing 194
Hypoglycemic agents 89

I

Ibuprofen 188
Imidazole 204
Imipenem 152
Imipenem-cilastatin 169, 190
Imipramine hydrochloride 191
Immunoglobulin 32, 33, 189, 195, 346, 352, 381
    intravenous 195
Immunomodulators 198, 243
Immunostimulant 213
Immunosuppressant drug 34, 45, 106, 238
Immunosuppressive drugs 60
Indinavir 123, 192, 268, 275
Indomethacin 193, 409
Influenza vaccine 289
Inhaled bronchodilator 380
Inhaled corticosteroid 57
Inhibitors 112, 377
Inosine
    monophosphate dehydrogenase inhibitor 259
    pranobex 198
Inotrope 10, 30, 62, 130, 133
Insulin 135, 194, 279
    oral hypoglycemics 370
Integrase inhibitor 131
Intestinal motility agents 54
Ionotropic drugs 130, 276
Ipratropium bromide 196
Iron 62, 75, 127, 137, 154, 369
    chelators 110
Isoniazid 105, 149, 197
Isoprinosine 198
Isosorbide dinitrate 199

Itraconazole 39, 151, 200, 413
Ivermectin 201, 213

K

Kanamycin 202
Kaolin 90
Ketamine 203
Ketoconazole 39, 106, 114, 151, 155, 204, 215, 225, 244, 275, 349
Ketorolac 325
Ketotifen 205

L

Labetalol 206
Lactulose 207
Lamivudine 208
Lamotrigine 209
Lansoprazole junior 210
Ledipasvir 211
Leukotriene inhibitor 255
Leuprolide acetate 212
Levamisole hydrochloride 213
Levetiracetam 214
Levocetirizine 215
Levofloxacin 216
Levosalbutamol 217
Levothyroxine 218
Lidocaine 274
Lignocaine hydrochloride 219
Lincomycin 98, 220
Linezolid 221
Lipid-lowering agent 43
Lisinopril 222
Lithium 59, 174, 223, 246, 398
Live vaccines 32–34, 147, 181, 189, 243, 346, 352, 381, 408
Live-attenuated virus vaccines 195
Liver enzymes, drugs affecting 25, 71
Loop diuretic 59, 167, 189
Lopinavir 224
Loratadine 225
Lorazepam 226
Losartan 227
Lovastatin 40

M

Macrolide 19, 22, 46
 antibiotics and antifungals 377
Magnesium sulfate 228
Mannitol 229
Mebendazole 230

Mefenamic acid 231
Mefloquine hydrochloride 232
Melatonin 233
Meropenem 234
Metformin 86, 131, 235
Methadone 1, 123, 236
Methimazole 237
Methotrexate 51, 96, 238, 240, 280, 293, 312, 313, 344
Methylcobalamin 239
Methylene blue 241
Methylphenidate 242
Methylprednisolone 243
Methylxanthine 8, 61, 383
Metoclopramide 187
 hydrochloride 244
Metoprolol 245, 400
Metronidazole 47, 230, 246
Mexiletine 247
Micafungin 248
Midazolam 140, 192, 249, 264, 349, 362
Milrinone 250
Miltefosine 251
Mineralocorticoid 158
Minocycline 252
Minoxidil 253
Mometasone 254
Monoamine oxidase inhibitors 26, 42, 107, 117, 126, 133, 135, 164, 187, 191, 257, 306, 334
Monobactam 47
Monoclonal antibody 357
Montelukast sodium 255
Morphine 274
 sulfate 256
Moxifloxacin 258
Mucolytic 260
Muscarinic antagonist 196
Muscle relaxant 48, 104, 249, 257, 266, 267
Mycophenolate 95, 363, 405
Myelopoiesis, drugs affecting 45

N

N-acetylcysteine 260
Nalidixic acid 261
Naloxone hydrochloride 262
Naproxen 263
Narcotic 153
 analgesic drug 296, 396
 antagonist 103, 262
Nelfinavir 123, 264, 285
Neomycin 336, 414
 sulfate 265
Neostigmine 266

Nephrotoxic drugs 7, 27, 55, 64, 82, 97, 157, 171, 202, 229, 265, 267, 302, 318, 378, 407
Nephrotoxicity 18
Netilmicin sulfate 267
Neuraminidase
    blocking drug 421
    inhibitor 289
Neuromuscular blockers 228
    drugs 64, 292, 341, 373, 410
Neuromuscular drugs 386
Neurotoxic drugs 105
Neutropenia 111
Nevirapine 23, 268
Niacin 393
Niclosamide 269
Nifedipine 248, 270
Nitazoxanide 271
Nitrates 178, 187
Nitrazepam 272
Nitrofuran 273
Nitrofurantoin 273
Nitroglycerin 144
Nitroimidazole 246
Nitroprusside 274
Nizatidine 275
Non-nucleoside reverse transcriptase inhibitor 140
Nonsteroidal anti-inflammatory drugs 3, 59, 91, 115, 121, 157, 180, 184, 188, 193, 222, 223, 231, 263, 282, 298, 316, 322, 348, 398, 401
Nonstimulant 42
Norepinephrine 276, 367, 394
Norfloxacin 277
Nucleoside reverse transcriptase inhibitor 141, 372
Nucleotide
    analog 351
    reverse transcriptase inhibitor 208
Nutritional supplement 182
Nystatin 278

O

Octreotide 279
Ofloxacin 280
Olanzapine 99, 281
Olmesartan 282
Omalizumab 283
Omeprazole 285, 374
Ondansetron hydrochloride 286
Opioid 115, 168, 303
    agonist 305
    analgesic 236

Oral anticoagulants 190, 374
Oral antidiabetic agents 205
Oral contraceptives 28, 102, 218, 259, 290, 388, 389, 404, 412
Oral hypoglycemics 235
Oral rehydration salt 287
Orlistat 141
Ornidazole 288
Oseltamivir 289
Osmotic laxative 317
Ototoxic drugs 171, 265, 267
Ototoxicity 18
Oxazolidinone 221
Oxcarbazepine 290

P

P450 enzyme system 370
P450 inducers 321
P450 inhibitors 321
Palonosetron 291
Pancuronium 98, 292
Pantoprazole 293
Para-amino salicylic acid 240, 294
Paracetamol 295
Paraldehyde 296
Paromomycin sulfate 297
Pefloxacin 298
Penicillamine 369
Penicillin 24, 25, 28, 51, 52, 154, 252, 301, 313, 325, 327, 366, 382
    G aqueous 299
    G benzathine 300
    V potassium 301
Penicillinase-resistant penicillin 102
Pentamidine 302
Pentazocine hydrochloride 303
Permethrin 304
Pernicious anemia 239
Pethidine hydrochloride 305
Pheniramine maleate 306
Phenobarb 244
Phenobarbital 100
Phenobarbitone 106, 116, 163, 175, 227, 287, 355, 384
    sodium 307
Phenothiazine derivative 93, 328, 329, 400
Phenoxymethylpenicillin 301
Phenytoin 15, 66, 89, 94, 100, 106, 116, 120, 158, 163, 197, 244, 247, 328, 374, 384, 390, 397, 401, 412, 413, 417
    sodium 309

Phosphate binder 363
Phosphodiesterase inhibitors 30, 199
Physostigmine 310
Pimozide 311
Piperacillin 312
Piperacillin-tazobactam 313
Piperazine 314
Piracetam 315
Piroxicam 316
Polyethylene glycol 317
Polymyxin
  B 318, 407
  group 104
Polypeptide 318
Polyvalent 33
Potassium
  channel blocking agent 20
  chloride 319, 391
Potassium-sparing diuretic 371, 398
Potentiate neuromuscular blockade 340
Pralidoxime 320
Praziquantel 12, 321
Prednisolone 322
Pregabalin 323
Primaquine 324
Primidone 163
  enhance 116
Probenecid acid 6, 24, 25, 28, 29, 51, 52, 67, 72, 75, 79-81, 84, 86, 118, 134, 169, 234, 298, 312, 313, 325, 366, 388, 419
Procainamide 349
  hydrochloride 326
Procaine penicillin 327
Prochlorperazine 328
Prokinetic drug 132
Promethazine hydrochloride 329
Propranolol 328, 330
Propylthiouracil 332
Prostaglandin
  E1 16
  synthetase inhibiting drugs 41
Protamine 333
Protease inhibitors 22, 40, 109, 119, 131, 144, 192, 210, 264, 268, 356, 362
Proton pump inhibitor 99, 210, 344
Pseudoephedrine 334
Pulmonary surfactant 376
Pulmonary vasodilator 250
Pyrantel pamoate 314, 335

Pyridostigmine 336
Pyridoxine 337
Pyrimethamine 240
Pyrimethamine-sulfadoxine 338

Q

QT interval
  drugs affecting 50, 186
  drugs causing prolonged 132
  drugs prolonging 21, 88, 93, 97, 246
QTC prolongation 361
  drugs 232
Quinacrine 324
Quinidine 17, 187, 340
Quinine 17, 264
  dihydrochloride 341
  sulfate 342
Quinolone 19, 104, 261, 273, 277, 423
Quinupristin 343

R

Rabeprazole 344
Rabies
  human monoclonal antibody 345
  immunoglobulin 346
Racecadotril 347
Ramipril 348
Ranitidine 349, 374
Rasburicase 350
rDNA monoclonal antibody 345
Recombinant urate oxidase 350
Remdesivir 351
Renin-angiotensin system
  drugs affecting 142
  inhibitors 3
Respiratory depression 303
Respiratory stimulant 61, 135
Respiratory syncytial virus 352
Retrovir 422
Reverse transcriptase inhibitor 123
Ribavirin 45, 123, 353
Riboflavin 354
Rifabutin 116, 268
Rifampicin 40, 106, 116, 118, 131, 227, 268, 342, 355, 379, 384
Rifampin 158, 287, 362
Ritonavir 224, 268, 356, 364
Rituximab 357
Rizatriptan benzoate 358
Roxithromycin 359

S

Salbutamol 360
Salicylates 15
Salmeterol 361
Saquinavir 118, 268, 285, 362
Scabicidal drug 304
Sedation 303
   general anesthetic for 203
Sedative 87, 88, 92, 93, 103, 128, 186, 205, 233, 249, 256, 296, 308, 329, 399
Selective serotonin reuptake inhibitors 115, 161
Serotonergic drug 241, 257, 291
Serotonin
   agonist 358
   syndrome 291
Sevelamer 363
Sildenafil 40, 192, 364
Simethicone 365
Simvastatin 40
Sirolimus 248
Sodium
   benzoate 366
   bicarbonate 135, 367
   nitroprusside 368
   phenylacetate 366
   picosulfate 369
   valproate 152, 395
Sofosbuvir oral 211
Somatostatin analog 279
Somatropin 370
Sorbitol 208
Spironolactone 371
Stavudine 372, 422
Steroids 49, 56, 68, 94, 185, 218, 397
   activity 49
Stimulant 26, 242
   laxative 369
Streptomycin 336, 373
Succinylcholine 336
Sucralfate 137, 374
Sulbactam 29
Sulfonamide 401
Sulfone group 118
Sumatriptan 375
Supplement 69, 319
Sympathomimetic drugs 9, 41, 135, 360
Synthetic opiate 153
Synthetic sugar 207

T

Tachycardia 361
Tacrolimus 377, 390
Teicoplanin 378
Terbinafine 247
   hydrochloride 379
Terbutaline 380
Terfenadine 140, 264, 362
Tetanus immunoglobulin 381
Tetracycline 369, 423
   derivative 136
   hydrochloride 382
Theophylline 12, 68, 96, 237, 258, 261, 332, 383, 385, 420
Thiabendazole 385
Thiamine 386
Thiazide 63, 184, 207
Thiobarbiturate 387
Thiopental 387
Thyroxine 218, 363
Ticarcillin disodium 388
Tigecycline 389
Tinidazole 390
Tiotropium 391
Tizanidine 61
Tobramycin 392
Tocopherol 393
Tolazoline hydrochloride 394
Topiramate 329, 395
Torsades de pointes 129
Tourette syndrome 176
Tramadol 396
Triamcinolone 397
Triamterene 151, 398
Triazole 200
   antifungal drug 416
Triclofos sodium 399
Tricyclic antidepressants 115, 159, 183, 187
Trifluoperazine hydrochloride 400
Trimethoprim 118
   sulfamethoxazole 401
Triprolidine 402
   hydrochloride 402
Triptorelin 403
Tubocurarine 98
Tumor necrosis factor-α receptor blocker 147

U

Uricosuric drug 325
Ursodeoxycholic acid 404

V

Valganciclovir 405
Valproate 66, 134, 190, 234, 366, 406

Vancomycin 18, 267, 312, 313
  hydrochloride 407
Varicella 5
Varicella-zoster
  immunoglobulin 408
  infection 5
Vasoconstrictors 10, 115
Vasodilator 16, 30, 199, 274, 368
Vasodilatory drugs 199
Vasopressin 409
  analog 115
Vecuronium 410
Verapamil 22, 70, 411
Vigabatrin 412
Vinca alkaloid 413
Vincristine 298
  sulfate 413
Vitamin 14, 38, 163, 415
  A 63, 414
  B_1 386
  B_{12} 239, 294
    deficiency 239
  B_2 414
  B_6 337
  C 38
    oral 113
  D 63
    supplements 14
  D_3 supplement 94
  fat-soluble 374
  K 415
Voriconazole 416

W

Warfarin 69, 82, 96, 102, 120, 201, 210, 216, 246, 258, 277, 280, 287, 344, 349, 389, 390, 393, 401, 418
  sodium 178
West syndrome 4

X

Xanthine 164
  oxidase inhibitors 15, 198

Z

Zafirlukast 420
Zalcitabine 419
Zanamivir 421
Zidovudine 23, 169, 372, 405, 419, 422
Zinc 137
  sulfate 423